MOUNT SINAI
EXPERT GUIDES

Obstetrics and Gynecology

T0257320

MOUNT SINAI EXPERT GUIDES

Obstetrics and Gynecology

EDITED BY

Rhoda Sperling
Icahn School of Medicine at Mount Sinai
New York, NY, USA

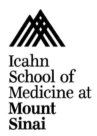

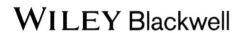

Registered Office(s)
John Wiley & Sons, Inc., 111 River Street, Hoboken, NJ 07030, USA
John Wiley & Sons Ltd, The Atrium, Southern Gate, Chichester, West Sussex, PO19 8SQ, UK

Editorial Office
9600 Garsington Road, Oxford, OX4 2DQ, UK

For details of our global editorial offices, customer services, and more information about Wiley products visit us at www.wiley.com.

Wiley also publishes its books in a variety of electronic formats and by print-on-demand. Some content that appears in standard print versions of this book may not be available in other formats.

Library of Congress Cataloging-in-Publication Data
Names: Sperling, Rhoda, editor.
Title: Obstetrics and gynecology / edited by Rhoda Sperling.
Description: Hoboken, NJ : Wiley-Blackwell, 2020. | Series: Mount Sinai expert guides | Includes bibliographical references and index.
Identifiers: LCCN 2020010613 (print) | LCCN 2020010614 (ebook) | ISBN 9781119450115 (library binding) | ISBN 9781119450108 (adobe pdf) | ISBN 9781119450078 (epub)
Subjects: LCSH: Obstetrics–Handbooks, manuals, etc. | Gynecology–Handbooks, manuals, etc.
Classification: LCC RG531 .O27 2020 (print) | LCC RG531 (ebook) | DDC 618.2–dc23
LC record available at https://lccn.loc.gov/2020010613
LC ebook record available at https://lccn.loc.gov/2020010614

Cover image: © Raycat/Getty Images
Cover design by Wiley

Set in 8.5/12pt FrutigerLTStd by Aptara Inc., New Delhi, India

Printed and bound by CPI Group (UK) Ltd, Croydon, CR0 4YY

10 9 8 7 6 5 4 3 2 1

Contents

Part 3: REPRODUCTIVE ENDOCRINOLOGY

Part 4: GYN ONCOLOGY

Part 5: FAMILY PLANNING

Contributors

Omara Afzal, DO
Department of Obstetrics, Gynecology and
 Reproductive Science
Icahn School of Medicine at Mount Sinai,
 New York, NY

Devora Aharon, MD
Reproductive Medicine Associates of
 New York
Division of Reproductive Endocrinology and
 Infertility
Icahn School of Medicine at Mount Sinai,
 New York, NY

Charles Ascher-Walsh, MD
Division of Female Pelvic Medicine and
 Reconstructive Surgery
Department of Obstetrics, Gynecology and
 Reproductive Science
Icahn School of Medicine at Mount Sinai,
 New York, NY

Ann Marie Beddoe, MD
Division of Gynecologic Oncology
Department of Obstetrics, Gynecology and
 Reproductive Science
Icahn School of Medicine at Mount Sinai,
 New York, NY

Eric P. Bergh, MD
Maternal-Fetal Medicine Subspecialist
UT Health – McGovern Medical School
Division of Maternal-Fetal Medicine,
 Houston, TX

Veerle Bergink, MD, PhD
Department of Psychiatry and Department of
 Obstetrics, Gynecology and Reproductive
 Science
Icahn School of Medicine at Mount Sinai,
 New York, NY

Neha R. Bhardwaj, MD, MS
Division of Family Planning
Department of Obstetrics, Gynecology and
 Reproductive Science
Icahn School of Medicine at Mount Sinai,
 New York, NY

Angela Bianco, MD
Division of Maternal-Fetal Medicine
Department of Obstetrics, Gynecology and
 Reproductive Science
Icahn School of Medicine at Mount Sinai,
 New York, NY

Catherine A. Bigelow, MD
Maternal-Fetal Medicine Subspecialist
Minnesota Perinatal Physicians
Allina Health, Minneapolis, MN

Stephanie V. Blank, MD
Division of Gynecologic Oncology
Department of Obstetrics, Gynecology and
 Reproductive Science
Icahn School of Medicine at Mount Sinai,
 New York, NY

Karen F. Brodman, MD
Department of Obstetrics, Gynecology and
 Reproductive Science
Icahn School of Medicine at Mount Sinai,
 New York, NY

Danielle Brooks, MD
Department of Medicine
Division of Endocrinology, Diabetes, and
 Metabolism
Icahn School of Medicine at Mount Sinai,
 New York, NY

Lois Brustman, MD
Division of Maternal-Fetal Medicine
Department of Obstetrics, Gynecology and
 Reproductive Science
Icahn School of Medicine at Mount Sinai, New
 York, NY

Laudy Burgos, LCSW
Department of Social Work Services
MSH, NERA-Undergraduate Behavioral Health
 Fellowship Program
Icahn School of Medicine at Mount Sinai,
 New York, NY

Francesco Callipari, MD
Department of Obstetrics, Gynecology and
 Reproductive Science
Icahn School of Medicine at Mount Sinai,
 New York, NY

Woojin Chong, MD
Urogynecologist, Inspira Health, Vineland, New
 Jersey, NJ
Division of Female Pelvic Medicine and
 Reconstructive Surgery
Department of Obstetrics, Gynecology and
 Reproductive Science
Icahn School of Medicine at Mount Sinai, New
 York, NY

Garfield Clunie, MD
Maternal-Fetal Medicine
The Brooklyn Hospital Center
Division of Maternal-Fetal Medicine
Icahn School of Medicine at Mount Sinai,
 New York, NY

Carmel J. Cohen, MD
Division of Gynecologic Oncology
Department of Obstetrics, Gynecology and
 Reproductive Science
Icahn School of Medicine at Mount Sinai,
 New York, NY

Katherine A. Connolly, MD
Division of Maternal-Fetal Medicine
Department of Obstetrics and Gynecology
University of California, San Francisco, CA

Alan B. Copperman, MD
Reproductive Medicine Associates of New York
Division of Reproductive Endocrinology and
 Infertility
Icahn School of Medicine at Mount Sinai,
 New York, NY

Lisa Dabney, MD
Division of Female Pelvic Medicine and
 Reconstructive Surgery
Department of Obstetrics, Gynecology and
 Reproductive Science
Icahn School of Medicine at Mount Sinai, New
 York, NY

Gillian Dean, MD, MPH
Planned Parenthood Federation of America
Division of Family Planning
Department of Obstetrics, Gynecology and
 Reproductive Science
Icahn School of Medicine at Mount Sinai,
 New York, NY

Andrew Ditchik, MD
Department of Obstetrics and Gynecology
Elmhurst Hospital Center, Queens, NY
Department of Obstetrics, Gynecology and
 Reproductive Science
Icahn School of Medicine at Mount Sinai,
 New York, NY

Matthew Dominguez, MD
Department of Psychiatry
Icahn School of Medicine at Mount Sinai,
 New York, NY

Janine A. Doneza, MD
Robotic and Minimally Invasive Gynecologic
 Surgery
MIGS/Urogynecology Fellowship Program
 Fibroid Center
Bronxcare Hospital, Bronx, NY,
Icahn School of Medicine at Mount Sinai,
 New York, NY

Peter Dottino, MD
Division of Gynecologic Oncology
Department of Obstetrics, Gynecology and
    Reproductive Science
Icahn School of Medicine at Mount Sinai,
    New York, NY

Keith Eddleman, MD
Division of Maternal-Fetal Medicine
Department of Obstetrics, Gynecology and
    Reproductive Science
Icahn School of Medicine at Mount Sinai,
    New York, NY

John A. Fantl, MD
Division of Female Pelvic Medicine and
    Reconstructive Surgery
Department of Obstetrics, Gynecology and
    Reproductive Science
Icahn School of Medicine at Mount Sinai,
    New York, NY

Suzanne S. Fenske, MD
Department of Obstetrics, Gynecology and
    Reproductive Science
Icahn School of Medicine at Mount Sinai,
    New York, NY

Lauren Ferrara, MD
Division of Maternal-Fetal Medicine
Department of Obstetrics, Gynecology and
    Reproductive Science
Icahn School of Medicine at Mount Sinai,
    New York, NY

Geetha N. Fink, MD, MPH
Division of Family Planning
Department of Obstetrics, Gynecology and
    Reproductive Science
Icahn School of Medicine at Mount Sinai,
    New York, NY

Eric Flisser, MD
Reproductive Medicine Associates of New York
Division of Reproductive Endocrinology and
    Infertility
Icahn School of Medicine at Mount Sinai,
    New York, NY

Faith J. Frieden, MD
Department of Obstetrics, Gynecology and
    Reproductive Science
Icahn School of Medicine at Mount Sinai,
    New York, NY

Elissa Gretz Friedman, MD
Department of Obstetrics, Gynecology and
    Reproductive Science
Icahn School of Medicine at Mount Sinai,
    New York, NY

Frederick Friedman Jr., MD
Department of Obstetrics, Gynecology and
    Reproductive Science
Icahn School of Medicine at Mount Sinai,
    New York, NY

Eric M. Ganz, MD
Department of Obstetrics, Gynecology and
    Reproductive Science
Icahn School of Medicine at Mount Sinai,
    New York, NY

Sharon Gerber, MD
Division of Family Planning
Department of Obstetrics, Gynecology and
    Reproductive Science
Icahn School of Medicine at Mount Sinai,
    New York, NY

Jeannette Guziel, MD
Hematology/Medical Oncology
Kaiser Permanente
Southern California Permanente Medical Group,
    Woodland Hills, CA

Anne Hardart, MD
Division of Female Pelvic Medicine and
    Reconstructive Surgery
Department of Obstetrics, Gynecology and
    Reproductive Science
Icahn School of Medicine at Mount Sinai,
    New York, NY

Nola S. Herlihy, MD
Reproductive Endocrinology and Infertility
IVIRMA, New Jersey, NJ

Karina Hoan, MD
FMIGS Faculty, Division of Minimally Invasive
    Gynecology
The Portland Clinic, Portland, OR

Adam Jacobs, MD
Division of Family Planning
Department of Obstetrics, Gynecology and
    Reproductive Science
Icahn School of Medicine at Mount Sinai,
    New York, NY

Nina S. Jacobson, MD
Division of Female Pelvic Medicine and
    Reconstructive Surgery
Department of Obstetrics and Gynecology
Jersey Shore University Medical Center, Neptune
    City, NJ

Tamara Kolev, MD
Department of Obstetrics, Gynecology and
    Reproductive Science
Icahn School of Medicine at Mount Sinai,
    New York, NY

Anna Kremer, MD
Department of Obstetrics, Gynecology and
    Reproductive Science
Icahn School of Medicine at Mount Sinai,
    New York, NY

Rashmi Kudesia, MD, MSc
Houston Methodist Hospital, CCRM Fertility,
    Houston, TX

Tatyana Kushner, MD
Department of Medicine
Division of Liver Diseases
Icahn School of Medicine at Mount Sinai,
    New York, NY

Carol Levy, MD
Department of Medicine
Division of Endocrinology, Diabetes, and
    Metabolism
Icahn School of Medicine at Mount Sinai,
    New York, NY

Holly C. Loudon, MD, MPH
Department of Obstetrics, Gynecology and
    Reproductive Science
Icahn School of Medicine at Mount Sinai,
    New York, NY

Britt Lunde, MD, MPH
Division of Family Planning
Department of Obstetrics, Gynecology and
    Reproductive Science
Icahn School of Medicine at Mount Sinai,
    New York, NY

Laura MacIsaac, MD, MPH
Division of Family Planning
Department of Obstetrics, Gynecology and
    Reproductive Science
Icahn School of Medicine at Mount Sinai,
    New York, NY

Rachel Masch, MD, MPH
Division of Family Planning
Department of Obstetrics, Gynecology and
    Reproductive Science
Icahn School of Medicine at Mount Sinai,
    New York, NY

Peter G. McGovern, MD
Division of Reproductive Endocrinology and
    Infertility
Department of Obstetrics, Gynecology and
    Reproductive Science
Icahn School of Medicine at Mount Sinai,
    New York, NY

Maria Teresa Mella, MD
Department of Obstetrics, Gynecology and
    Reproductive Science
Icahn School of Medicine at Mount Sinai,
    New York, NY

Keerti Murari, MD
Department of Medicine
Division of Endocrinology and Metabolism
Yale School of Medicine, New Haven, CT

Navya Nair, MD, MPH
Division of Gynecologic Oncology
Department of Obstetrics and Gynecology
Louisiana State University School of Medicine,
New Orleans, LA

Taraneh Gharib Nazem, MD
Reproductive Medicine Associates of New York
Division of Reproductive Endocrinology and
Infertility
Icahn School of Medicine at Mount Sinai,
New York, NY

Annacecilia Peacher, MD
Division of Female Pelvic Medicine and
Reconstructive Surgery
Department of Obstetrics, Gynecology and
Reproductive Science
Icahn School of Medicine at Mount Sinai,
New York, NY

Elena Pereira, MD
Gynecologic Oncology
Department of Obstetrics and Gynecology
Donald and Barbara Zucker School of Medicine at
Hofstra/Northwell Health, New York, NY

Jamal Rahaman, MD
Division of Gynecologic Oncology
Department of Obstetrics, Gynecology and
Reproductive Science
Icahn School of Medicine at Mount Sinai,
New York, NY

Andrei Rebarber, MD
Maternal Fetal Medicine Associates
New York, NY
Division of Maternal-Fetal Medicine
Department of Obstetrics, Gynecology and
Reproductive Science
Icahn School of Medicine at Mount Sinai,
New York, NY

Patricia Rekawek, MD
Maternal-Fetal Medicine
New York University Long Island School of
Medicine, NYU Winthrop Hospital, Mineola, NY

V. Ord Sarabanchong, MD, MPH
Department of Obstetrics, Gynecology and
Reproductive Science
Icahn School of Medicine at Mount Sinai,
New York, NY

Fahimeh Sasan, DO
Department of Obstetrics, Gynecology and
Reproductive Science
Icahn School of Medicine at Mount Sinai,
New York, NY

Melissa Schwartz, MD
Division of Gynecologic Oncology
Department of Obstetrics, Gynecology and
Women's Health
Saint Louis University School of Medicine,
St. Louis, MO

Lucky Sekhon, MD
Reproductive Medicine Associates of New York
Division of Reproductive Endocrinology and
Infertility
Icahn School of Medicine at Mount Sinai,
New York, NY

Kathryn L. Shaia, MD, MHA
Duke Fertility Center
Division of Reproductive Endocrinology and
Infertility
Department of Obstetrics and Gynecology
Duke University School of Medicine, Durham, NC

Amanda M. Silbermann, MD
Department of Obstetrics and Gynecology
New York University School of Medicine,
New York, NY

Marti Soffer, MD
Division of Maternal Fetal-Medicine
Department of Obstetrics and Gynecology
Massachusetts General Hospital, Boston, MA

Rhoda Sperling, MD
Department of Obstetrics, Gynecology and
Reproductive Science
Department of Medicine, Division of Infectious
Diseases
Icahn School of Medicine at Mount Sinai,
New York, NY

Daniel E. Stein, MD
Reproductive Medicine Associates of New York
Division of Reproductive Endocrinology and
  Infertility
Icahn School of Medicine at Mount Sinai,
  New York, NY

Joanne L. Stone, MD
Division of Maternal-Fetal Medicine
Department of Obstetrics, Gynecology and
  Reproductive Science
Icahn School of Medicine at Mount Sinai,
  New York, NY

Noel Strong, MD
Division of Maternal-Fetal Medicine
Department of Obstetrics, Gynecology and
  Reproductive Science
Icahn School of Medicine at Mount Sinai,
  New York, NY

Jian Jenny Tang, MD
Department of Obstetrics, Gynecology and
  Reproductive Science
Icahn School of Medicine at Mount Sinai,
  New York, NY

Dyese Taylor, MD
Department of Obstetrics, Gynecology and
  Reproductive Science
Icahn School of Medicine at Mount Sinai,
  New York, NY

Amy Tiersten, MD
Department of Medicine
Division of Hematology and Medical Oncology
Icahn School of Medicine at Mount Sinai,
  New York, NY

Shannon Tomita, MD
Division of Gynecologic Oncology
Department of Obstetrics, Gynecology and
  Reproductive Science
Icahn School of Medicine at Mount Sinai,
  New York, NY

Luciana Vieira, MD
Division of Maternal-Fetal Medicine
Department of Obstetrics, Gynecology and
  Reproductive Science
Icahn School of Medicine at Mount Sinai,
  New York, NY

Brian Wagner, MD
Division of Maternal-Fetal Medicine
Department of Obstetrics, Gynecology and
  Reproductive Science
Icahn School of Medicine at Mount Sinai,
  New York, NY

Elizabeth Yoselevsky, MD
Division of Maternal-Fetal Medicine
Department of Obstetrics, Gynecology, and
  Reproductive Biology
Brigham and Women's Hospital, Boston, MA

Series Foreword

Now more than ever, immediacy in obtaining accurate and practical information is the coin of the realm in providing high quality patient care. The Mount Sinai Expert Guides series addresses this vital need by providing accurate, up-to-date guidance, written by experts in formats that are accessible in the patient care setting: websites, smartphone apps, and portable books. The Icahn School of Medicine, which was chartered in 1963, embodies a deep tradition of preeminence in clinical care and scholarship that was first shaped by the founding of the Mount Sinai Hospital in 1855. Today, the Mount Sinai Health System, comprised of seven hospitals anchored by the Icahn School of Medicine, is one of the largest health care systems in the United States, and is revolutionizing medicine through its embracing of transformative technologies for clinical diagnosis and treatment. The Mount Sinai Expert Guides series builds upon both this historical renown and contemporary excellence. Leading experts across a range of disciplines provide practical yet sage advice in a digestible format that is ideal for trainees, mid-level providers, and practicing physicians. Few medical centers in the United States could offer this type of breadth while relying exclusively on its own physicians, yet here no compromises were required in offering a truly unique series that is sure to become embedded within the key resources of busy providers. In producing this series, the editors and authors are fortunate to have an equally dynamic and forward-viewing partner in Wiley Blackwell, which together ensures that health care professionals will benefit from a unique, first-class effort that will advance the care of their patients.

Scott Friedman MD
Series Editor
Dean for Therapeutic Discovery
Fishberg Professor and Chief, Division of Liver Diseases
Icahn School of Medicine at Mount Sinai
New York, NY, USA

Preface

Designed for both trainees and practitioners, this Expert Guide explores the wide breadth of topics that define the discipline of obstetrics and gynecology. This Expert Guide is dedicated to Dr. Michael Brodman, Chair of the Department of Obstetrics, Gynecology and Reproductive Sciences at the Icahn School of Medicine at Mount Sinai; his tireless efforts have built a strong, innovative, and diverse faculty whose expertise are now showcased in these chapters.

Rhoda Sperling, MD
Department of Obstetrics, Gynecology and Reproductive Science
Department of Medicine
Division of Infectious Diseases
Icahn School of Medicine at Mount Sinai,
New York, NY

About the Companion Website

This series is accompanied by a companion website:

www.wiley.com/go/sperling/mountsinai/obstetricsandgynecology

The website includes:
- Advice for patients
- Case studies with interactive MCQs
- ICD codes
- Color versions of images

PART 1

Obstetrics

CHAPTER 1

Multiple Gestations

Katherine A. Connolly[1] and Joanne L. Stone[2]

[1] Division of Maternal-Fetal Medicine, Department of Obstetrics and Gynecology, University of California, San Francisco, CA
[2] Division of Maternal-Fetal Medicine, Department of Obstetrics, Gynecology and Reproductive Science, Icahn School of Medicine at Mount Sinai, New York, NY

OVERALL BOTTOM LINE
- The incidence of twin gestation has risen due to advancing maternal age and the use of assisted reproductive techniques (ART).
- There are increased risks of a twin gestation, including preterm labor, preterm delivery, low birth weight, fetal growth restriction, gestational diabetes, preeclampsia, and need for cesarean delivery.
- Twin gestations require increased surveillance due to these increased risks.

Background
Definition of disease
- Twin gestation refers to an intrauterine gestation of two fetuses.

Disease classification
- Dizygotic twins occur after ovulation and fertilization of two different oocytes. This type of twins has two placentas and two amniotic sacs (Figure 1.1).
- Monozygotic twins result from ovulation and fertilization of one single oocyte, with subsequent division. Depending on what day the embryo splits, these monozygotic twins are further classified as the following:
  - Dichorionic/diamniotic (Day 1–3)
  - Monochorionic/diamniotic (Day 4–8) (Figure 1.2)
  - Monochorionic/monoamniotic (Day 8–13)
  - Conjoined twins (Day 13–15)

Incidence/prevalence
- The natural incidence of twins is 1/80.
- The incidence of multiple gestation increased by 76% from 1980 to 2009 due to ART and has since stabilized.
- Twins now account for 3% of live births.

Economic impact
- Twin gestations are associated with higher cost, which is mostly related to the increased rate of preterm delivery. The cost of a premature infant is up to 10 times greater than that of a term infant in the first year.

Mount Sinai Expert Guides: Obstetrics and Gynecology, First Edition. Edited by Rhoda Sperling.
© 2020 John Wiley & Sons Ltd. Published 2020 by John Wiley & Sons Ltd.
Companion Website: www.wiley.com/go/sperling/mountsinai/obstetricsandgynecology

Predictive/risk factors

Risk factor	Contribution
Assisted reproductive technology	Accounts for 1/3 of all twin pregnancies
Maternal age	Fourfold increase from age 15 to age 35
Family history	Increased risk of dizygotic twins

Prevention

> **BOTTOM LINE/CLINICAL PEARLS**
> * The incidence of twin gestation has stabilized over time as the number of embryos transferred with ART has decreased. Single embryo transfer has become an increasingly common practice.

Screening
* Ultrasound in the first or early second trimester is essential in diagnosing twin gestation and establishing chorionicity (Figures 1.1 and 1.2).

Primary prevention
* Single embryo transfer to decrease the number of twin gestations that result from in vitro fertilization is an important prevention method. Splitting of an embryo into a monozygotic twin gestation, whether spontaneous or after ART, is not preventable.

Secondary prevention
* After a twin gestation is diagnosed, a multifetal pregnancy reduction procedure can be performed, resulting in a single fetus and improved pregnancy outcomes.
* Multifetal pregnancy reduction to a singleton gestation is associated with higher birth weights and lower rates of preterm deliveries.

Diagnosis

> **BOTTOM LINE/CLINICAL PEARLS**
> * The diagnosis of twins is made with ultrasound.
> * This ultrasound should be done in the first or early second trimester in order to most accurately establish chorionicity, which has important implications for the pregnancy.

Typical presentation
* Twin gestation may be suspected if uterine size measures larger than would be expected for a given gestational age.
* Diagnosis can be confirmed only with ultrasound.

Clinical diagnosis
History
* Age
* Family history of twin gestation
* Use of ART

Physical examination
- Clinical examination of uterine size with bimanual exam and measurement of fundal height

Laboratory diagnosis

List of diagnostic tests
- The risk of aneuploidy is higher in dizygotic twins. The mathematical probability that a single fetus is affected is doubled in a twin gestation.
  - The chance that a 33-year-old with twins has one fetus with Down syndrome is equivalent to the chance that a 35-year-old has a singleton fetus with Down syndrome.
- All pregnant patients are counseled on options for genetic screening (serum screening such as sequential or quad screen) or diagnostic testing (chorionic villus sampling or amniocentesis).
- Even in a singleton pregnancy, serum screening is never diagnostic, but this screening is even further limited in twin gestations.
  - Analyte levels in maternal serum for twins are estimated using mathematical models.
  - Analyte levels in maternal serum from each fetus are averaged together, possibly normalizing the levels and masking an affected fetus.
  - First trimester serum screening combined with nuchal translucency measurements identifies 75–85% of pregnancies with Down syndrome and 66% of pregnancies with trisomy 18 in twins.
  - Second trimester serum screening identifies 63% of pregnancies with Down syndrome in twins.
- Noninvasive prenatal screening (NIPS), which analyzes cell-free fetal DNA in maternal serum, is not recommended for multiple gestations.
- Invasive testing with chorionic villus sampling (CVS) or amniocentesis remain the only two options for diagnostic testing.
  - CVS samples the chorionic villi and may be performed as early at 9 weeks.
    - CVS may be more technically challenging in a twin gestation. There is an approximately 1% rate of sampling error, meaning that one fetus was sampled twice.
  - Amniocentesis is performed by sampling the amniotic fluid and is done after 15 weeks.
    - To avoid sampling error, once a needle is inserted into the first amniotic sac, indigo carmine is injected into this sac, which results in blue colored fluid. This needle is then removed and a second needle inserted into the second sac. If the fluid is clear, it is confirmed that the second sac has been entered. If the fluid is blue, this indicates that the same sac has just been entered a second time.
    - There is approximately a 1.8% pregnancy loss rate prior to 24 weeks after amniocentesis in twins.

List of imaging techniques
- Ultrasound is the primary imaging modality used in the surveillance of all pregnancies, including twin gestation.

Potential pitfalls/common errors made regarding diagnosis of disease
- Ultrasound should be performed in the first or early second trimester for the most accurate determination of chorionicity. It is essential that chorionicity is accurately established, as monochorionic twins and dichorionic twins are at risk for different complications and need to be monitored and managed differently.

Treatment

Treatment rationale
- There have been several interventions that have been studied in an attempt to decrease the rate of preterm delivery in twins that have not found to be beneficial:
  - Prophylactic cerclage: not beneficial, not recommended
  - Cerclage for short cervix: not only not beneficial but actually DOUBLES the rate of spontaneous preterm delivery and is therefore not recommended

- Bed rest: not beneficial, not recommended
- Prophylactic tocolytics: not beneficial, not recommended
- Prophylactic pessary: not beneficial, not recommended
- Prophylactic use of progesterone: not beneficial, not recommended
- Twin pregnancies require increased surveillance to detect signs of preterm labor. There are several beneficial interventions if a patient is found to be in preterm labor that are discussed in the following sections.

When to hospitalize

- There are several indications for hospitalization of twins:
  - Preterm labor, advanced cervical exam, preeclampsia/gestational hypertension, bleeding, fetal growth restriction
  - Twins are at higher risk for all of the aforementioned complications, but once they are diagnosed, they are often managed similarly to the way singletons are managed.

Managing the hospitalized patient

- Management of preterm labor in twin gestation:
  - Tocolytics: Data are limited in twin gestations, though a 48-hour course to enable the administration of corticosteroids seem to be beneficial in twins as well. First-line agents include calcium channel blockers and nonsteroidal anti-inflammatory agents (indomethacin).
  - Corticosteroids: Administration of steroids between 24 and 34 weeks has been shown to decrease the incidence of neonatal death, respiratory distress syndrome, intraventricular hemorrhage, and necrotizing enterocolitis in singleton gestations. Based on this evidence, the National Institutes of Health recommends that they should be administered in multiple gestations as well.
  - Magnesium sulfate: Administration has been shown to reduce the incidence of cerebral palsy when given prior to delivery when it is occurs less than 32 weeks.

Table of treatment

Treatment	Comments
Medical	When a patient with twins is admitted for preterm labor, administration of corticosteroids (if between 24–34 weeks), tocolytics (if between 24–34 weeks), and magnesium sulfate prior to delivery (if less than 32 weeks) is recommended.
Surgical	Cerclage is not recommended in twin gestations, as it leads to worse outcomes. There is a higher rate of cesarean delivery in twin gestations, although vaginal delivery is possible if the presenting fetus (typically fetus A) is in cephalic presentation.
Radiological	The use of ultrasound is essential to the management of twin gestation. Early ultrasound to establish chorionicity, then second trimester anatomic survey, and then serial growth ultrasounds to look for growth restriction or twin to twin transfusion syndrome are employed.
Psychological (includes cognitive, behavioral, etc., therapies)	Mothers who give birth to twins are at increased risk of postpartum depression; therefore, it is important to administer a depression scale at their postpartum visit and treat as necessary.

Prevention/management of complications

- Prevention is aimed at early identification of complications for which twins are at risk.
  - Preterm delivery: cervical length screening to identify patients at risk for preterm delivery is reasonable in order to optimize outcomes with steroids and magnesium sulfate if preterm delivery is imminent.

- Preeclampsia: blood pressure should be taken at each visit and patients counseled on signs and symptoms of preeclampsia.
- Gestational diabetes: all patients should be screened for gestational diabetes and early screen should be considered in patients with risk factors.
- Twin to twin transfusion syndrome: this complication is unique to monochorionic twins. Screening for this is with ultrasound that is performed every 2 weeks starting at 16 weeks in monochorionic gestations.
- Growth discordance/restriction: all twin gestations should be followed with serial growth ultrasounds to detect differences in weight or selective growth restriction.

CLINICAL PEARLS
- Chorionicity is best established in the first or early second trimester.
- Twin gestations are at an increased risk for spontaneous abortion, genetic abnormalities, growth restriction, preeclampsia, gestational diabetes, and cesarean delivery and patients should be counseled accordingly.
- Multifetal pregnancy reduction has been shown to improve outcomes and may be offered to patients with multiple gestation.

Prognosis

BOTTOM LINE/CLINICAL PEARLS
- Twins are at increased risk for preterm delivery and the neonatal complications that accompany it. Twin gestations delivery earlier on average, even with treatment of preterm labor.
- The following table compares delivery timing and infant morbidity in singleton versus twin gestation.

Outcomes in singleton versus twin gestations

	Singletons	Twins
Mean gestational age at delivery	38.7 weeks	35.3 weeks
Mean birth weight	3296 g	2336 g
Percentage who deliver <32 weeks	1.6	11.4
Percentage who deliver <37 weeks	10.4	58.8
Rate of cerebral palsy (per 1000 live births)	1.6	7

Reading list

American College of Obstetricians and Gynecologists. Multifetal gestations: twin, triplet and higher-order multifetal pregnancies. Practice bulletin no. 169. *Obstet Gynecol* 2016;e131-46.

Society for Maternal Fetal Medicine Publications Committee. Prenatal aneuploidy screening using cell-free DNA. Consult series no. 36. *Am J Obstet Gynecol* 2015;212:711-6.

Stone J, Ferrara L, Kamrath J, et al. Contemporary outcomes with the latest 1000 cases of multifetal pregnancy reduction (MPR). *Am J Obstet Gynecol* 2008 Oct;199(4):408.e1-4. doi: 10.1016/j.ajog.2008.05.020

Suggested websites

American College of Obstetricians and Gynecologists. www.acog.org
Society for Maternal-Fetal Medicine. www.smfm.org

Guidelines
National society guidelines

Title	Source	Date/full reference
Multifetal gestations: twin, triplet, and higher-order multifetal pregnancies	American College of Obstetricians and Gynecologists	American College of Obstetricians and Gynecologists. Multifetal gestations: twin, triplet and higher-order multifetal pregnancies. Practice bulletin no. 169. *Obstet Gynecol* 2016;e131-46.

Images

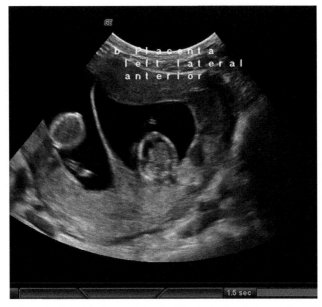

Figure 1.1 "Twin peak" or Lambda sign characteristic of a dichorionic diamniotic gestation. This sonographic sign is used to help establish chorionicity. Another sonographic feature of a dichorionic diamniotic gestation is two placentas. If the fetal sex is discordant, the pregnancy is dichorionic.

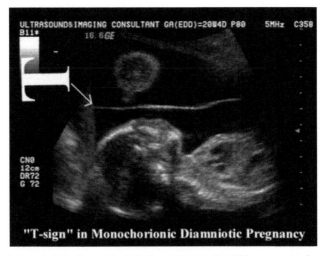

Figure 1.2 "T sign" characteristic of monochorionic diamniotic gestation. This sonographic feature is 100% sensitive and >98% specific for the diagnosis of monochorionic gestation.

Additional material for this chapter can be found online at:
www.wiley.com/go/sperling/mountsinai/obstetricsandgynecology

This includes multiple choice questions, advice for patients, and ICD codes.

CHAPTER 2

Preeclampsia/Eclampsia

Patricia Rekawek[1] and Brian Wagner[2]
[1] Maternal-Fetal Medicine, New York University Long Island School of Medicine, NYU Winthrop Hospital, Mineola, NY
[2] Division of Maternal-Fetal Medicine, Department of Obstetrics, Gynecology and Reproductive Science, Icahn School of Medicine at Mount Sinai, New York, NY

OVERALL BOTTOM LINE

- Preeclampsia is a disorder characterized by the development of hypertension and either proteinuria or end-organ dysfunction after 20 weeks gestation in a previously normotensive woman.
- Preeclampsia should be differentiated from other hypertensive disorders of pregnancy including chronic hypertension, gestational hypertension, preeclampsia superimposed on chronic hypertension, hemolysis elevated liver enzymes and low platelets (HELLP) syndrome, and eclampsia.
- Women with preeclampsia are at increased risk of the development of end-organ damage including placental abruption, kidney injury, hepatic failure, pulmonary edema, cardiac failure, stroke, and eclampsia. Additionally, these women are at increased risk for future cardiovascular disease.
- Pregnancy complications may include fetal growth restriction, preterm delivery, and stillbirth.
- Delivery remains the treatment for preeclampsia.

Background
Definition of disease
- Preeclampsia is a progressive disease defined as the new onset of hypertension and either proteinuria or other signs of end-organ dysfunction after 20 weeks gestation in a previously normotensive patient.
- Hypertension is defined as systolic blood pressure (BP) ≥ 140 mm Hg or diastolic BP ≥ 90 mm Hg on two occasions at least 4 hours apart and proteinuria is defined as ≥ 0.3 g in a 24-hour urine collection or a ratio of urine protein to creatinine of > 0.3 mg/dL.

Disease classification
- Some clinical findings increase the risk of morbidity and mortality and these indicate a severe form of preeclampsia, known as preeclampsia with severe features.
- These findings include severe range blood pressure, defined as systolic BP ≥ 160 mm Hg or diastolic BP ≥ 110 mm Hg on two occasions at least 4 hours apart and/or thrombocytopenia, impaired liver function, renal insufficiency, pulmonary edema, and cerebral or visual disturbances (see disease severity classification).

Incidence/prevalence
- Worldwide, 4.6% of pregnancies are complicated by preeclampsia.
- The prevalence of preeclampsia in the United States is approximately 3.4%; however, this varies by gestational age.

Mount Sinai Expert Guides: Obstetrics and Gynecology, First Edition. Edited by Rhoda Sperling.
© 2020 John Wiley & Sons Ltd. Published 2020 by John Wiley & Sons Ltd.
Companion Website: www.wiley.com/go/sperling/mountsinaiobstetricsandgynecology

- Variances in prevalence are likely due to differences in maternal age and percentage of nulliparous pregnant women among worldwide populations.

Etiology
- A clear cause for preeclampsia has yet to be elucidated.
- It is thought that preeclampsia may be due to placental and maternal vascular dysfunction. Although incompletely understood, it is thought that impaired remodeling of uterine spiral arteries leads to reduced placental perfusion.
- This leads to increased inflammation, increased production of antiangiogenic factors, and resultant maternal endothelial cell damage that manifest in the signs and symptoms of preeclampsia.

Pathology/pathogenesis
- The pathophysiology of preeclampsia involves abnormal placental development. Spiral arteries abnormally invade the myometrium, which creates hypoxic trophoblast tissue, thereby resulting in a state of placental oxidative stress.
- Placental villous angiogenesis is thereby altered resulting in increased secretion of placental antiangiogenic factors such as soluble fms-like tyrosine kinase (sFlt-1) and endoglin.
- This further leads to widespread maternal vascular dysfunction, which leads to end-organ damage and manifests clinically as hypertension, proteinuria, or signs of renal/liver/cerebral damage.

Predictive/risk factors

Risk factor	Relative risk
History of preeclampsia	7.19
Antiphospholipid antibodies	9.72
Pregestational diabetes	3.56
Nulliparity	2.91
Family history of preeclampsia	2.90

Prevention

> **BOTTOM LINE/CLINICAL PEARLS**
> - Low-dose aspirin (81 mg) has been shown to be the only effective pharmacologic agent that reduces the risk of preeclampsia.
> - Recent studies have shown that the effect of aspirin on preventing preeclampsia in high-risk pregnancies is greatest when initiated at less than 16 weeks gestation and that the optimal dose is 100–150 mg.
> - Anticoagulation does not prevent recurrence.

Screening
- Women at high risk for preeclampsia include the following:
  - Previous pregnancy with preeclampsia; most significantly with early onset and with adverse outcome
  - Multifetal gestation
  - Chronic hypertension
  - Type 1 or type 2 diabetes mellitus

- Chronic kidney disease
- Autoimmune disorders such as antiphospholipid syndrome or systemic lupus erythematous

Primary prevention

- Low-dose aspirin (81 mg) during pregnancy has been shown to modestly reduce the risk of preeclampsia and adverse pregnancy outcomes in high-risk women.
  - These include multifetal gestation, type 1 or 2 diabetes, chronic hypertension, autoimmune disease, and chronic kidney disease.
- Recent data suggest that doses up to 150 mg of aspirin may be more effective at reducing risk of recurrent preeclampsia.
- Obese women who lose weight prior to becoming pregnant may reduce their risk of developing preeclampsia.

Secondary prevention

- Low-dose aspirin (81 mg) during pregnancy has been shown to modestly reduce the risk of recurrent preeclampsia and adverse pregnancy outcomes especially in patients with early onset and severe disease.
- Weight loss in obese women between pregnancies may reduce the risk of recurrent disease.

Diagnosis

> **BOTTOM LINE/CLINICAL PEARLS**
> - Clinical symptoms of preeclampsia include persistent and/or severe headache, visual abnormalities, upper abdominal or epigastric pain, altered mental status, and dyspnea or retrosternal chest pain.
> - Exam findings may include generalized hyperreflexia, peripheral edema, pulmonary edema, or oliguria (urine output < 500 mL/24 hours).
> - Laboratory findings include proteinuria, elevated creatinine level, thrombocytopenia, elevated transaminase levels, hemolysis, and/or hemoconcentration.

Differential diagnosis

Differential diagnosis (see Algorithms 2.1 and 2.2)	Features
Chronic hypertension	Defined as systolic blood pressure ≥ 140 mm Hg and/or diastolic ≥ 90 mm Hg, present before 20 weeks gestation and persists longer than 12 weeks postpartum
Chronic hypertension with superimposed preeclampsia	New onset of either proteinuria or end organ dysfunction after 20 weeks in women with chronic hypertension
Gestational hypertension	Hypertension developing after 20 weeks gestation in a previously normotensive woman with no proteinuria and no signs of end-organ damage
HELLP syndrome	Defined as hemolysis, elevated liver enzymes, and low platelets. This is characterized as a more severe form of preeclampsia, although it can be diagnosed without hypertension or proteinuria.
Eclampsia	Grand mal seizures in a woman with preeclampsia

Algorithm 2.1 Diagnostic algorithm for preeclampsia
Preeclampsia

Systolic blood pressure ≥ 140 mm Hg or diastolic blood pressure ≥ 90 mm Hg on two occasions at least four hours apart after 20 weeks gestation in a previously normotensive patient.
- If systolic BP ≥ 160 mm Hg or diastolic blood pressure is ≥ 110 mm Hg, confirmation within minutes is sufficient.

AND

Proteinuria
- ≥ 0.3 g in a 24-hour urine specimen or
- Urine protein to creatinine ratio ≥ 0.3 mg/Dl
- Urine dip ≥ 1+, if quantitative measurements are unavailable

OR

New-onset hypertension with the onset of any of the following (with or without proteinuria)
- Serum transaminase concentration ≥ 2 times upper limit of normal range
- Thrombocytopenia defined as platelets < 100°000/microL
- Serum creatinine > 1.1 mg/dL or doubling of serum creatinine concentration
- Liver transaminase levels at least twice the upper limit of normal
- Pulmonary edema
- Cerebral or visual symptoms

Data from American College of Obstetricians and Gynecologists, Task Force on Hypertension in Pregnancy. Hypertension in pregnancy. Report of the American College of Obstetricians and Gynecologists' Task Force on Hypertension in Pregnancy. *Obstet Gynecol* 2013;122:1122.

Algorithm 2.2 Diagnostic algorithm for preeclampsia with severe features
Preeclampsia with severe features (based on the presence of one or more of the following)

Severe blood pressure elevation
- Systolic blood pressure ≥ 160 mm Hg and/or diastolic blood pressure ≥ 110 mm Hg on two occasions at least 4 hours apart while patient is on bedrest.

Symptoms of central nervous system dysfunction
New-onset cerebral or visual disturbance, such as:
- Photopsia, scotomata, cortical blindness, retinal vasospasm
- Severe headache or headache that persists and progresses despite analgesia
- Altered mental status

Hepatic abnormality
- Severe persistent right upper quadrant or epigastric pain unresponsive to medication and not accounted for by an alternative diagnosis; or
- Serum transaminase concentration ≥ 2 times upper limit of normal range

Thrombocytopenia
- < 100°000 platelets/microL

Renal abnormality
- Progressive renal insufficiency such as serum creatinine > 1.1 mg/dL; or
- Doubling of serum creatinine concentration in absence of other renal disease

Pulmonary edema

Adapted from Hypertension in pregnancy: Report of the American College of Obstetricians and Gynecologists' Task Force on Hypertension in Pregnancy. *Obstetic Gynecol* 2013;122:1122.

Typical presentation

- The typical presentation of preeclampsia is of a nulliparous patient with new-onset hypertension and proteinuria ≥ 34 weeks gestation. The degree of maternal hypertension and proteinuria or additional signs of end-organ damage can be quite variable.

Clinical diagnosis

History

- The clinician should inquire about symptoms suggestive of preeclampsia. These clinical symptoms include persistent and/or severe headache not responsive to analgesia, visual abnormalities (blurred vision, scotomata, photophobia, or temporary blindness), upper abdominal or epigastric pain, altered mental status, or dyspnea or retrosternal chest pain.

Physical examination

- Physical examination findings include tenderness to palpation of epigastrium, generalized hyperreflexia, peripheral edema, pulmonary edema, oliguria, or gross neurologic deficits to suggest stroke.

Disease severity classification

- The disease is classified as preeclampsia with severe features if the following occur:
  - Mild range blood pressures with signs/symptoms of end-organ injury (+/-proteinuria):
    - Thrombocytopenia (<100°000 platelets/microL)
    - Impaired liver function (serum transaminase concentration ≥ 2 times upper limit of normal)
    - Progressive renal insufficiency (serum creatinine > 1.1 mg/dL or doubling of serum creatinine in absence of other renal disease)
    - Pulmonary edema
    - New-onset neurologic or visual disturbances
    - Severe persistent right upper quadrant or epigastric pain unresponsive to medication
  - Severe hypertension defined as systolic BP ≥ 160 mm Hg and/or diastolic BP ≥ 110 mg Hg with proteinuria and/or signs of end-organ injury as noted previously.

Laboratory diagnosis

List of diagnostic tests

- Proteinuria
  - Persistent ≥ 1+ (30 mg/dL) on paper test strip
  - Confirmed by random urine ratio of protein to creatinine ≥ 0.3 mg/dL
  - Diagnostic test is ≥ 0.3 g protein in a 24-hour urine collection
- Elevated creatinine
  - Creatinine level > 1.1 mg/dL or doubling from baseline
- Thrombocytopenia
  - Platelet count < 100°000/microL
- Elevated transaminase levels
  - Twice the upper limit of normal
- Hemolysis
  - Schistocytes and helmet cells on peripheral blood smear
- Hemoconcentration

List of imaging techniques
- Fetal ultrasound is used to assess for adequate growth as preeclampsia can result in reduced uteroplacental perfusion and subsequent fetal growth restriction.
  - Testing of fetal well-being can be performed including a biophysical profile.
  - Umbilical artery Doppler is used to measure the impedance of flow in the umbilical arteries that results from abnormalities in uteroplacental development. This can be used to guide management particularly in fetuses with growth restriction. Absent and reversed end-diastolic flow is associated with a poor perinatal prognosis.
- Maternal echocardiography can be used to assess for changes in cardiac function and morphology as the disease progresses in severity.
- Maternal right upper quadrant (RUQ) sonography can be used to assess liver capsule if hematoma is suspected.

Potential pitfalls/common errors made regarding diagnosis of disease
- Delay in diagnosis can result in significant maternal and/or fetal morbidity and mortality.
- Atypical presentations should be considered. This includes those with severe features of preeclampsia without hypertension, which can occur in up to 15% of patients with HELLP syndrome and in some with eclampsia.

Treatment
Treatment rationale
- Definitive treatment of preeclampsia is delivery. This prevents progression of disease and resultant maternal and/or fetal morbidity and mortality.
  - All women diagnosed with preeclampsia at $\geq$ 37 weeks should undergo delivery.
  - All women diagnosed with preeclampsia with severe features at $\geq$ 34 weeks should undergo delivery.
  - In a tertiary care setting, expectant antepartum management is an option for women diagnosed with preeclampsia before these gestational ages.
- Antihypertensive therapy is indicated for treatment of severe hypertension to prevent maternal cerebrovascular complications (see table of treatment).
- Antenatal glucocorticoids, to promote fetal lung maturity, are recommended for women with a diagnosis of preeclampsia < 34 weeks.
- Magnesium sulfate is recommended intrapartum and postpartum for seizure prophylaxis for women with preeclampsia with severe features.
- See also Algorithm 2.3.

When to hospitalize
- Hospitalization is indicated for women with the diagnosis of preeclampsia with severe features who are being expectantly managed and remote from term (<34 weeks gestational age).

Managing the hospitalized patient
- The hospitalized patient is managed by serial blood pressure assessment, serial laboratory assessment, and monitoring for features of severe disease.
- Fetal well-being should be assessed with a combination of tests (nonstress test, biophysical profile, umbilical artery Doppler, fetal growth) as dictated by the clinical picture.

Table of treatment

Treatment	Side effects
Medical	
Acute management of severe hypertension	
Labetalol IV 10–20 mg over 2 minutes; 20–80 mg every 20 to 30 minutes to maximum 300 mg	Avoid in asthma, heart disease, or congestive heart failure May cause neonatal bradycardia
Hydralazine IV 5 mg over 1 to 2 minutes; 5–10 mg every 20 to 40 minutes	Associated with increase in maternal hypotension
Nifedipine orally 10 mg; repeat in 30 minutes	Causes reflex tachycardia and overshoot hypotension Concern for neuromuscular blockade and severe hypotension when combined with magnesium sulfate
Longer-term blood pressure control	
Labetalol 100 mg orally bid; increase by 100 mg twice-daily as needed; maximum dose 2400 mg daily	
Nifedipine extended release 30 to 60 mg orally qd; maximum dose 120 mg daily	
Methyldopa 250 mg orally bid to tid; maximum dose 3000 mg daily	
Hydralazine 10 mg orally qid; 200 mg maximum dose	
Seizure prophylaxis	
Magnesium sulfate 4 g IV loading dose followed by 2 g IV per hour	Contraindicated in myasthenia gravis Side effects include diaphoresis, flushing, warmth, nausea/vomiting
Delivery	
Preeclampsia without severe features	Delivery indicated at 37 weeks
Preeclampsia with severe features	Delivery indicated at 34 weeks or earlier in the case of worsening progression of disease (consultation with maternal-fetal medicine specialist recommended)

Prevention/management of complications
- **Magnesium toxicity:** This is uncommon in women with adequate renal function. Toxicity correlates with level of serum magnesium concentration:
  - Loss of deep tendon reflexes occurs at 7 to 10 mEq/L
  - Respiratory paralysis at 10 to 13 mEq/L
  - Cardiac conduction is altered at > 15 mEq/L
  - Cardiac arrest occurs at > 25 mEq/L
  - Calcium gluconate is administered as an antidote to severe cardiac toxicity related to hypermagnesemia

Algorithm 2.3 Management and treatment of preeclampsia
Diagnosis of preeclampsia
What is the gestational age?
    <24 weeks – consider termination of pregnancy

    ≥37 weeks – recommend delivery; antihypertensive therapy and magnesium sulfate for seizure prophylaxis as needed for severe features

    24–37 weeks

Is there evidence of severe disease or contraindications to expectant management?

No – outpatient expectant management; twice-weekly office visits to assess maternal and fetal status

Yes – **Admit**

Admit for preeclampsia with severe features?

Is the maternal and fetal status stable? Are there contraindications to expectant management?

No – delivery

Yes – daily assessment of maternal and fetal status; antenatal corticosteroids; magnesium sulfate during initial assessment

Worsening of maternal and/or fetal status?

Yes – delivery; recommend magnesium sulfate for seizure prophylaxis; antihypertensives as needed

No – continue expectant management; plan for delivery at 34 weeks

---

CLINICAL PEARLS
- Delivery remains the definitive treatment of preeclampsia. This depends on the severity of preeclampsia, maternal/fetal condition, and gestational age at diagnosis. Delivery is recommended at $\geq$ 37 weeks. Close outpatient expectant management can be performed if diagnosed at earlier gestational ages.
- Delivery is recommended in preeclampsia with severe features at $\geq$ 34 weeks. Expectant management is an option for women diagnosed at earlier gestational ages. This requires hospitalization and close assessment of maternal and fetal status to monitor for worsening disease that would necessitate delivery.
- To prevent maternal cerebrovascular complications, antihypertensive therapy is indicated for treatment of severe hypertension.
- To prevent seizures/eclampsia, magnesium sulfate is recommended for seizure prophylaxis intrapartum and postpartum in women with severe features.

Prognosis

BOTTOM LINE/CLINICAL PEARLS
- There is an associated increased risk of preeclampsia in subsequent pregnancies.
- The American Heart Association regards a history of preeclampsia or pregnancy-induced hypertension as a major risk for development of cardiovascular disease in the future.

Natural history of untreated disease
- With untreated disease, preeclampsia can result in maternal/fetal morbidity and mortality. This includes development of end-stage organ damage, possible seizure, stroke, or renal failure and obstetrical complications including fetal growth restriction, preterm delivery, placental abruption, and stillbirth.

Prognosis for treated patients
- Even when adequately treated, there is a risk of recurrent preeclampsia and related complications in subsequent pregnancies and long-term maternal health risks.

Follow-up tests and monitoring
- In subsequent pregnancies, lab assessment of renal and liver function and level of proteinuria should be evaluated early and repeat as the clinical situation warrants.

- Comprehensive gynecologic care in the future should include assessment of cardiovascular risk factors and risk reducing interventions should be recommended.
  - Risk reducing interventions include healthy diet, smoking avoidance, management of hypertension, type 2 diabetes, and dyslipidemia, physical activity, weight loss, and aspirin therapy.

Reading list

American College of Obstetricians and Gynecologists. ACOG committee opinion no. 560: Medically indicated late-preterm and early-term deliveries. *Obstet Gynecol* 2013;121:908.

American College of Obstetricians and Gynecologists. ACOG practice bulletin no. 202: Gestational hypertension and preeclampsia. *Obstet Gynecol* 2019;133:e1-25.

American College of Obstetricians and Gynecologists. Emergent therapy for acute-onset, severe hypertension during pregnancy and the postpartum period. ACOG committee opinion No. 767. *Obstet Gynecol* 2019;133:e174-80.

American College of Obstetricians and Gynecologists Committee on Obstetric Practice. Committee Opinion No. 623: Emergent therapy for acute-onset, severe hypertension during pregnancy and the postpartum period. *Obstet Gynecol* 2015 Feb;125(2):521-5.

American College of Obstetricians and Gynecologists, Task Force on Hypertension in Pregnancy. Hypertension in pregnancy. Report of the American College of Obstetricians and Gynecologists' Task Force on Hypertension in Pregnancy. *Obstet Gynecol* 2013;122:1122.

Hauth JC, Ewell MG, Levine RJ, et al. Pregnancy outcomes in healthy nulliparas who developed hypertension. Calcium for Preeclampsia Prevention Study Group. *Obstet Gynecol* 2000;95:24.

Heard AR, Dekker GA, Chan A, et al. Hypertension during pregnancy in South Australia, part 1: pregnancy outcomes. *Aust N Z J Obstet Gynaecol* 2004;44:404.

Koopmans CM, Bijlenga D, Groen H, et al. Induction of labour versus expectant monitoring for gestational hypertension or mild pre-eclampsia after 36 weeks' gestation (HYPITAT): a multicentre, open-label randomised controlled trial. *Lancet* 2009;374:979.

National Collaborating Centre for Women's and Children's Health. *Hypertension in pregnancy: The management of hypertensive disorders during pregnancy.* London: RCOG Press; 2010.

Safe Motherhood Initiative. Maternal safety bundle for severe hypertension in pregnancy. ACOG; April 2018. Available from: https://www.acog.org/-/media/Districts/District-II/Public/SMI/v2/HTNSlideSetApril2018.pdf?dmc=1&ts= (accessed 18 February 2020).

Spong CY, Mercer BM, D'Alton M, et al. Timing of indicated late-preterm and early-term birth. *Obstet Gynecol* 2011;118:323.

Suggested websites

American College of Obstetricians and Gynecologists. www.acog.org

Society for Maternal-Fetal Medicine. www.smfm.org

Guidelines
National society guidelines

Title	Source	Date/full reference
Task Force on Hypertension in Pregnancy. Report of the American College of Obstetricians and Gynecologists' Task Force on Hypertension in Pregnancy.	American College of Obstetricians and Gynecologists	American College of Obstetricians and Gynecologists, Task Force on Hypertension in Pregnancy. Report of the American College of Obstetricians and Gynecologists' Task Force on Hypertension in Pregnancy. *Obstet Gynecol* 2013;122:1122.
Gestational hypertension and preeclampsia. ACOG practice bulletin no. 202.	American College of Obstetricians and Gynecologists	American College of Obstetricians and Gynecologists. ACOG practice bulletin no. 202: Gestational hypertension and preeclampsia. *Obstet Gynecol* 2019;133:e1-25.

International society guidelines

Title	Source	Date/full reference
Hypertension in pregnancy: the management of hypertensive disorders during pregnancy.	National Collaborating Centre for Women's and Children's Health	National Collaborating Centre for Women's and Children's Health. *Hypertension in pregnancy: The management of hypertensive disorders during pregnancy.* London: RCOG Press; 2010.

Evidence

Type of evidence	Title and comment	Date/full reference
Multicenter, randomized placebo-controlled trial	Do women with pre-eclampsia, and their babies, benefit from magnesium sulphate? The Magpie Trial: a randomised placebo-controlled trial. Comment: This trial demonstrated that magnesium sulfate reduces the risk of eclampsia by half without harmful maternal/fetal effects.	Altman D, Carroli G, Duley L, et al. Magpie Trial Collaboration Group. Do women with pre-eclampsia, and their babies, benefit from magnesium sulphate? The Magpie Trial: a randomised placebo-controlled trial. *Lancet* 2002 Jun 1;359(9321):1877-90.
Randomized, placebo-controlled trial	Magnesium sulfate in women with mild preeclampsia: a randomized controlled trial. Comment: This trial showed that use of magnesium sulfate did not impact disease progression in women with preeclampsia without severe features.	Livingston JC, Livingston LW, Ramsey R, et al. Magnesium sulfate in women with mild preeclampsia: a randomized controlled trial. *Obstet Gynecol* 2003;101(2):217.
Multicenter, randomized controlled trial	Induction of labour versus expectant monitoring for gestational hypertension or mild pre-eclampsia after 36 weeks' gestation. Comment: This trial showed that for women who have nonsevere hypertension at 34–37 weeks gestation, immediate delivery might reduce small risk of maternal outcomes at expensive of increasing neonatal respiratory distress syndrome. Expectant monitoring until 37 weeks can therefore be justified until clinical situation deteriorates.	Koopmans CM, Bijlenga D, Groen H, et al. Induction of labour versus expectant monitoring for gestational hypertension or mild pre-eclampsia after 36 weeks' gestation (HYPITAT): a multicentre, open-label randomised controlled trial. *Lancet* 2009;374:979.
Meta-analysis	Recurrence of hypertensive disorders of pregnancy: an individual patient data metaanalysis. Comment: This meta-analysis performed in 2015 of individual patient data from 75°000 women with preeclampsia found that 16% developed recurrent preeclampsia and 20% developed hypertension in a subsequent pregnancy.	Van Oostwaard MF, Langenveld J, Schuit E, et al. Recurrence of hypertensive disorders of pregnancy: an individual patient data metaanalysis. *Am J Obstet Gynecol* 2015;212(5):624.e1.
Meta-analysis	Cardiovascular sequelae of preeclampsia/eclampsia: a systematic review and meta-analyses. Comment: This meta-analysis demonstrated that women with a history of preeclampsia/eclampsia double their risk of future cerebrovascular disease and cardiovascular mortality.	McDonald SD, Malinowski A, Zhou Q, et al. Cardiovascular sequelae of preeclampsia/eclampsia: a systematic review and meta-analyses. *Am Heart J* 2008;156(5):918.

(Continued)

(Continued)

Type of evidence	Title and comment	Date/full reference
Systematic review and meta-analysis	The role of aspirin dose on the prevention of preeclampsia and fetal growth restriction: systematic review and meta-analysis. Comment: This meta-analysis showed that in women at high risk for development of preeclampsia, the maximal effect of aspirin occurs with initiation < 16 weeks gestation and the effect is dose dependent (with studies showing a dose of up to 150 mg associated with greater reduction in risk of preeclampsia and fetal growth restriction as compared to lower doses).	Roberge S, Nicolaides K, Demers S, et al. The role of aspirin dose on the prevention of preeclampsia and fetal growth restriction: systematic review and meta-analysis. *Am J Obstet Gynecol* 2017 Feb;216(2):110-20. Epub 2016 Sep 15.

CHAPTER 3

Gestational Diabetes

Marti Soffer[1], Catherine A. Bigelow[2], and Garfield Clunie[3]

[1] Division of Maternal Fetal-Medicine, Department of Obstetrics and Gynecology, Massachusetts General Hospital, Boston, MA
[2] Maternal-Fetal Medicine Subspecialist, Minnesota Perinatal Physicians, Allina Health, Minneapolis, MN
[3] Maternal-Fetal Medicine, The Brooklyn Hospital Center, Division of Maternal-Fetal Medicine, Icahn School of Medicine at Mount Sinai, New York, NY

OVERALL BOTTOM LINE

- Gestational diabetes affects 6–7% of pregnancies in the United States.
- All women should be screened for gestational diabetes in pregnancy, with timing of screening dictated by patient-specific risk factors.
- Patients diagnosed with gestational diabetes should be encouraged to follow dietary restriction, with the addition of oral hypoglycemics or insulin as needed for optimal glycemic control.
- Well-controlled gestational diabetes leads to good maternal and fetal outcomes.
- Women with gestational diabetes mellitus (GDM) should have postpartum glucose testing to guide long-term assessment of glycemic status.

Background

Definition of disease

- Gestational diabetes is the diagnosis or recognition of abnormal glucose tolerance in the setting of pregnancy.

Incidence/prevalence

- Traditionally, GDM has a 6–7% prevalence in the US, range 1–25%, with increasing rates over time, likely because of higher maternal age and body mass index (BMI).
- In the US, rates are higher among African American, Pacific Islander, Native American, and South or East Asian populations as compared to white women.

Economic impact

- In 2007, GDM in mothers of ~180 000 delivered newborns was associated with $636 million in increased medical costs.

Etiology

- Normal pregnancy is characterized by hyperplasia of the insulin-secreting pancreatic beta cells, increased insulin secretion, and an early increase in insulin sensitivity followed by progressive insulin resistance.
- If a woman's pancreas cannot overcome this insulin resistance, gestational diabetes occurs.

Pathology/pathogenesis

- Maternal insulin resistance is normal, starting in the second trimester and reaching a peak in the third trimester.

Mount Sinai Expert Guides: Obstetrics and Gynecology, First Edition. Edited by Rhoda Sperling.
© 2020 John Wiley & Sons Ltd. Published 2020 by John Wiley & Sons Ltd.
Companion Website: www.wiley.com/go/sperling/mountsinai/obstetricsandgynecology

- It occurs from placental secretion of diabetogenic hormones like growth hormone (GH), corticotropin releasing hormone (CRH), human placental lactogen (hPL), and progesterone.
- Normally, this state is developmentally advantageous to the growing fetus; the insulin resistance leads to increased lipolysis preferentially giving the fetus glucose and amnio acids and preserving protein.
- It is unknown why certain patients are unable to compensate for this increased insulin resistance.

Predictive/risk factors

Risk factor	Odds ratio
Nonwhite ethnicity	1.5–2x increased risk of GDM
Prior pregnancy with GDM	33–66% will have GDM in subsequent pregnancy
Family history of DM	RR 1.68
Pregravid BMI >30	RR 2.9
Multiple gestation	OR 1.3

Retakran and Shah 2016; Solomon et al. 1997

Prevention

BOTTOM LINE/CLINICAL PEARLS
- Weight loss among overweight or obese women prior to pregnancy can reduce risk of GDM.
- Exercise programs (both high and low intensity) have not been proven to decrease the risk.
- Smoking cessation may reduce risk for GDM.

Screening
- All pregnant women should be screened for GDM, ideally between 24–28 weeks gestation.
- Early screening for undiagnosed type 2 DM is indicated for patients with risk factors including prior pregnancy with GDM, known impaired glucose metabolism, and obesity.
- Screening is done with either a two-step approach or a one-step approach.
  - Two step (most common in the US): screening with administration of a 50 g oral glucose solution followed by a 1-hour glucose test. Those screening positive then undergo a 100 g 3-hour fasting diagnostic glucose tolerance test.
  - One step: administration of 75 g 2-hour oral glucose solution for screening and diagnosis
- Patients with GDM are at increased risk for preeclampsia, and therefore normal BP monitoring and lab assessment should be done as well as patient education to monitor for signs and symptoms of preeclampsia.
- Postpartum screening is done 6 weeks postpartum with a 75 g glucose tolerance test.

Primary prevention
- Weight loss among women with pregravid BMI >25

Secondary prevention
- Weight loss
- Smoking cessation
- Possible exercise

Diagnosis

BOTTOM LINE/CLINICAL PEARLS
- Diagnosis of gestational diabetes is based on laboratory findings (see Algorithm 3.1).
- If the two-step approach is used, a 1-hour result greater than 130–140 (practice and study dependent) should prompt diagnostic workup with a 3-hour glucose tolerance test.
  - If the result from the 1-hour test is 200 or greater, the diagnosis of GDM is made and no further testing is required.
  - Three-hour results with two positive values gives the diagnosis of GDM. Cut-offs vary between studies to determine diagnostic thresholds.
- If the one-step approach is used, any single elevated value on the 2-hour glucose tolerance test yields a diagnosis (>92 fasting, >180 1 hr, >153 2 hr).

Typical presentation
- The diagnosis of GDM is laboratory based and does not typically present with symptoms.

Clinical diagnosis
History
- A patient with prior history of large babies (>4500 g) or prior history of gestational diabetes would prompt workup for current pregnancy affected by GDM.

Physical examination
- Should a patient lack prenatal care, exam may give clues to suggest GDM.
  - Fetal size greater than dates
  - Estimated fetal weight >97th percentile

Algorithm 3.1 Algorithm for diagnosis of overt diabetes and gestational diabetes in the pregnant population

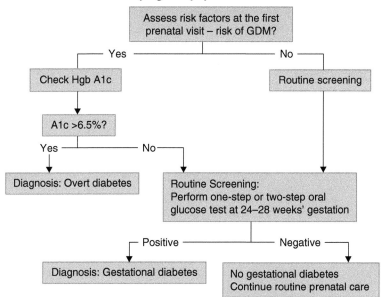

Disease severity classification
- GDMA1 – diet-controlled gestational diabetes
  - These patients have the same baseline risk of stillbirth as women without diabetes
- GDMA2 – medication-controlled gestational diabetes
  - These patients have an elevated risk of stillbirth based on some studies

Laboratory diagnosis

List of diagnostic tests
- Two step (most common in the US): screening with administration of a 50 g oral glucose solution followed by a 1-hour glucose test. Those screening positive then undergo a 100 g 3-hour fasting diagnostic glucose tolerance test.
- One step: administration of 75 g 2-hour oral glucose solution for screening and diagnosis

Treatment

Treatment rationale
- Once diagnosed, patients should be evaluated by nutrition and a high risk provider. They should be given information about healthy eating and exercise. They should be monitored with glucose fingersticks every morning fasting and 1 hour postprandial. If fingersticks are well controlled (generally <95 fasting and <140 postprandial), the patient can be managed for the duration of her pregnancy with tight diet control.
- If patients are not meeting their goal, medical management should be initiated. There is no threshold at which clinicians should initiate medical management, whether with oral or injectable medication.
- Oral medication is often used initially for patients given the greater ease of use. Glyburide and metformin are increasingly used, though they have not been approved by the Food and Drug Administration for this indication.
- Insulin is the recommended first line treatment. If insulin is used, it is easily titrated to reach glycemic control. Starting dose is 0.7–1 unit/kg daily (based on the trimester of pregnancy) given in divided doses.
- Often, patients who require increasing doses of medication based on their glycemic logs will continue to need higher doses of oral medication, be switched to insulin, or require higher doses of insulin as their insulin resistance increases throughout the third trimester.
- Patients with GDMA1 (diet controlled) may continue pregnancy until 41 weeks gestation.
- Patients with GDMA2 (medication controlled) should be delivered by 39 weeks gestation given the increased risk for stillbirth. This timing may also decrease the risk for shoulder dystocia compared to later delivery.
- Postpartum screening and management is recommended for women with gestational diabetes. See Algorithm 3.2.

When to hospitalize
- Should a patient be noncompliant with medications and their glucose logs are erratic, it is reasonable to admit a patient for direct observed therapy.
- Should a patient have a diagnosis of GDM but preexisting type 2 DM is suspected, a patient's fingersticks may be increasingly erratic as pregnancy continues. In this case, hospitalization may be warranted for tight control.
- Diabetic ketoacidosis (DKA) is a life-threatening emergency but is uncommon in patients with GDM. However, in the setting of extreme stress, it is possible. Should this be suspected, hospitalization and management with a multidisciplinary team including endocrinology and maternal-fetal medicine is warranted.

Managing the hospitalized patient
- Fingerstick testing should continue to be performed, including fasting and 1 hour postprandial.
- Coordination of care with endocrinology may be appropriate.

Algorithm 3.2 Management of postpartum screening results

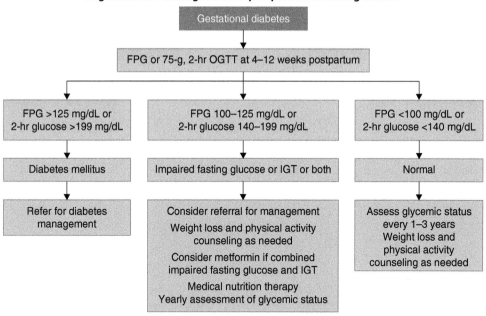

FPG, fasting plasma glucose; OGTT, oral glucose tolerance test; IGT, impaired glucose tolerance.

Table of treatment

Treatment	Comments
Conservative	Dietary control; initial therapy for all patients, continued therapy in patients meeting glucose goals
Medical	Glyburide 2.5–5 mg/day with max 20 mg/day Metformin 500–1000 mg BID Insulin 0.7–1 kg/day in divided doses, titrated to requirements
Psychological	Social work coordination may be of use given the high health literacy required for diabetes management and the large stress of checking fingersticks, logging, and presenting for appointments.

Prevention/management of complications
- Noncompliance – patients who are noncompliant with fingersticks, medications, or visits may warrant hospitalization. They should also be counseled on the complications of untreated GDM.
- Prevention of further obstetric/fetal complications is achieved through regular testing starting at 32 weeks among women who are controlled with medication. These women are also delivered by 39 weeks gestation (vs 41 weeks gestation for those who are diet controlled).

CLINICAL PEARLS
- Start with diet and exercise alone.
- Medication requirements tend to increase as pregnancy continues.
- Strict blood glucose control is needed to prevent adverse outcomes.

Prognosis

> **BOTTOM LINE/CLINICAL PEARLS**
> * Well controlled GDM is associated with good obstetric outcomes both for mother and baby.
> * Most women are normoglycemic after delivery; however, they are at increased risk for recurrent GDM, impaired glucose tolerance, or overt diabetes within the next 5 years.
> * Ideally patients should be screened postpartum to assess glycemic control.

Natural history of untreated disease
* Fetal: Macrosomia (weight >4000 g), shoulder dystocia, polyhydramnios, fetal demise, birth injury, neonatal hypoglycemia, and NICU admission
* Maternal: cesarean delivery, preeclampsia, postpartum hemorrhage, third- and fourth-degree perineal lacerations

Follow-up tests and monitoring
* Patients on medications for control should undergo antenatal fetal surveillance starting at 32 weeks. Frequency and type of testing varies by institution.
* At 6 weeks postpartum, patients should be screened with a 75 g glucose tolerance test to assess for impaired fasting glucose, impaired glucose tolerance or overt diabetes mellitus.

Reading list
Albrecht SS, Kuklina EV, Bansil P, et al. Diabetes trends among delivery hospitalizations in the U.S., 1994–2004. *Diabetes Care* 2010;33:768.

American College of Obstetricians and Gynecologists. *Gestational diabetes mellitus.* Practice bulletin no. 190. Published 2018, reaffirmed 2019. *Obstet Gynecol* 2018 Feb;131(2):e49-e64.

American College of Obstetricians and Gynecologists. Gestational diabetes mellitus. Practice bulletin no. 190. *Am J Obstet Gynecol* 2018;131:e49-e64.

Bardenheier BH, Elixhauser A, Imperatore G, et al. Variation in prevalence of gestational diabetes mellitus among hospital discharges for obstetric delivery across 23 states in the United States. *Diabetes Care* 2013;36:1209.

Catalano PM, McIntyre HD, Cruickshank JK, et al. The hyperglycemia and adverse pregnancy outcome study: associations of GDM and obesity with pregnancy outcomes. *Diabetes Care* 2012;35(4):780-6.

Dabelea D, Snell-Bergeon JK, Hartsfield CL, et al. Increasing prevalence of gestational diabetes mellitus (GDM) over time and by birth cohort: Kaiser Permanente of Colorado GDM Screening Program. *Diabetes Care* 2005;28:579.

Dall TM, Yang W, Halder P, et al. The economic burden of elevated blood glucose levels in 2012: diagnosed and undiagnosed diabetes, gestational diabetes mellitus, and prediabetes. *Diabetes Care* 2014 Dec;37(12):3172-79.

Ferrara A. Increasing prevalence of gestational diabetes mellitus: a public health perspective. *Diabetes Care* 2007;30 Suppl 2:S141.

Getahun D, Nath C, Ananth CV, et al. Gestational diabetes in the United States: temporal trends 1989 through 2004. *Am J Obstet Gynecol* 2008;198:525.e1.

HAPO Study Cooperative Research Group, Metzger BE, Lowe LP, et al. Hyperglycemia and adverse pregnancy outcomes. *New Engl J Med* 2008;358(19):1991-2002.

Hartling L, Dryden DM, Guthrie A, et al. *Screening and diagnosing gestational diabetes mellitus.* Evidence report/technology assessment no. 210. (Prepared by the University of Alberta Evidence-based Practice Center under Contract No. 290-2007-10021-I.) AHRQ Publication No. 12(13)-E021-EF. Rockville, MD: Agency for Healthcare Research and Quality; October 2012. Available from: https://effectivehealthcare.ahrq.gov/products/gestational-diabetes-screening-diagnosis/research. (accessed 10 February 2020).

Kim SY, Saraiva C, Curtis M, et al. Fraction of gestational diabetes mellitus attributable to overweight and obesity by race/ethnicity, California, 2007–2009. *Am J Public Health* 2013;103:e65.

Moyer VA, US Preventive Services Task Force. Screening for gestational diabetes mellitus: US Preventive Services Task Force recommendation statement. *Ann Intern Med* 2014;160:414.

Retnakran R, Shah BR. Impact of twin gestation and fetal sex on maternal risk of diabetes during and after pregnancy. *Diabetes Care* 2016;Aug:39(8):e110-1.

Society of Maternal-Fetal Medicine (SMFM) Publications Committee. SMFM statement: pharmacological treatment of gestational diabetes. *Am J Obstet Gynecol* 2018;218(5):B2-B4.

Solomon CG, Willett WC, Carey VJ, et al. A prospective study of pregravid determinants of gestational diabetes mellitus. *JAMA* 1997;278(13):1078.

Suggested website

Effective Health Care Program. http://www.effectivehealthcare.ahrq.gov/reports/final.cfm

Guidelines

National society guidelines

Title	Source	Date/full reference
Gestational diabetes mellitus. ACOG practice bulletin no. 190	American College of Obstetricians and Gynecologists	February 2018 (reaffirmed 2019) *Obstet Gynecol* 2018 Feb;131(2):e49-e64.
Pharmacological treatment of gestational diabetes	Society of Maternal-Fetal Medicine	*Am J Obstet Gynecol* 2018 May;218(5):B2-B4.

Evidence

Type of evidence	Title and comment	Date/full reference
Randomized controlled trial (RCT)	Australian Carbohydrate Intolerance Study Comment: first large-scale study to demonstrate benefit of treatment of GDM	Crowther CA, Hiller JE, Moss JR, et al. Effect of treatment of gestational diabetes mellitus on pregnancy outcomes. Australian Carbohydrate Intolerance Study in Pregnant Women (ACHOIS) Trial Group. *N Engl J Med* 2005;352:2477-86.
RCT	Comment: Multicenter trial to demonstrate benefit of treatment of GDM	Landon MB, Spong CY, Thorn E, et al. A multicenter, randomized trial of treatment for mild gestational diabetes. Eunice Kennedy Shriver National Institute of Child Health and Human Development Maternal-Fetal Medicine Units Network. *N Engl J Med* 2009;361:1339-48.
Prospective blinded study	Comment: Multicenter blinded study of >28 000 women to determine adverse obstetric outcomes associated with incremental increases in hyperglycemia	HAPO Study Cooperative Research Group, Metzger BE, Lowe LP, et al. Hyperglycemia and adverse pregnancy outcomes. *N Engl J Med* 2008;358(19):1991-2002.

Additional material for this chapter can be found online at:
www.wiley.com/go/sperling/mountsinai/obstetricsandgynecology

This includes a case study.

CHAPTER 4

Viral Infections and Pregnancy

Catherine A. Bigelow[1] and Lauren Ferrara[2]
[1] Maternal-Fetal Medicine Subspecialist, Minnesota Perinatal Physicians, Allina Health, Minneapolis, MN
[2] Division of Maternal-Fetal Medicine, Department of Obstetrics, Gynecology and Reproductive Science, Icahn School of Medicine at Mount Sinai, New York, NY

OVERALL BOTTOM LINE
- Acute viral illness in pregnancy includes a wide differential with multiple potential fetal outcomes.
- Maternal serologies should be sent to evaluate the pregnant patient with symptoms of acute viral illness.
- If serum testing is concerning for acute infection, diagnostic testing for intrauterine infection with amniocentesis and viral polymerase chain reaction (PCR) may be indicated.
- The pregnant patient with a new diagnosis of HIV requires multidisciplinary care.
- Fetal and neonatal/childhood outcomes are variable based on timing and acuity of certain viral illnesses in pregnancy.

Background

Definition of disease
- Viral infections in pregnancy cause a constellation of symptoms in the pregnant patient, which vary by pathogen.

Incidence/prevalence
- Cytomegalovirus (CMV) is the most common viral illness in pregnancy, with an incidence of 0.7–4% of primary CMV infection in previously seronegative pregnant women in the United States.
- Comprehensive medical care for the HIV-positive pregnant patient has drastically reduced perinatal transmission.
- The introduction of Zika virus has made attention worldwide as only 20% of women may be symptomatic but there can be significant fetal malformations related to exposure.
- Measles, also known as rubeola, was previously declared eliminated in 2000 but is now increasing in the United States, with 31 states reporting confirmed outbreaks and 1282 individual cases confirmed in 2019.

American College of Obstetricians and Gynecologists 2015; Centers for Disease Control and Prevention 2020

Etiology
- Each viral infection in pregnancy is caused by a unique organism, which leads to characteristic maternal and fetal clinical manifestations. For details, please refer to the table under "Differential Diagnosis."

Pathology/pathogenesis
- Immunologic changes in pregnancy increase the risk of certain infectious diseases.
- The virus may transmit across the placenta and have significant manifestations in the fetus including intrauterine growth restriction and congenital malformations.

Mount Sinai Expert Guides: Obstetrics and Gynecology, First Edition. Edited by Rhoda Sperling.
© 2020 John Wiley & Sons Ltd. Published 2020 by John Wiley & Sons Ltd.
Companion Website: www.wiley.com/go/sperling/mountsinai/obstetricsandgynecology

Predictive/risk factors
- Risk factors will be based primarily on risk of exposure. Some examples include:
  - Parvovirus – working with young children
  - HIV – high-risk behaviors or healthcare workers
  - Zika – travel to endemic areas or sexual contact with someone who has traveled
  - Measles – travel or contact with someone who lives in a high-risk community with low rates of vaccination

Prevention

> **BOTTOM LINE/CLINICAL PEARLS**
> - Barrier contraception and preexposure prophylaxis (PrEP) decrease the sexual transmission of HIV.
> - Vaccination against rubella, hepatitis B, and varicella prevents the development of the disease when administered prior to pregnancy.
> - No interventions have been demonstrated to prevent the development of herpes simplex virus (HSV), CMV, or parvovirus.
> - Avoid travel to Zika endemic areas. Use barrier contraception with partners who may have traveled to these areas.

Screening
- The American College of Obstetricians and Gynecologists (ACOG) recommends routine screening for HIV, hepatitis B, varicella, and rubella at the first prenatal visit.
- Due to recent outbreaks of measles in certain high-risk populations and regions of the United States, pregnant women with suspected measles exposure should have serologic testing, with treatment based on serology results.
- Routine serologic screening for CMV or parvovirus is not recommended, as there is neither a vaccine for prevention nor an effective therapy available for primary infection.
- Routine genital cultures are not recommended to screen for HSV.
- Screening for Zika should be considered if a patient has travelled to an endemic area.

Primary prevention
- Routine vaccination against rubella (measles-mumps-rubella vaccine, MMR), varicella (varicella zoster vaccine, Varivax), and hepatitis B have greatly decreased the incidence of primary infection with these viruses.
- HIV infection is prevented with barrier contraception use (to prevent sexual transmission) and educational campaigns against shared needle use (to prevent parenteral transmission).
- Antiretroviral medications may be used pre- or postexposure to decrease the risk of HIV transmission in patients who are at high risk for HIV infection.
- There are no primary prevention strategies against CMV, parvovirus, or HSV infections.
- Avoidance of travel to Zika endemic areas will minimize risk of exposure. When travel cannot be avoided, appropriate clothing should be worn and use of DEET containing mosquito repellents can help to minimize exposure.

Secondary prevention
- Recurrent HSV infection may be prevented by taking valacyclovir prophylaxis during pregnancy, which is typically administered after 36 weeks gestational age.

Diagnosis

> **BOTTOM LINE/CLINICAL PEARLS**
> - The clinician should inquire about prodromal symptoms, rashes, recent or planned travel, high-risk behaviors, or sick contacts in order to narrow the differential diagnosis in the pregnant patient presenting with an acute viral illness.
> - Rash, lymphadenopathy, or genital lesions may narrow the diagnosis.
> - Maternal serum screening tailored to likely infections should be the first laboratory investigations sent. If positive, many infections require confirmatory PCR testing of amniotic fluid to evaluate for fetal infection.
> - A detailed fetal anatomic survey should be performed to evaluate for fetal abnormalities or hydrops fetalis.

Differential diagnosis

Differential diagnosis	Features
Cytomegalovirus (CMV)	Maternal: Typically asymptomatic. May experience fever, myalgias, malaise. Fetal: Intrauterine growth restriction, polyhydramnios, nonimmune hydrops fetalis, periventricular calcifications, echogenic bowel, microcephaly, hepatic calcifications, enlarged cisterna magna. Neonatal: Sensorineural hearing loss, hepatosplenomegaly, chorioretinitis, periventricular intracranial calcifications, thrombocytopenia, microcephaly, intellectual disability.
Parvovirus B19	Maternal: Reticular truncal rash ("erythema infectiosum") and peripheral arthropathy; 20% of adults are asymptomatic. Fetal: Spontaneous abortion, nonimmune hydrops fetalis, stillbirth. Neonatal: No apparent long-term adverse effects.
Rubella (German measles)	Maternal: Mild viral prodrome (low-grade fever, malaise, sore throat). Maculopapular erythematous rash starting on the face and spreading to trunk and extremities. Fetal: Spontaneous abortion, stillbirth, intrauterine growth restriction. Neonatal: Congenital cataracts, cardiac malformations, radiolucent bone disease, sensorineural hearing loss, extramedullary hematopoiesis ("blueberry muffin" lesions).
Measles (rubeola)	Maternal: Viral prodrome (high fever up to 105°F, malaise) with conjunctivitis, coryza, and cough. Maculopapular erythematous rash starting on the face and spreading to trunk and extremities. Pregnant women are at increased risk of hospitalization and pneumonia, diarrhea, and encephalitis. Fetal: Spontaneous abortion, stillbirth, low birth weight, preterm birth Neonatal: Rash within 10 days of birth, wide spectrum of disease
Human immunodeficiency virus (HIV)	Maternal: Up to 60% asymptomatic. Acute retroviral syndrome (fever, lymphadenopathy, pharyngitis, maculopapular rash, myalgia/arthralgia, weight loss, headache), mucocutaneous ulcers. Fetal: No antenatal findings. Neonatal: Typically asymptomatic.
Herpes simplex virus (HSV)*	Maternal: Painful genital ulcers, dysuria, fever, tender inguinal lymphadenopathy, headache, myalgias, urinary retention. Fetal: No antenatal findings. Neonatal: Thrombocytopenia, mucocutaneous vesicles or scarring, transaminitis, conjunctivitis, hypotension, jaundice, disseminated intravascular coagulation, apnea.

Differential diagnosis	Features
Varicella zoster virus (VZV)	Maternal: 10–20% of pregnant women develop pneumonia (with mortality up to 40%). Encephalitis, fever, malaise, and maculopapular rash that becomes vesicular. Fetal: Limb hypoplasia, microcephaly. Neonatal: Skin scarring, chorioretinitis, microcephaly.
Hepatitis B	Maternal: Anorexia, nausea, malaise. More rarely, jaundice or fulminant hepatitis. Fetal: No antenatal findings. Neonatal: Typically asymptomatic.
Zika	Maternal: Often asymptomatic. May present with fever, rash, arthralgias. Fetal: May have no findings in utero but sonographic signs may include: microcephaly, ventriculomegaly, intracerebral calcifications

* Symptoms related to primary HSV infection

Typical presentation
- Please refer to the table "Differential Diagnosis" for typical presentations of these viral infections in the mother and the fetus.

Clinical diagnosis
History
- Clinicians should ask about prodromal symptoms, travel, rash, and sick contacts, along with high-risk behaviors that may increase the risk of acute hepatitis or HIV infection.
- Clinicians should verify the patient's immunization history.
- Ultrasound reports to document fetal status or abnormalities should be reviewed when seeing the patient in consultation.

Physical examination
- The clinician should check vital signs for fever. A complete head, eyes, ears, nose, and throat (HEENT) evaluation (including oropharyngeal and lymph node evaluation) and checking for characteristic rashes may guide the diagnosis of many acute viral illnesses (including type of lesions present, distribution, and time course). An abdominal examination is necessary to identify hepatic tenderness or hepatomegaly with acute hepatitis infection. A careful pelvic exam is necessary for the diagnosis of primary HSV to identify and culture ulcerative lesions.

Laboratory diagnosis
List of diagnostic tests
- CMV IgM + IgG with avidity testing – if positive, amniotic fluid CMV PCR
- Parvovirus B19 IgM + IgG – if positive, amniotic fluid Parvovirus B19 PCR
- Rubella IgM + IgG, viral culture – if positive, CVS or amniotic fluid rubella PCR
- Measles IgG – if negative and documented high risk exposure, treatment should be administered empirically
- HIV 1/2 antibody screening – if positive, RT-PCR viral load for confirmation
- HSV PCR (preferred), viral culture or direct fluorescent antibody testing
- VZV PCR from base of vesicle or VZV culture from vesicular fluid – if positive, amniotic fluid or fetal blood VZV PCR

- Complete hepatitis B serologies (hepatitis B surface antibody and antigen, hepatitis B core IgM + IgG and antigen, hepatitis B e antigen) – if positive, send HBV DNA and hepatitis B genotype
- Zika IgM – if positive, send serum PCR. Can consider amniocentesis though sensitivity is not well described

List of imaging techniques
- Detailed fetal ultrasound is recommended when there is suspicion for acute CMV, parvovirus, varicella, rubella, or Zika infection in pregnancy to evaluate for fetal effects (see table for fetal findings).
- Right upper quadrant ultrasound may be beneficial in the setting of acute hepatitis infection to rule out other etiologies of transaminitis.
- There are no recommended imaging studies for acute HIV or HSV infection.

Potential pitfalls/common errors made regarding diagnosis of disease
- There are rarely errors made regarding the diagnosis of an acute viral infection in pregnancy, as diagnosis is laboratory based.
- Errors in diagnosis are related to the false-positive and false-negative rates for each given laboratory test.
- The largest pitfall is not considering viral infections as part of our differential diagnosis for entities like intrauterine growth restriction or certain fetal anomalies.

Treatment
Treatment rationale
- Many viral illnesses in pregnancy are self-limited and only supportive care is required.
- For the fetus with presumed fetal anemia, ultrasound assessment of the middle cerebral artery (MCA) peak systolic velocity should be assessed. If MCA-PSV is >1.5 multiples of the median (MoM), percutaneous umbilical blood sampling and fetal transfusion are recommended to correct fetal anemia mediated by acute viral infection.
- Treatment for hepatitis B is indicated with an HBV DNA viral load of >200 000 units/mL to decrease the risk of vertical transmission. First-line treatment of hepatitis B in pregnancy is tenofovir disoproxil fumarate, a nucleotide reverse transcriptase inhibitor. Lamivudine may be considered as a second-line agent.
- Initiation of antiretroviral therapy (ART) is indicated for all HIV-positive pregnant women to suppress the viral load and decrease the rate of vertical transmission during pregnancy. The first-line regimen should be a triple drug regimen that includes a dual nucleos(t)ide reverse transcriptase inhibitor (NRTI) backbone and either a protease inhibitor or an integrase inhibitor. The choice of drug should be determined in concert with an infectious disease specialist with clinical expertise in HIV care.
- Intrapartum IV zidovudine (AZT) should be used to treat HIV-positive women with a viral load >1000 copies/mL or unknown viral load to decrease the risk of vertical transmission at the time of delivery.

When to hospitalize
- Although many women with acute parvovirus are asymptomatic, in cases of women with aplastic anemia hospitalization may be indicated for workup as well as possible transfusion.
- In the case of HIV infection, for women who demonstrate noncompliance with their medication, admission may be recommended for direct observation therapy.

Table of treatment

Treatment	Comments
Conservative	
Supportive care	Recommended for patients with acute CMV, parvovirus B19, Zika, or rubella, as these are typically self-limited and there is not maternal medical therapy available.
Medical	
Antiretroviral (ARV) medication for HIV	ARVs may require specific monitoring (serum chemistry, viral load, CD4 count), which should be discussed with an infectious disease specialist and tailored to the regimen.
Antiviral medications may be used to decrease vertical transmission of hepatitis B, varicella, and herpes simplex.	Hepatic function and hepatitis viral load should be monitored with tenofovir treatment for hepatitis B. No monitoring is needed for use of acyclovir to treat varicella or herpes.
Intravenous immunoglobulin (IVIG) may be administered for the seronegative patient with measles exposure	Some patients will require pretreatment with acetaminophen or nonsteroidal anti-inflammatory drugs (NSAIDs) to prevent inflammatory symptoms. Frequently, antihistamines with or without glucocorticoids are given before IVIG infusion. Pretreatment monitoring of hematologic parameters, renal function, and metabolic status may be indicated.
Radiological	Serial obstetric ultrasounds for fetal growth and to evaluate for congenital infections/anomalies are recommended with acute infection during pregnancy. See "Differential Diagnosis."
Other	For the fetus with suspected anemia and hydrops fetalis, percutaneous umbilical blood sampling (PUBS) and fetal transfusion may be required during the acute phase of infection.

Prevention/management of complications
- Antiretroviral therapy for maternal HIV infection has been associated with intrauterine growth restriction – patients on ARVs should have serial growth ultrasounds throughout the pregnancy.

> **CLINICAL PEARLS**
> - Obstetric ultrasound and measurement of the MCA Doppler predicts fetal anemia. In fetuses with elevated MCA Dopplers and acute parvovirus infection, fetal blood sampling, and intrauterine transfusion may be indicated.
> - Hepatitis B should be treated with maternal viral loads of >200 000 units/mL to decrease the risk of vertical transmission.
> - HIV in pregnancy should be treated with antiretroviral therapy to decrease the risk of vertical transmission. The use of zidovudine (AZT) at the time of delivery depends on viral load and maternal medication compliance.
> - Obstetric ultrasound for assessment of fetal head size and intracranial anatomy is recommended for patients with acute CMV, VZV, or Zika infection in pregnancy.

Prognosis

> **BOTTOM LINE/CLINICAL PEARLS**
> - Most viral illnesses in pregnancy are self-limited and will resolve with supportive care only, with good maternal prognosis.

> • Fetal prognosis is variable and will depend on timing and type of acute viral illness.
> • Women with hepatitis B or HIV in pregnancy should be monitored in conjunction with an infectious disease specialist to evaluate for disease progression, which may affect treatment decisions and long-term prognosis.

Natural history of untreated disease
- Most viral illnesses in pregnancy are self-limited and will resolve with supportive care only.
- Acute varicella infection can progress to varicella pneumonia, which is rare but may be life threatening in the pregnant patient.
- Maternal-to-fetal transmission of acute parvovirus B19 ranges from 17–33%.
- Parvovirus-related hydrops fetalis and fetal anemia portends a poor prognosis with high rates of fetal demise, ranging up to 40–70%.
- Acute hepatitis B can progress to chronic hepatitis B, which may lead to cirrhosis, hepatocellular carcinoma, and death.
- Untreated HIV can lead to progressive immunologic decline and the acquired immunodeficiency syndrome (AIDS) and opportunistic infections.
- Risk of transmission for Zika ranges from 1–10% with increased risk for fetal implications if exposure is in the first trimester.

Prognosis for treated patients
- Maternal prognosis is good for self-limited viral infections in pregnancy.
- Fetal prognosis is variable and depends on timing and type of viral infection in pregnancy.
- Fetuses that undergo intrauterine transfusion for parvovirus-related anemia have a good prognosis without long-term neurologic sequelae if hydrops fetalis is not present.

Follow-up tests and monitoring
- For women with hepatitis B, hepatic function tests and viral load should be monitored, as worsening disease may affect the decision to initiate antiviral therapy.
- HIV should be monitored in conjunction with an infectious disease specialist – routine monitoring includes checking HIV viral load, CD4 count, and screening for illnesses related to immunosuppression.

Reading list
American College of Obstetricians and Gynecologists. Cytomegalovirus, parvovirus B19, varicella zoster, and toxoplasmosis in pregnancy. Practice bulletin no. 151. *Obstet Gynecol* 2015;1-16.
Centers for Disease Control and Prevention. *Measles cases and outbreaks*. Atlanta, GA: CDC; 2020. Available from: https://www.cdc.gov/measles/cases-outbreaks.html (accessed 14 February 2020).
Connor EM, Sperling RS, Gelber R, et al. Reduction of maternal-infant transmission of human immunodeficiency virus type 1 with zidovudine treatment. Pediatric AIDS Clinical Trials Group Protocol 076 Study Group. *N Engl J Med* 1994;331(18):1173.
Honein MA, Dawson AL et al. Birth defects among fetuses and infants of US women with evidence of possible Zika virus infection during pregnancy. *JAMA* 2017;317(1):59-68.
Kilpatrick SJ, Papile LA, Macones GA, et al., eds. Chapter 5: prepregnancy care. In *Guidelines for perinatal care*. 8th ed. Washington, DC and Itasca, IL: American College of Obstetrics and Gynecology and American Academy of Pediatrics; 2017:131-47.
Panel on Treatment of HIV-Infected Pregnant Women and Prevention of Perinatal Transmission. *Recommendations for use of antiretroviral drugs in pregnant HIV-1-infected women for maternal health and interventions to reduce perinatal HIV transmission in the United States*. Available from: http://aidsinfo.nih.gov/contentfiles/lvguidelines/PerinatalGL.pdf (accessed 17 January 2020).
von Kaisenberg CS, Jonat W. Fetal parvovirus B19 infection. *Ultrasound Obstet Gynecol* 2001;18:280-8.

Suggested websites

Centers for Disease Control and Prevention. www.cdc.gov
American College of Obstetrics and Gynecology. www.acog.org

Guidelines
National society guidelines

Title	Source	Date/full reference or URL
Cytomegalovirus, parvovirus B19, varicella zoster, and toxoplasmosis in pregnancy: ACOG practice bulletin no. 151	ACOG Comment: Overview of diagnosis and management of specific infections in pregnancy	*Obstet Gynecol* 2015 Jun;125(6):1510-25.
Diagnosis and management of congenital cytomegalovirus infection	Society for Maternal-Fetal Medicine (SMFM)	*Am J Obstet Gynecol* 2016 Jun;214(6):B5-B11
Viral hepatitis in pregnancy: ACOG practice bulletin no. 86	ACOG	2007 – reaffirmed 2018. *Obstet Gynecol* 2007;110:941–55.
Gynecologic care for women and adolescents with human immunodeficiency virus: ACOG practice bulletin no. 167	ACOG	October, 2016 – reaffirmed 2019. *Obstet Gynecol* 2016;128:e89–110
Management of pregnant and reproductive-aged women during a measles outbreak: ACOG practice advisory	ACOG	2019 https://www.acog.org/Clinical-Guidance-and-Publications/Practice-Advisories/Management-of-Pregnant-and-Reproductive-Age-Women-during-a-Measles-Outbreak

Evidence

Type of evidence	Title and comment	Date/full reference
Randomized controlled trial (RCT)	Reduction of maternal-infant transmission of human immunodeficiency virus type 1 with zidovudine treatment Comment: double-blind placebo-controlled RCT demonstrating a decrease in vertical transmission when zidovudine (AZT) is administered to HIV-infected women at the time of delivery	Connor EM, Sperling RS, Gelber R, et al. Reduction of maternal-infant transmission of human immunodeficiency virus type 1 with zidovudine treatment. Pediatric AIDS Clinical Trials Group Protocol 076 Study Group. *N Engl J Med* 1994;331(18):1173.

CHAPTER 5

Placenta Previa and Morbidly Adherent Placenta

Elizabeth Yoselevsky[1], Katherine A. Connolly[2], and Noel Strong[3]
[1] Division of Maternal-Fetal Medicine, Department of Obstetrics, Gynecology, and Reproductive Biology, Brigham and Women's Hospital, Boston, MA
[2] Division of Maternal-Fetal Medicine, Department of Obstetrics and Gynecology, University of California, San Francisco, CA
[3] Division of Maternal-Fetal Medicine, Department of Obstetrics, Gynecology and Reproductive Science, Icahn School of Medicine at Mount Sinai, New York, NY

OVERALL BOTTOM LINE
- Placenta previa is a condition in which the placenta completely or partially covers the internal cervical os. Patients should be screened for placenta previa using ultrasonography. It is associated with risk of bleeding, which can be massive and life threatening and patients are counseled to practice pelvic rest and contact their providers in case of bleeding. Cesarean delivery is required for patients diagnosed with placenta previa that does not resolve.
- Morbidly adherent placenta (MAP) is a spectrum of disorders characterized by abnormal attachment of the placenta to the uterine wall or beyond. This disorder is further subclassified based on the degree of invasion of the placenta. Placenta accreta describes a placenta that is abnormally adherent to the uterine myometrium. Placenta increta describes a placenta that invades into the myometrium. Placenta percreta describes a placenta that invades through the myometrium and serosa of the uterus and possibly into adjacent organs such as the bowel or bladder.
- MAP is diagnosed with ultrasonography and occasionally with magnetic resonance imaging. Attempts to detach the placenta from the uterine wall can cause life-threatening hemorrhaging so often a cesarean hysterectomy is performed at time of delivery.

Background
Definition of disease
- Placenta previa: placental tissue that extends partially or completely over the internal cervical os
- MAP: when part of or all the placenta invades into and is inseparable from the uterine wall or surrounding organs

Incidence/prevalence
- Placenta previa: 3.5–4.6 per 1000 births
- MAP: as high as 1 in 533 births

Etiology
- Placenta previa: etiology unknown; theorized that alteration to the endometrium in the fundus of the uterus causes the placenta to grow toward more favorable tissue in the lower uterus; alteration to the endometrium may be caused by surgeries or prior miscarriages
- MAP: etiology unknown, known to be associated with damage to the myometrium

---

Mount Sinai Expert Guides: Obstetrics and Gynecology, First Edition. Edited by Rhoda Sperling.
© 2020 John Wiley & Sons Ltd. Published 2020 by John Wiley & Sons Ltd.
Companion Website: www.wiley.com/go/sperling/mountsinai/obstetricsandgynecology

Pathology/pathogenesis
- Placenta previa can be asymptomatic. It may also present with painless vaginal bleeding thought to be caused by cervical dilation or expansion of the lower uterine segment, both of which can disrupt the placental attachment.

Predictive/risk factors for morbidly adherent placenta

Risk factor	Risk of MAP
Prior cesarean delivery (CD)	
1 prior CD	0.3%
2 prior CD	0.6%
3 prior CD	2.7%
Presence of placenta previa with prior CD:	
0 prior CD	1–5%
1 prior CD	11–25%
2 prior CD	35–47%
3 prior CD	40%
4 + prior CD	50–67%

Prevention

> **BOTTOM LINE/CLINICAL PEARLS**
> - Women with a history of uterine surgery, such as cesarean deliveries or myomectomies, are at risk for abnormally adherent placentas so avoiding surgery may prevent the development of a placenta accreta.

Screening
- Placenta previa: Placentas are localized during routine ultrasounds performed during pregnancy for assessment of fetal anatomy or gestational age. If placental location is unknown, ultrasound should be considered in any woman who presents after 20 weeks gestation with vaginal bleeding.
- MAP: During routine ultrasounds, placentas are examined for characteristics that may suggest abnormal adherence to the uterine wall.

Primary prevention
- Cesarean delivery and other intrauterine surgical procedures have been shown to be associated with abnormal placentation such as a previa or accreta, therefore avoiding these surgeries may help decrease the chance of having an abnormal placenta.

Diagnosis

> **BOTTOM LINE/CLINICAL PEARLS**
> - Placenta previa:
>   - Painless vaginal bleeding after 20 weeks may be suggestive of placenta previa.
>   - Placenta previa is diagnosed with ultrasonography – if the placenta covers the internal os of the cervix it is considered a previa; if the placental edge is within 2 cm of the internal os, it is considered low lying.

- MAP:
  - Generally asymptomatic during pregnancy though may be associated with vaginal bleeding if also a placenta previa.
  - MAP is diagnosed with ultrasonography – signs of accreta include irregular vascular spaces within the placenta with or without turbulent blood flow, thinning of the myometrium overlying the placenta, protrusion of the placenta into the bladder, increased vascularity at the uterus–bladder interface.
  - Magnetic resonance imaging may be used to supplement ultrasonography in determining the placental boundaries and presence or absence of invasion into maternal tissue.
  - Ultimately, MAP is diagnosed after pathological examination determines the extent of invasion into the uterine wall.

Differential diagnosis

Differential diagnosis	Features
Placental abruption	A portion of the placenta prematurely detaches causing abdominal pain and bleeding, placenta not overlying the cervical os, may see fetal distress on monitoring or contractions
Vasa previa	Fetal blood vessels course over the cervical os, may cause bleeding that is life threatening to the fetus

Typical presentation

- Often placenta previas are asymptomatic. A placenta previa may be suspected in any patient who experiences painless vaginal bleeding in the second or third trimester.
- MAP may be asymptomatic throughout the antenatal course. If associated with a placenta previa, the accreta may cause painless bleeding in the second or third trimester. The main clinical presentation is at the time of delivery when the placenta does not cleanly detach from the uterus after delivery of the neonate and can lead to massive hemorrhage.

Clinical diagnosis

History

- Placenta previa: Clinicians should inquire about any vaginal bleeding in the second or third trimester if the patient does not have an ultrasound documenting placental location.
- MAP: Clinicians should inquire about a patient's history of uterine surgeries to assess if the patient is at increased risk of a morbidly adherent placenta.

Physical examination

- Placenta previa: Clinicians should avoid digital vaginal exam if placenta previa is suspected.

Disease severity classification

- Any placenta that is morbidly adherent to the uterus by invading into the uterine wall is described as a placenta accreta. There are further subcategories of placenta accreta that describe how invasive the placenta is. Placenta increta describes a placenta that invades only into the myometrium, whereas a placenta percreta describes a placenta that invades through the myometrium and serosa of the uterus and possibly into adjacent organs such as the bowel or bladder.

Laboratory diagnosis

List of diagnostic tests

- Patients with placenta previas and/or MAP should have updated complete blood counts to monitor for anemia and active type and screen specimens once inpatient so cross-matched blood can be readily available.

List of imaging techniques

- Placenta previa: Transvaginal ultrasound is sufficient for diagnosing placenta previa.
- MAP: Transvaginal ultrasound should be used initially to diagnose a morbidly adherent placenta. Magnetic resonance imaging may be useful if ultrasonography is inconclusive or to better delineate the extent of placental invasion, especially if adherent to the posterior uterus that may be difficult to assess on ultrasound.

Potential pitfalls/common errors made regarding diagnosis of disease

- Placenta previas should be periodically monitored with ultrasound as they may resolve later in the pregnancy at the uterus grows and placenta remodels.

Treatment

Treatment rationale

- Placenta previa: Once a placenta previa has been diagnosed, a woman is advised to avoid having anything in the vagina that could disrupt the placenta such as sexual intercourse or digital vaginal examinations. If the antenatal course is not complicated by bleeding, a planned cesarean delivery is usually performed between 36 and 37 weeks.
- MAP: There is no treatment for MAP but steps can be taken to minimize maternal morbidity. Prenatal anemia should be corrected if present. Surgical planning with a multidisciplinary team of maternal-fetal medicine specialists, anesthesiologists, neonatologists, and other surgeons should be performed. If placenta accreta is diagnosed prenatally, a planned cesarean delivery should occur between 34 and 36 weeks. The usual treatment is cesarean hysterectomy; however, uterine conservation with delayed removal of the placenta is possible if massive hemorrhage is not occurring and the patient is a good candidate for such conservative management.

When to hospitalize

- Patients with placenta previas or MAP are usually hospitalized after their first episode of vaginal bleeding. Once proven to be stable without additional bleeding, they may be discharged home. If these patients experience a second bleed, many clinicians opt to keep the patients hospitalized until delivery.

Managing the hospitalized patient

- Patients hospitalized with placenta previas or accretas should be treated as preoperative patients until deemed stable. This entails having the patient on an NPO diet and with an active type and screen, cross-matched blood readily available, two large bore IV lines placed, and continuous fetal and contraction monitoring. Once a patient has proven to be stable without further vaginal bleeding, she can usually resume normal activities such as having a normal diet, ambulating and having intermittent fetal and contraction monitoring. An active type and screen and cross-matched blood should always be available. If the fetus is < 34 weeks gestational age, a course of betamethasone is given for fetal lung maturity in the event premature delivery is indicated.

Table of treatment
Placenta previa

Treatment	Comments
Conservative	If the vaginal bleeding associated with a placenta previa is self-limited, the mother shows no signs of hemodynamic shock and the fetus shows no signs of distress, the patient may be observed.
Surgical	If a placenta previa causes a life-threatening hemorrhage or the fetus shows signs of distress, cesarean delivery is indicated. Otherwise, a planned cesarean delivery should take place between 36 and 37 weeks gestation.

Morbidly adherent placenta

Treatment	Comments
Conservative	After cesarean delivery, a placenta may be left in situ to avoid hysterectomy. Placental tissue can sometimes be later removed hysteroscopically. Caution should be taken as a placenta left in situ may cause delayed life-threatening hemorrhage, resulting in emergent surgery and hysterectomy.
Surgical	A planned cesarean hysterectomy from 34 to 36 weeks is recommended and ideally takes place in a tertiary care center with a multidisciplinary team and intensive care unit in the event of massive hemorrhage.
Radiological	Interventional radiology may place intravascular balloon catheters into the internal iliac arteries prior to cesarean delivery to decrease perfusion of the uterus after delivery.

Prevention/management of complications
- Early diagnosis is critical with placenta previas and MAP. Patients with placenta previas should be counseled to avoid sexual intercourse or any examination that may disrupt the placenta.
- For delivery planning for patients with MAP, a multidisciplinary approach should be taken involving maternal-fetal medicine specialists, anesthesiologists, neonatologists, possibly urologists, general surgeons, and interventional radiologists to plan the surgical approach to the case.

> **CLINICAL PEARLS**
> - Do not perform a vaginal exam in a patient with a known placenta previa.
> - It is important to determine the placenta location for all patients during routine ultrasound.
> - Special care should be taken to examine the placental–myometrial border in patients with placenta previa or with prior cesarean delivery.

Prognosis

> **BOTTOM LINE/CLINICAL PEARLS**
> - Patients with placenta previa and MAP are much more likely to experience clinically significant bleeding than patients with normal placentas. Maternal mortality related to a placenta previa is estimated to be less than 1% in countries with adequate medical resources. Maternal mortality is increased with MAP compared to patient without MAP.

Follow-up tests and monitoring
- For patients with placenta previa or suspected MAP on ultrasound, serial follow-up ultrasounds should be performed to assess fetal growth and to continue to monitor the placenta location and check for invasion. MRI can be considered if placenta percreta is suspected or if the ultrasound is unclear and the MRI will aid in the multidisciplinary approach.

Reading list

Ananth CV, Smulian JC, Vintzileos AM. The association of placenta previa with history of cesarean delivery and abortion: a metaanalysis. *Am J Obstet Gynecol* 1997;177(5):1071.

Clark, SL. Placenta previa and abruptio placentae. In: Creasy RK, Resnik R eds. *Maternal fetal medicine: Principles and practice*. Philadelphia: WB Saunders; 1999:616.

Faiz AS, Ananth CV. Etiology and risk factors for placenta previa: an overview and meta-analysis of observational studies. *J Matern Fetal Neonatal Med* 2003;13(3):175.

Knuttien MG, Jani A, Gaba, RC, et al. Balloon occlusion of the hypogastric arteries in the management of placenta accreta: A case report and review of the literature. *Semin Intervent Radiol* 2012 Sep;29(3):161-8.

Wu S, Kocherginsky M, Hibbard JU. Abnormal placentation: twenty-year analysis. *Am J Obstet Gynecol* 2005;192: 1458-61.

Suggested websites

American College of Obstetricians and Gynecologists. www.acog.org

Society for Maternal-Fetal Medicine. www.smfm.org

Guidelines
National society guidelines

Title	Source	Date/full reference
Placenta accreta	Society for Maternal-Fetal Medicine	Publications committee, Society for Maternal-Fetal Medicine. Placenta accreta. *Am J Obstet and Gynecol* 2010;203:430-9.

Additional material for this chapter can be found online at:
www.wiley.com/go/sperling/mountsinai/obstetricsandgynecology

This includes a case study, multiple choice questions, advice for patients, and ICD codes.

CHAPTER 6

Gastrointestinal Disorders and Pregnancy

Eric P. Bergh[1] and Maria Teresa Mella[2]

[1] Maternal-Fetal Medicine Subspecialist, UT Health – McGovern Medical School, Division of Maternal-Fetal Medicine, Houston, TX
[2] Department of Obstetrics, Gynecology and Reproductive Science, Icahn School of Medicine at Mount Sinai, New York, NY

OVERALL BOTTOM LINE
- Recognize and treat common gastrointestinal (GI) complaints in pregnancy
- Recognize and treat common disorders of the upper GI tract
- Recognize and treat common disorders of the small bowel and colon
- Recognize and treat hepatic, gallbladder, and pancreatic disorders

---

Background
- Diagnosis and evaluation of GI disorders is complicated by normal anatomical, physiologic, and functional changes that occur in pregnancy. Although many common complaints are not life threatening, the clinician should be aware of several pregnancy-specific disorders of the GI tract that may have significant maternal and fetal morbidity.

Disease classification
- Disorders of the GI tract may be classified by location: upper and lower GI tracts, as well as hepatic, gallbladder, and pancreatic disorders.
- Conditions may also be classified according to duration: acute versus chronic disorders.
- Conditions that are limited to pregnancy include hyperemesis gravidarum, intrahepatic cholestasis of pregnancy, preeclampsia, hemolysis elevated liver enzymes and low platelets (HELLP) syndrome, and acute fatty liver of pregnancy.

Incidence/prevalence
- The incidence and prevalence of GI disorders in pregnancy is specific to each disease state. Although some degree of nausea/vomiting, constipation, and heartburn is experienced by a majority of women, fewer women will experience chronic debilitating or life-threatening disease.

Physiologic changes in pregnancy
- Physiologic changes in pregnancy include decreased GI motility secondary to hormonal effects and an enlarging uterus.
- Decreased lower esophageal sphincter tone leads to frequent gastroesophageal reflux or "heartburn."
- Decreased contractility of the gallbladder, reduced emptying, and increased lithogenicity of bile increase risk for gallstone disease and pancreatitis in pregnancy.
- Increased absorption of sodium and water retention in the colon leads to worsening constipation.
- Hemorrhoids are a common complaint in pregnancy secondary to constipation and increased venous pressure below the growing uterus.

Mount Sinai Expert Guides: Obstetrics and Gynecology, First Edition. Edited by Rhoda Sperling.
© 2020 John Wiley & Sons Ltd. Published 2020 by John Wiley & Sons Ltd.
Companion Website: www.wiley.com/go/sperling/mountsinai/obstetricsandgynecology

Pathology/pathogenesis of pregnancy-specific GI disorders

- Hyperemesis gravidarum is an exaggerated response to rising serum levels of pregnancy-related hormones, in particular β-human chorionic gonadotropin (β-hCG). The presentation is severe, intractable nausea and vomiting that are not responsive to dietary modification and antiemetics and often persist beyond 16 weeks gestation.
- Intrahepatic cholestasis of pregnancy (IHCP) occurs when bile acids are cleared incompletely. The resulting accumulation of serum bile acids results in pruritis (typically the palms of the hands and/or soles of the feet and worse at night) and/or jaundice. Although the exact cause of IHCP is unknown, rising serum bile acids and gestational age beyond the late preterm and/or early term increase the risk for spontaneous stillbirth.
- Preeclampsia and HELLP are both associated with varying degrees of vascular dysfunction leading to end-organ damage.
- Acute fatty liver of pregnancy occurs when microvesicular fat accumulates within hepatocytes, disrupting normal maternal liver function. Inherited defects in maternal and fetal mitochondrial beta-oxidation of fatty acids (long-chain 3-hydroyacyl CoA dehydrogenase [LCHAD] deficiency) may predispose some women to this disorder.

Incidence

GI disorder	Incidence
Some degree of nausea and vomiting	Variable
Constipation	Variable
Hemorrhoids	Variable
Hyperemesis gravidarum	0.3–3:100 pregnancies (Interventions 2015)
Intrahepatic cholestasis of pregnancy	Population dependent
Acute fatty liver of pregnancy	1:10 000 pregnancies (Nelson et al. 2013)
Appendicitis	1:800–1:1500 pregnancies (Andersen and Nielsen 1999; Mourad et al. 2000)
Cholecystitis	1:1000 pregnancies (Cunningham 2014)
Pancreatitis	1:3450 pregnancies (Eddy et al. 2008)
HELLP syndrome	1:1000 pregnancies (Stone 1998)

Prevention

- Prevention is generally aimed at adapting diet and lifestyle to physical changes associated with pregnancy.
- For women with chronic inflammatory bowel disease, continued suppression of colitis is achieved with adherence to most prepregnancy maintenance therapies.

Screening

- Women with a history of bariatric surgery (particularly those associated with malabsorption [i.e. Roux-en-Y bypass]) should have early screening for gestational diabetes in pregnancy, frequent evaluation of serum nutrition/vitamin status, and serial ultrasounds in the pregnancy to monitor for adequate fetal growth.
- Women with a history of inflammatory bowel disease should have evaluation of serum as well as fecal biomarkers to aid with assessment of disease activity.

Primary prevention

- Reduce portion size and increase meal frequency to prevent nausea/vomiting from reduced stomach capacity due to enlarging uterus.
- Adhere to well-balanced diet. Avoid fatty foods.
- Ensure adequate hydration to prevent constipation that occurs due to increased colonic absorption.
- In both ulcerative colitis and Crohn's disease, levels of calcium, B12, and iron should be monitored. Folic acid supplementation may help reduce incidence of anemia and neural tube defects.
- Daily aspirin (81 mg) for patients at high risk for preeclampsia.
- Take prenatal vitamins with food, not on an empty stomach.

Secondary prevention

- Nausea and vomiting may be treated with avoidance of triggers and diet modification (small meals, frequent snacking). High-protein, salty, and bland foods and carbonated beverages are encouraged in addition to ginger-containing foods. Pyridoxine and doxylamine are first-line oral medications for mild symptoms. Patients with moderate to severe symptoms may also benefit from H1-antagonists, dopamine antagonists, or serotonin antagonists. Patients with hyperemesis gravidarum will often require multiple oral agents including occasional courses of glucocorticoids to control symptoms.
- Adequate hydration, high fiber diet, and stool softeners (Colace) are frequent treatments for constipation in pregnancy.
- Hemorrhoids are typically treated with medical management (topical agents) although severe disease may require surgical management in pregnancy.
- Behavioral modifications such as taking prenatal vitamins with food or elevating the head of the bed to reduce symptoms of reflux esophagitis. Oral antacids, H2-blockers, and proton pump inhibitors are generally considered safe for treatment in pregnancy.
- Medical management with 5-ASA derivatives (sulfasalazine), corticosteroids, and immunomodulating agents are mainstays of therapy for inflammatory bowel disease.

Diagnosis

- Diagnosis of GI disorders in pregnancy requires a detailed medical, surgical, and obstetric history. Particular attention should be paid to current gestational age, onset and character of pain, as well as composition and quality of emesis or bowel movements. The differential diagnosis should include disorders specific to pregnancy as well as obstetric causes of abdominal pain.
- Due to anatomical changes brought on by the enlarging gravid uterus, right lower quadrant pain associated with appendicitis in the nonpregnant patient is shifted cephalad with continued appendiceal displacement.
- Alterations in complete blood count, complete metabolic panel, hepatic function panel, and pancreatic enzymes (amylase/lipase) will help to guide diagnosis. Total bile acids should be sent when intrahepatic cholestasis of pregnancy is suspected although elevated serum levels may lag several weeks behind onset of symptoms.
- Multiple imaging modalities are employed in the diagnosis of GI disorders in pregnancy. Abdominal and pelvic ultrasound and magnetic resonance imaging (MRI) are considered safe in pregnancy. Abdominal X-ray and computed tomography (CT) scan with IV and PO contrast are frequently employed in the diagnosis of GI disorders in pregnancy and pregnancy-specific protocols can reduce fetal exposure to <5 rad (the level below which there is no perceived adverse effect) (Brent 1989). Gadolinium contrast is not recommended in pregnancy with the exception of rare circumstances.
- Diagnostic and therapeutic endoscopy, flexible sigmoidoscopy, magnetic resonance cholangiopancreatography (MRCP), endoscopic retrograde cholangiopancreatography (ERCP), and colonoscopy may all be performed when indicated in pregnancy.

Non-GI sources of abdominal pain in pregnancy

Differential diagnosis	Features
Abruption	Severe abdominal pain that is central and located above the uterus. Typically presents with or without vaginal bleeding and tetanic uterine contractions on abdominal palpation.
Preterm labor	Colicky abdominal or back pain that is associated with cervical shortening or dilation and may be associated with nausea/vomiting, vaginal bleeding, or leakage of fluid from ruptured membranes.
Ovarian torsion	Unilateral pelvic or abdominal pain that comes and goes and may present after several days of symptoms. Pelvic and abdominal examination may reveal adnexal fullness. On ultrasound, typically associated with ovarian mass/cyst with surrounding edema.
Urolithiasis	Colicky pain that radiates from the flank to the groin and may be reproducible as either costovertebral tenderness or lower quadrant abdominal tenderness. Typically presents with intractable pain and hematuria, often with hydronephrosis on the affected side on renal ultrasound.
Pyelonephritis	Flank pain that may radiate to the abdomen associated with fever, leukocytosis, nausea, and vomiting. Often with symptoms of dysuria or history of urinary tract infection (UTI) (positive urine culture) in pregnancy.
Degenerating fibroid	Abdominal/pelvic pain in a patient with a history of fibroids or ultrasound (US) diagnosis of necrotic fibroid with liquefaction. Often occurs in the setting of low-grade fever.
Uterine rupture	Severe abdominal pain that is typically midline and associated with shock and hypotension with or without vaginal bleeding. Fetal parts may be palpated above the uterine fundus and there is extrauterine free fluid with nonreassuring fetal status on abdominal ultrasound.

Differential diagnosis of nausea/vomiting in pregnancy

Differential diagnosis	Features
Hyperemesis gravidarum	Severe nausea/vomiting with signs of starvation and dehydration unresponsive to typical diet modification that persists beyond 16 weeks.
Appendicitis	Nausea/vomiting, persistent abdominal pain (right lower quadrant [RLQ] or right upper quadrant [RUQ] pain) often with low-grade fever and leukocytosis. Findings on abdominal US, MRI, or CT abdomen/pelvis consistent with appendicitis
Cholelithiasis	RUQ pain associated with nausea/vomiting, fever, and leukocytosis. Abdominal ultrasound reveals cholelithiasis, biliary sludge, common bile duct dilation, gallbladder wall thickening.
Pancreatitis	Epigastric pain associated with nausea/vomiting, fever, and tachycardia. Serologies typically show significantly elevated serum pancreatic enzymes and hypocalcemia.
Intestinal obstruction	Abdominal pain, nausea/vomiting, often with a history of abdominal/pelvic surgery, endometriosis or inflammatory bowel disease. Most often occurs with changes in size of the uterus. Abdominal X-ray, CT, and MRI all aid in diagnosis of intestinal obstruction.
Acute fatty liver of pregnancy	Nausea/vomiting that occurs late in gestation and associated with epigastric pain and jaundice. May occur in setting of hypertension or preeclampsia. Progressive liver failure leads to varying degrees of hypoglycemia, transaminitis, and coagulopathy.

Typical presentation

- GI disorders in pregnancy may have a variable presentation. Due to the fact that nausea/vomiting may normally wax and wane throughout gestation, many disorders may go undiagnosed or patients may experience a delayed diagnosis. For this reason, clinical suspicion should remain high even when complaints appear benign.
- Presentation for many disorders includes nausea/vomiting and abdominal pain. These are presented in the previous table.
- Preeclampsia and HELLP syndromes are pregnancy-specific disorders that often involve abnormal liver dysfunction and occur after 20 weeks gestation. In addition to RUQ pain, these disorders may also present with hypertension, scotoma, and headache and abnormal coagulation/metabolic profile. Patients with acute fatty liver of pregnancy often have signs/symptoms of preeclampsia in addition to nausea/vomiting and jaundice.
- Intrahepatic cholestasis of pregnancy typically occurs in the second or third trimester and presents with intolerable generalized or focal pruritis on the hands and soles that is worse at night.
- Chronic inflammatory bowel disease may flare in pregnancy and may/may present with nausea/vomiting, abdominal, rectal or perianal discomfort, and blood stools or diarrhea.

Clinical diagnosis

History

- Medical, surgical, obstetric, and gynecologic history should be reviewed in detail when assessing GI complaints in pregnancy. This is in addition to any chronic medications that the patient is taking or recently prescribed antibiotics. Furthermore, diet and history of travel and sick contacts should be explored. Review of systems should include gastrointestinal symptoms as well as neurologic, hematologic, and genitorurinary complaints.

Physical examination

- Thorough abdominal examination, checking for uterine tenderness to exclude obstetric sources of abdominal pain.
- Rectal examination to evaluate hemorrhoids
- Special attention should be made to evaluate pain secondary to deep palpation as the growing uterus may elevate the anterior abdomen off an inflamed viscera thus masking peritoneal signs and rebound.
- Auscultation for bowel sounds
- Pelvic exam to check for cervical dilation in cases of undiagnosed preterm labor or abruption.
- Tocodynamometry to evaluate for the presence and regularity of uterine contractions
- Check for bilateral costovertebral tenderness as pyelonephritis and hydronephrosis secondary to urinary tract obstruction may produce back pain referred to the abdomen.
- Bedside ultrasound should be performed to check for fetal status, amniotic fluid level, and for any extrauterine free fluid.

Disease severity classification

- GI disorders can generally be classified by acuity.
  - Common disorders with benign maternal course often managed as an outpatient: nausea/vomiting, gastroesophageal reflux, constipation, hemorrhoids, intrahepatic cholestasis of pregnancy
  - Chronic GI disorders occasionally managed with inpatient therapy: inflammatory bowel disease flare, hyperemesis gravidarum
  - GI disorders best managed in consultation with a surgical service: cholecystitis, appendicitis, pancreatitis, intestinal obstruction, Ogilvie syndrome

Laboratory diagnosis

List of diagnostic tests

- In general, it is reasonable to order the following laboratory tests in the evaluation of abdominal pain in pregnancy.
- Complete blood count with differential/basic metabolic panel (appropriate for all patients with a GI complaint)
- Hepatic function panel, pancreatic enzymes (amylase/lipase) (Order in cases of suspected upper GI pathology including nausea/vomiting, hypertensive spectrum disorders [preeclampsia/HELLP/fatty liver of pregnancy], pancreatitis or hepatobiliary disease)
- Urinalysis/urine microscopy/urine culture (Order in cases of suspected UTI, pyelonephritis, or nephrolithiasis)
- Coagulation profile (prothrombin time [PT], activated partial thromboplastin time [aPTT], fibrinogen) (Order in cases of hypertensive spectrum disorder, placental abruption, fetal demise)
- Type and screen (Order in cases of suspected surgical/obstetric emergency or vaginal bleeding)

List of imaging techniques

- We recommend beginning with bedside abdominal/pelvic ultrasound in all pregnant patients to evaluate for common pregnancy-specific abnormalities that may be benign (i.e. fibroids) or life-threatening (i.e. massive placental abruption).
- A more formal abdominal, pelvic, or renal ultrasound may be ordered to further evaluate the adnexa, appendix, gallbladder, or kidneys.
- When ultrasound is nondiagnostic and abdominal pathology suspected, MRI is particularly useful in the diagnosis of appendicitis.
- Abdominal X-ray and CT scan with IV and PO contrast are frequently employed in the diagnosis of GI disorders in pregnancy, especially at institutions that do not have ready access to MRI. As stated previously, pregnancy-specific protocols can reduce fetal exposure to <5 rad (the level below which there is no perceived adverse effect) (Brent 1989). Gadolinium contrast should be avoided in pregnancy.

Potential pitfalls/common errors made regarding diagnosis of disease

- Diagnosis of appendicitis may be missed or delayed in pregnancy secondary to:
  - Cephalad displacement of pain above the RLQ in the second and third trimesters
  - Muted abdominal pain due to elevation of parietal peritoneum off inflamed viscera by enlarged uterus
  - Mild leukocytosis (up to 15k cells/microL) (Kuvin and Brecher 1962) often encountered in normal pregnancy
  - Symptoms of nausea/vomiting often encountered in normal pregnancy

Treatment

- Hyperemesis gravidarum: fluid resuscitation, symptom control with antiemetic, transition to PO intake and behavior/diet modification to achieve maintenance.
- Intrahepatic cholestasis of pregnancy: first-line treatment is ursodeoxycholic acid with or without diphenhydramine for symptoms relief. Pregnancy may be managed until late preterm or early term in consultation with maternal fetal medicine and pending reassuring fetal status (ACOG 2013).
- Preeclampsia with significant liver disease (doubling of serum transaminases above the upper limit of normal) or patients with HELLP syndrome are managed with prompt delivery.
- Cholecystitis and appendicitis: first-line treatment is surgical management.

When to hospitalize

- Hyperemesis gravidarum: inability to tolerate PO intake, severe metabolic abnormalities
- Preeclampsia with significant liver disease (doubling of serum transaminases above the upper limit of normal) or patients with HELLP syndrome should be managed as an inpatient.
- Cholecystitis, appendicitis, pancreatitis: initial hospitalization until surgical clearance for discharge

Managing the hospitalized patient

- Inpatient management of patients with hyperemesis gravidarum consists of thiamine and electrolyte repletion, intravenous fluid hydration, and initiation of antiemetic regimen that adequately controls symptoms so that PO intake may resume. In cases of severe symptoms uncontrolled by medication, patients should be given the option of termination if within the legal limit of gestational age.
- Management of colitis flare is generally performed in consultation with a gastroenterology service. Treatment consists of fluid hydration, calcium supplementation, pain control, bowel rest, and resumption of maintenance therapy with possible addition of corticosteroids or immunomodulating agents.
- Surgical emergencies should be managed in consultation with a surgical service. In general, mainstays of therapy beyond surgical exploration include fluid hydration, bowel rest, and pain control.

CLINICAL PEARLS

- GI disorders in pregnancy are varied and include a large differential, including several disorders that are specific to pregnant patients.
- GI disorders may have an atypical presentation during pregnancy secondary to physiologic and anatomic changes that occur with advancing gestation.
- History taking, physical exam, serologies, and radiologic studies are all crucial to a thorough patient evaluation and accurate diagnosis.

Reading list

American College of Obstetricians and Gynecologists. Nonmedically indicated early-term deliveries. Committee opinion no. 561. *Obstet Gynecol* 2013;121:911-5.

Andersen B, Nielsen TF. Appendicitis in pregnancy: diagnosis, management and complications. *Acta Obstet Gynecol Scand* 1999;78(9):758-62.

Belfort MA, Saade G, Foley MR, et al. *Critical care obstetrics*. 5th ed. Hoboken, NJ: Blackwell Publishing; 2010.

Berghella V. *Evidence based guidelines*. 2nd ed. New York: Informa Healthcare; 2012.

Brent RL. The effect of embryonic and fetal exposure to x-ray, microwaves, and ultrasound: counseling the pregnant and nonpregnant patient about these risks. *Semin Oncol* 1989;16(5):347-68.

Cunningham FG, Leveno KJ, Bloom SL, et al. *Williams obstetrics*. 24th ed. New York: McGraw-Hill Education; 2014.

Eddy JJ, Gideosen MD, Song JY, et al: Pancreatitis in pregnancy. *Obstet Gyncol* 2008;112:1075-81.

Gabbe SG, Niebyl J, Simpson J, et al. *Obstetrics normal and problem pregnancies*. 7th ed. New York: Elsevier; 2017.

Interventions for nausea and vomiting in early pregnancy. *Cochrane Database Syst Rev* 2015 Sep 8;(9).

Kuvin SF, Brecher G. Differential neutrophil counts in pregnancy. *New Eng J Med* 1962;266:877-8.

Mourad J, Elliott JP, Erickson L, Lisboa L. Appendicitis in pregnancy: new information that contradicts long-held clinical beliefs. *Am J Obstet Gynecol* 2000;182(5):1027-9.

Nelson DB, Yost NP, Cunningham FG. Acute fatty liver of pregnancy: clinical outcomes and expected duration of recovery. *Am J Obstet Gynecol* 2013 Nov;209(5):456.e1-7.

Resnik R, Creasy R, Iams J, et al. *Creasy & Resnik's maternal-fetal medicine*. 7th ed. Philadelphia: Elsevier Saunders; 2014.

Stone JH. HELLP Syndrome: Hemolysis, Elevated liver enzymes, and low platelets. *JAMA* 1998;280(6):559-62.

Additional material for this chapter can be found online at:
www.wiley.com/go/sperling/mountsinai/obstetricsandgynecology

This includes a case study and advice for patients.

CHAPTER 7

Ultrasound in Pregnancy

Eric P. Bergh[1] and Angela Bianco[2]

[1] Maternal-Fetal Medicine Subspecialist, UT Health – McGovern Medical School, Division of Maternal-Fetal Medicine, Houston, TX
[2] Division of Maternal-Fetal Medicine, Department of Obstetrics, Gynecology and Reproductive Science, Icahn School of Medicine at Mount Sinai, New York, NY

OVERALL BOTTOM LINE
- Ultrasound evaluation of the fetus and placenta has revolutionized the field of obstetrics.
- Clinicians should be familiar with the indications for transvaginal and transabdominal ultrasound.
- Invasive ultrasound guided procedures can be used for diagnosis and for therapy.

Background

Ultrasound has revolutionized the field of obstetrics. It has proven critical to determining accurate pregnancy dating and in the diagnosis of fetal anomalies, multiple gestations, fetal malpresentation, cervical shortening, and abnormal placentation. Furthermore, ultrasound-guided procedures have allowed for the development of improved genetic diagnoses as well as intrauterine fetal therapies.

Indications

- Confirm or establish the gestational age of a pregnancy
- Confirm pregnancy order (i.e. number of fetuses)
- Screening for fetal anatomic abnormalities
- Assessment of fetal growth and well-being
- Detection of cervical shortening to identify patients at risk for preterm birth
- Screen for abnormal placentation
- Ultrasound-guided procedures and 3D/4D ultrasound may be employed for diagnostic or treatment purposes in pregnancy

Procedure (transvaginal ultrasound)

- Ideal for obtaining high resolution images of early pregnancy, cervix, and adnexal structures
- May be performed in any trimester
- Optimal images obtained when the bladder is empty (patient should void prior to procedure)
- The patient should be positioned in dorsal lithotomy.
- *Calculate gestational age* (prior to 14 weeks): Crown-rump length measurement of fetus is obtained in the midsagittal plane (Figure 7.1).
- *Calculate nuchal translucency* (between 11 to 14 weeks): Measurement of the translucent space beneath the skin of the neck, when viewed in the midsagittal plane. Measurements above the 97th percentile may be associated with increased risk for fetal aneuploidy (i.e. chromosomal abnormalities) (Figure 7.2).
- *Calculate cervical length* (between 12–28 weeks): Average of three measurements of the cervix (internal to external os), taken in the midsagittal plane with an empty bladder (Figure 7.3). Cervical length

---

Mount Sinai Expert Guides: Obstetrics and Gynecology, First Edition. Edited by Rhoda Sperling.
© 2020 John Wiley & Sons Ltd. Published 2020 by John Wiley & Sons Ltd.
Companion Website: www.wiley.com/go/sperling/mountsinai/obstetricsandgynecology

screening is generally performed in patients with evidence of cervical shortening or a history of prior preterm birth. Patients with a shortened cervix may be candidates for progesterone therapy or cervical cerclage to prevent preterm birth.

- *Evaluate adnexal structures*: Sweeping laterally in the sagittal plane allows for identification and characterization of the bilateral adnexa. Cysts, masses, and possible ectopic gestations can be visualized.
- *Identify abnormal placentation*: In the sagittal plane, the relationship of the placenta to the internal os of the cervix can be visualized.
  - A complete placenta previa is diagnosed when the placental edge covers the os (Figure 7.4).
  - A marginal placenta previa occurs when the distance from the leading edge of the placenta to the internal os is < 2 cm.
  - Patients with a history of prior cesarean delivery and a low-lying placenta or placenta previa are at high risk for morbidly adherent placenta (placenta accreta). Obliteration of the normal interface between the uterine myometrium and the bladder or the appearance of multiple vascular placental lakes should raise suspicion for adherent placenta (accreta).
  - Color Doppler ultrasound should be used to rule out vasa previa, which occurs when any fetal vessels traverse the internal os.

Procedure (transabdominal ultrasound)

- Ideal for evaluating the fetal anatomy in the second trimester and estimation of fetal growth in the third trimester as well as fetal presentation (cephalic or breech). In the thin patient, first trimester abdominal ultrasound is a useful technique for early pregnancy dating.
- Optimal images are obtained when the bladder is full. The distended bladder creates a sonographic "window" that allows improved penetration and visualization of abdominopelvic structures.
- The patient should be placed in dorsal supine position. Occasionally, left or right lateral tilt may be necessary to obtain specific images, particularly in the obese patient. If the patient has significant central adiposity, elevation of the pannus will improve sonographic images of the fetus and the abdominal viscera.
- In the second trimester, anatomical abnormalities seen via transabdominal ultrasound may raise suspicion for fetal aneuploidy or genetic syndromes.
- *Placentation*: If the placenta is low lying in appearance on transabdominal ultrasound, the distance of the leading edge to the cervix should be evaluated using vaginal ultrasound.
  - In multiple gestations, determination of chorionicity is best performed between weeks 10 and 14 (via transvaginal or transabdominal ultrasound).
    - Dichorionicity is suggested when the placentas are distinctly separate from each other or when fetal gender is discordant. When the placentas are adjacent, images of the insertion site of the amnion and chorion show a characteristic "lambda" sign with a thick intervening membrane (Figure 7.5).
    - A "T-sign" with a relatively thin interamniotic membrane is suggestive of monochorionicity (Figure 7.6).
- *Estimation of fetal size/weight*: performed by obtaining the following images to measure fetal biometries: Biparietal diameter, head circumference, abdominal circumference, femur length (Figures 7.7–7.9). Most ultrasound equipment is programmed to calculate fetal weight from biometric measurements although multiple online calculators exist for this purpose.
  - A fetus measuring below the 10th percentile is small for gestational age. Causes include inaccurate dating, constitutionally small fetus, infectious, genetic, and placental etiologies. A fetus measuring above the 90th percentile is large for gestational age. Most commonly, causes include inaccurate dating, uncontrolled maternal diabetes, or a fetus that is constitutionally large for gestational age.
  - In twins, a growth discordance of more than 20% may indicate problems of shared placentation or genetic causes and warrant increased monitoring.

- *Amniotic fluid*: The amniotic fluid index (AFI) the summation of the largest vertical pocket of fluid measured in each sonographic window when the maternal abdomen is divided into four quadrants. A normal range is typically 5–24 cm.
  - *Oligohydramnios*: Diagnosed when the AFI is < 5 cm. Causes include ruptured membranes, chronic nonsteroidal anti-inflammatory drugs (NSAID) usage, or fetal disorders of fluid production such as renal anomalies or lower urinary tract obstruction
  - *Polyhydramnios*: Diagnosed when the AFI measures > 24 cm. Causes are multiple but may be idiopathic or related to certain intraamniotic infections (cytomegalovirus, toxovirus, etc.), uncontrolled maternal diabetes mellitus, or disorders of fetal swallowing.
  - *Maximum vertical pocket (MVP)*: Often based on provider preference, the MVP may be used in place of the AFI. A normal MVP is any pocket of fluid measuring > 2 cm and < 8 cm (Figure 7.10). Oligohydramnios and polyhydramnios are diagnosed below and above these cutoffs.
- *Fetal well-being*:
  - *Pulsed-wave Doppler ultrasound*:
    - *Umbilical artery*: The ratio of systolic to diastolic blood flow in the umbilical artery can be investigated using doppler ultrasound. This is indicated in fetuses in which growth restriction is suspected. Abnormal or reversed diastolic flow in the umbilical artery indicates poor placental function and may be an indication for increased surveillance or early delivery
    - *Middle cerebral artery (MCA)*: Doppler ultrasound can be used to measure flow in the MCA. Abnormally increased flow is an indicator of low blood viscosity and likely fetal anemia.
  - *Biophysical profile (BPP)*:
    - The BPP is a scoring system to determine fetal well-being. A perfect score indicates low risk for fetal demise within 1 week of the procedure. A sonogram is performed for 30 minutes, during which time the following parameters are investigated:
      - Fetal breathing
      - Fetal movement
      - Fetal tone
      - Amniotic fluid volume

Ultrasound-guided procedures

The following procedures are all needle based and ultrasound guided and typically performed with the aid of an assistant.

- *Chorionic villus sampling*:
  - Needle-guided procedure to sample the placental chorionic villi for genetic diagnosis
  - May be performed electively due to patient preference, baseline risk for aneuploidy or genetic abnormality, or secondary to abnormal first trimester sonogram
  - Performed in the first trimester between 10–14 weeks gestation
  - May be performed via transabdominal or transvaginal approach
  - Complications include a pregnancy loss rate of approximately 1–2:1000 (Akolekar et al. 2015), which is variable and provider dependent
  - Prior to 10 weeks the procedure is associated with fetal limb reduction defects.
- *Amniocentesis*:
  - Needle-guided procedure to sample amniotic fluid for multiple diagnoses:
    - Collection of amniocytes (sloughed fetal skin cells) for genetic diagnosis
    - Evaluation of amniotic fluid for the presence of intraamniotic infections
    - Evaluation of amniotic fluid for the presence of markers of fetal lung maturity in cases of elective preterm birth
    - Evaluation of amniotic fluid for markers associated with neural tube and abdominal wall defects (elevated maternal serum alpha-protein and acetylcholinesterase)

- May be performed any time after 15 weeks, although most physicians will not perform beyond 23 weeks due to risk of ruptured membranes and possible iatrogenic preterm birth
- Associated with a 1:1000 (Akolekar et al. 2015) risk of fetal loss
- Complications may include intra-amniotic infection (associated with fever and abdominal pain), bleeding, and ruptured membranes, or fetal death.
  - In cases of intraamniotic infection, uterine evacuation is indicated due to subsequent risk for maternal sepsis.
  - In cases of rupture of membranes post amniocentesis, spontaneous resolution with resealing of the membranes can occur in up to 80–90% of cases provided there is no infection present.
- *Percutaneous umbilical cord sampling*
  - Needle-guided procedure to sample fetal blood most commonly for suspected anemia with simultaneous ability to perform intrauterine transfusion. Sampling and transfusion typically occurs from the umbilical vein, ideally at the site of the placental cord insertion. Intraperitoneal transfusion may also be performed in cases where safe access to the umbilical vein is not possible. Intrahepatic sampling and cardiocentesis are feasible but rarely performed secondary to technical challenges and high risk of complications associated with these approaches.
  - Performed when severe anemia suspected based on ultrasound findings of hydrops or elevated blood flow in the fetal middle cerebral artery. Typical etiologies include severe fetal infections (parvovirus) or Rh alloimmunization.
  - May be performed between 18 to 34 weeks
  - Complications include possible rupture of membranes, intrauterine infection, or rarely fetal death.
- Ultrasound-guided procedures that may be performed in pregnancy but that are beyond the scope of this chapter include:
  - Fetal reduction procedures for multiple gestation pregnancies
  - Termination of pregnancy
  - Laser ablation of abnormal placental vessels in cases of compromised twin pregnancies (twin-to-twin transfusion syndrome)
  - Advanced fetal therapy procedures:
    - Placement of bladder shunt for lower urinary tract obstruction
    - Placement of chest wall shunt in cases of fetal hydrothorax

3D/4D ultrasound

- Sophisticated ultrasound technology now provides images of structures in both 3D and 4D (live 3D images). Although not a routine technique, 3D/4D ultrasound is of particular use when evaluating certain congenital anomalies. These include:
  - Evaluation of the face and palate for clefts (Figure 7.11)
  - Evaluation of the fetal brain in conjunction with fetal magnetic resonance imaging (MRI) for neurologic abnormalities
  - Evaluation of the fetal spine for open neural tube defects
  - Evaluation of fetal extremities to assess for skeletal dysplasias and limb defects
  - Evaluation of the fetal heart for congenital disease and postnatal repair planning
- In the absence of suspected abnormality for which 3D/4D ultrasound may provide useful clinical information, routine "keepsake" ultrasounds are not recommended.

Reading list

Akolekar R, Beta J, Picciarelli G, et al. Procedure-related risk of miscarriage following amniocentesis and chorionic villus sampling: a systematic review and meta-analysis. *Ultrasound Obstet Gynecol* 2015;45:16.
American Institute of Ultrasound in Medicine. AIUM practice guideline for the performance of obstetric ultrasound examinations. *J Ultrasound Med* 2013;32(6):1083-1101.
Practice bulletin no. 175: Ultrasound in pregnancy. *Obstet Gynecol* 2016;128(6):e241-e256.

Suggested websites

American College of Obstetricians and Gynecologists. www.acog.org
Society for Maternal-Fetal Medicine. www.smfm.org
American Institute of Ultrasound in Medicine. www.aium.org
Perinatology. www.perinatology.com
The Fetus. https://sonoworld.com/thefetus/home.aspx

Guidelines
National society guidelines

Title	Source	Date/full reference
ACOG practice bulletin no. 175: Ultrasound in pregnancy	American College of Obstetricians and Gynecologists	*Obstet Gynecol* 2016;128(6):e241-e256.

International society guidelines

Title	Source	Date/full reference
American Institute of Ultrasound in Medicine (AIUM) practice guideline for the performance of obstetric ultrasound examinations	AIUM	*J Ultrasound Med* 2013;32(6):1083-1101.

Images

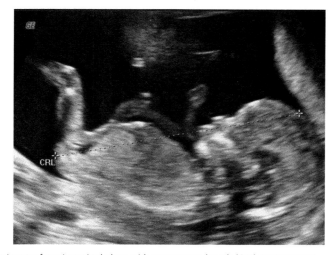

Figure 7.1 First trimester fetus in sagittal plane with crown-rump length (CRL) measurement.

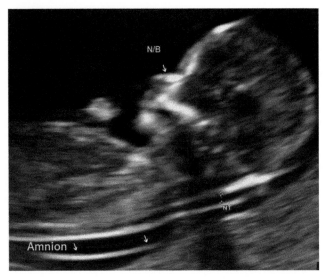

Figure 7.2 Nuchal translucency (NT) measurement with amnion/amniotic membrane and nasal bone (NB) visible in sagittal plane.

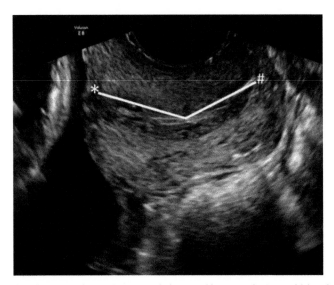

Figure 7.3 Cervical length measured using transvaginal ultrasound between the internal (*) and external (#) os.

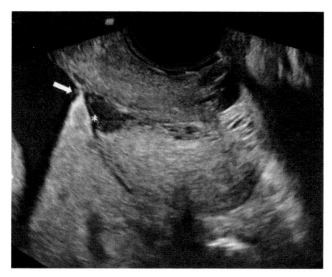

Figure 7.4 Transvaginal ultrasound image of cervix with placental edge (arrow) overlying the internal os of the cervix (*).

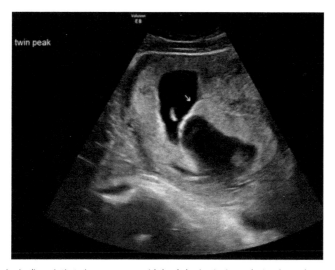

Figure 7.5 Dichorionic diamniotic twin pregnancy with lambda sign/twin peak sign (arrow).

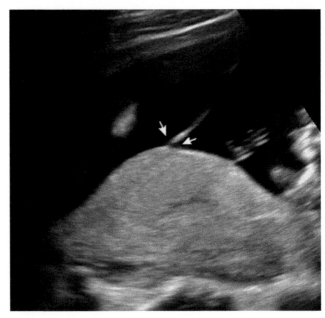

Figure 7.6 Monochorionic twin pregnancy with intervening membrane and "T" sign (arrows).

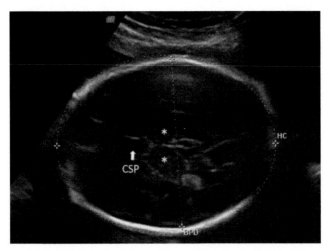

Figure 7.7 Axial view of the fetal cranium at the level of the cavum septum pellucidum (CSP) and thalami (*). The biparietal diameter (BPD) is measured from the outside of the near parietal bone to the inside of the far parietal bone. The head circumference (HC) is measured with an ellipse around the calvarium.

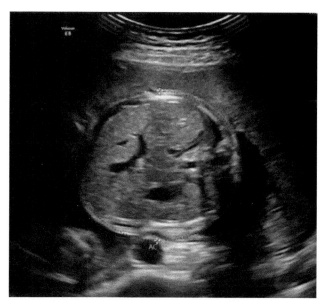

Figure 7.8 Axial view of the fetal abdomen at the level of the stomach (*) and the umbilical vein (UV). The abdominal circumference is measured with an ellipse around the fetal skin at this level.

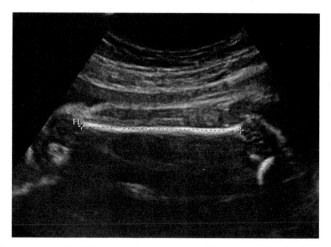

Figure 7.9 Longitudinal view of the fetal femur. The femur length (FL) is measured as the distance between the ends of the ossified diaphysis.

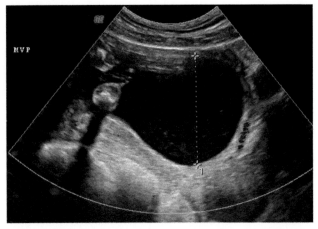

Figure 7.10 Maximal vertical pocket (MVP) measured between calipers. See color version on website.

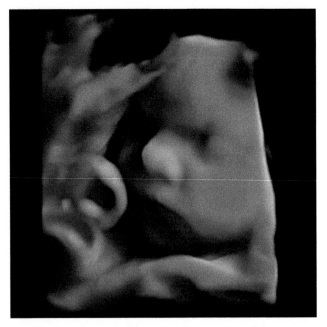

Figure 7.11 3D image of the third trimester fetal face. See color version on website.

Additional material for this chapter can be found online at:
www.wiley.com/go/sperling/mountsinai/obstetricsandgynecology

The following images are available in color: Figure 7.10 and Figure 7.11.

CHAPTER 8

Carrier Screening and Aneuploidy Screening

Luciana Vieira and Keith Eddleman
Division of Maternal-Fetal Medicine, Department of Obstetrics, Gynecology and Reproductive Science, Icahn School of Medicine at Mount Sinai, New York, NY

OVERALL BOTTOM LINE
- Pregnancy-related genetic testing includes carrier screening and aneuploidy screening.
- Carrier screening identifies genetic mutations that an asymptomatic individual can pass to their offspring.
- Advances in genomic medicine have led to the availability of expanded carrier screening panels for more than 280 diseases.
- Aneuploidy screening identifies fetuses at increased risk for chromosomal abnormalities and should be offered to all pregnant women.
- There are multiple options available for aneuploidy screening. Common testing algorithms are based on information derived from various sources including maternal serum levels of placental biomarkers, fetal ultrasound, and detection of fetal DNA in the maternal circulation.
- Carrier screening and aneuploidy screening identify "at-risk" fetuses. Invasive testing, chorionic villus sampling, and amniocentesis are utilized to confirm diagnoses.

Carrier screening
Background
- Carrier screening identifies genetic mutations that an asymptomatic individual can pass to their offspring.
- Carrier screening is available for a growing number of recessive and X-linked genetic disorders.
- Previously, a patient's race, ethnicity, or family history guided specific recommendations for carrier screening.
- As genomic medicine advances, there are expanded carrier panels including panels that screen for over 280 disorders.
- Quick turnaround time and lower costs have lead some commercial laboratories to offer this testing directly to consumers. In general, professional societies discourage this type of testing because it bypasses important pre- and posttest counseling information.
- Genetic counseling should explain the detection rate for a specific disorder, the positive predictive value of the results, and partner testing, as well as limitations of the screening.
- Carrier screening will typically not detect all mutations for a specific disease and as such, there remains a "residual risk." The residual risk for each disease is determined based on the mutations tested for the disease as well as ethnicity.
- Ideally, carrier screening should be part of preconception planning. If a woman is positive for a given disorder, the partner can be tested for that same disorder. If both partners are found to be carriers for the disorder, formal genetic counseling is indicated to review reproductive options (i.e. donor gametes,

---

Mount Sinai Expert Guides: Obstetrics and Gynecology, First Edition. Edited by Rhoda Sperling.
© 2020 John Wiley & Sons Ltd. Published 2020 by John Wiley & Sons Ltd.
Companion Website: www.wiley.com/go/sperling/mountsinai/obstetricsandgynecology

preimplantation genetic diagnosis, prenatal diagnosis) prior to conception. Confirmatory testing can take weeks to accomplish so having this done before conceiving will give the patient time to make informed reproductive decisions.

Indications and other considerations
- Ethnic-specific, panethnic, and expanded carrier screening are acceptable strategies for prepregnancy and prenatal carrier screening.
- However, in today's increasingly multiethnic/cross-cultural society, it is often difficult to precisely discern a patient's ancestry. For this reason, some couples will choose panethnic screening. The decision for which screening strategy is appropriate for a patient/couple is best made after reviewing the options and pretest counseling (refer to most recent American College of Obstetricians and Gynecologists [ACOG] for most recent guidelines pertaining to carrier frequency and residual risks, see key references at end of chapter).
- All patients who are considering pregnancy or are already pregnant, regardless of screening approach, should be offered carrier screening for cystic fibrosis, spinal muscular atrophy, thalassemias, and hemoglobinopathies.
- Fragile X premutation carrier screening is recommended for women with a family history of fragile X-related disorders, intellectual disability suggestive of fragile X syndrome, or women with a personal or family history ovarian insufficiency.
- Couples with consanguinity should be offered genetic counseling to discuss increased risks of recessive conditions.
- Patients should be informed that any recommendations for screening for a genetic condition is optional, and after informed consent and counseling, patient may decline to have the testing done.
- For patients or their partners who are found to be carriers for a disorder, providers should inform the couple of the implications for their relatives and recommend that they consider testing. Providers, however, should not disclose this information to relatives without consent from the patient (or her carrier partner, if that is the case).

Aneuploidy screening and diagnostic testing
Background
- Prenatal detection of common chromosomal abnormalities is the main goal of prenatal screening, because chromosomal anomalies occur in approximately 1 in 150 live births.
- An euploid fetus has two complete copies of each haploid autosome plus two sex chromosomes (46 in total). This is referred to as euploidy. Aneuploidy occurs when there is one or more extra or missing haploid chromosome(s), resulting in an unbalanced chromosome number in each cell (autosomal or sex chromosomal aneuploidy), or a complete extra set of all haploid chromosomes in multiples of 23 (i.e. triploidy, tetraploidy).
- Fetal chromosomal abnormalities commonly associated with increasing maternal age are trisomy 21, trisomy 18, trisomy 13, triple X syndrome, and Klinefelter's syndrome. Other risk factors for fetal aneuploidies include a history of prior aneuploidy and the presence of fetal anomalies.
- Down syndrome is the most common autosomal trisomy in live births, with a prevalence of 1 in 800. However, the most prevalent trisomy in the first trimester is actually trisomy 16.
- A positive screening test indicates an increased risk of Down syndrome or another aneuploidy but is not diagnostic. Generally, a "positive screen" is a cutoff determined by the laboratory to maximize the detection rate for a given disorder while minimizing the number of false positives. Many laboratories use the baseline risk of aneuploidy for a given age as the cutoff point for a positive screen. Conversely, a negative test does not completely rule out aneuploidy but rather decreases the baseline risk calculated by the screening test. It is not a diagnostic result.

Rationale and timing for testing

- Regardless of maternal age, both screening and invasive diagnostic testing for aneuploidy should be offered to all pregnant women. Ideally, this screening should be discussed and offered at the first pre-natal visit or prior to 20 weeks of gestation.
- When discussing options for aneuploidy screening, patients should be counseled about the differences between screening and invasive/diagnostic testing to allow them to make an informed choice.
- Patients should also be given information regarding the detection and false-positive rates and advantages, disadvantages, and limitations of each test in addition to the risks and benefits of diagnostic testing. It is also important to review the positive and negative predictive value in a given population or age group.
  - Pretest and posttest counseling is imperative to address the adjusted likelihood of an abnormal fetus following each test.
  - For patients with a family history of a chromosomal abnormality, genetic disorder, or congenital malformation, genetic counseling provided by a specialist in genetics or maternal-fetal medicine is recommended.

First trimester screening

- First trimester screening is performed between 11 0/7 weeks and 13 6/7 weeks gestation (crown-rump length measurement between 38–45 mm and 84 mm) (the serum portion of this screening test can be done as early as 9 weeks)
- The first trimesters screen includes an ultrasound to assess the thickness of the nuchal translucency (NT) in the fetus and maternal serum analytes, including human chorionic gonadotropin (hCG) – ideally, free β-hCG – and pregnancy-associated plasma protein A (PAPP-A). First trimester maternal serum AFP has also been incorporated into some screening protocols.
- Nuchal translucency refers to the fluid-filled space measured on the dorsal aspect of the fetal neck
  - NT >3 mm or more or above the 99th percentile for the crown-rump length is independently associated with fetal aneuploidy and structural malformations.
  - Credentialing of ultrasonographers in appropriate technique and ongoing quality review is imperative to maintain screening performance.
- A risk estimate is calculated using serum results, NT measurement as well as maternal age, prior history of aneuploidy, weight, race, and number of fetuses. However, this screening is not performed for gestations with more than two fetuses, and the detection rate is lower for twin gestations.
- Using both NT measurement and serum screening, the detection rate for Down syndrome ranges from 79–87% with a false-positive rate of 5%.
- Other markers for aneuploidy that can be evaluated in the first trimester include absence of nasal bone and abnormal ductus venosus waveform.
- Sonographers performing NT measurements must be certified and adhere to a strict protocol as determined by the Nuchal Translucency Quality Review Program (NTQR) or the Fetal Medicine Foundation (FMF) or other quality review mechanisms.

Second trimester screening

- Quadruple marker ("Quad") screen
  - The "quad" screen is performed after 15 0/7 weeks (range varies slightly dependent on the laboratory). This screening test includes four components of maternal serum: hCG, alpha-fetoprotein (AFP), dimeric inhibin A, unconjugated estriol.
  - This screening test does not include ultrasound findings in the reported result; however, online calculators (such as perinatology.com) allow for the modification of the reported risk based on ultrasound

findings. The quad screen also factors in maternal age, weight, race, presence of diabetes, and number of fetuses (up to two).
- The detection rate for Down syndrome ranges from 67–81% at a 5% false-positive rate with the quadruple screen.
- For best results, accurate gestational dating at time of serum sampling must be reported.
- Other second trimester screening tests
  - Penta screen
    - The penta screen includes hyperglycosylated hCG (also known as invasive trophoblast antigen) in addition to quad markers.
    - Performance has not been extensively evaluated; therefore, it is not widely used.
  - Triple screen
    - The triple screen measures hCG, AFP, and unconjugated estriol.
    - It has a lower sensitivity than quad screen and first trimester screening (69% at a 5% positive screening test result rate) and is rarely used.
- Maternal serum AFP screening
  - All women should be offered second trimester AFP to screen for neural tube defects.
  - Using a maternal AFP level of 2.0 or 2.5 MoM (multiples of the median) as the upper limit of normal, most laboratories report a detection rate of at least 90% for anencephaly and 80% for spina bifida, though the positive predictive value for an affected fetus is only 2 to 6%.
  - Many experts argue that when using the current state-of-the-art ultrasound equipment, ultrasound alone has a higher detection rate for neural tube defects than does maternal serum AFP. Although we support the use of ultrasound to detect fetal anomalies, maternal serum AFP remains the standard of care for the detection of open neural tube defects.

Combined first and second trimester screening
- Integrated
  - As part of the integrated first and second trimester screening, the patient undergoes first trimester NT measurement and analyte screening followed by second trimester quad screen but receives only a single test result that combines both later in second trimester
  - Although the Down syndrome detection rate is lower, the integrated screen can be done without the nuchal translucency measurement. This may be appropriate where a NT measurement by a certified ultrasonographer is not readily available.
  - Limitations include withholding results of first trimester screening and nonadherence to second blood draw (can be as high 25%)
- Sequential
  - With sequential first and second trimester screening, a patient is given preliminary risk estimate after first trimester screening (NT screening and serum analytes) is completed.
    - If result is "positive" or the risk of aneuploidy exceeds the laboratory-derived cutoff, the patient is notified and is offered further testing with invasive testing or cell-free DNA (cDNA) screening if she declines invasive testing.
    - If results are low risk or "negative," she is informed and proceeds to quad screening in the second trimester after which she receives a second result.
- Contingent
  - Contingent first and second trimester screening classifies aneuploidy risk as high, intermediate, or low based on results of first trimester screening.
  - Women with high risk results are offered early diagnostic procedure or cDNA screening. For those who are low risk, no further testing is performed.
  - Only women with intermediate risk results are offered second trimester screening (thus, fewer women go on to second trimester screening).

- Other considerations
  - Use of multiple screening tests independently results in an unacceptably high screen positive rate and is not recommended.
  - In patients who have only first trimester aneuploidy screening, maternal serum alpha-fetoprotein (MSAFP) should be performed as an isolated screening test for neural tube defects in the second trimester.

Ultrasonographic screening for aneuploidy

- Ultrasonographic screening for aneuploidy is routinely performed at the time of an anatomy scan at 18–22 weeks gestation.
- The anatomy ultrasound seeks to identify major structural defects and minor ultrasonographic "soft markers" of aneuploidy.
- Major structural anomalies associated with Down syndrome include cardiac anomalies and duodenal atresia.
- Soft markers include nonspecific findings such as echogenic intracardiac foci, thickened nuchal fold renal pelvis dilation echogenic bowel, ventriculomegaly, choroid plexus cysts (only associated with trisomy 18), and short femur length (refer to "ACOG Practice Bulletin No. 163: Screening for Fetal Aneuploidy" for a full list of soft markers and imaging criteria).
- Other soft markers include short humerus, sandal gap deformity, and clinodactyly.
- If a soft marker is noted, the patient's screening result should be multiplied by the appropriate likelihood ratio. If the result still falls below the cutoff for a "positive screen," then you can still call the patient "screen negative." However, if the modified result falls above the cutoff, then invasive testing should be offered.
- The role or modifiable risk of ultrasound soft markers in patients who have undergone noninvasive prenatal screening is unclear.

Cell-free fetal DNA screening for aneuploidy

- The latest technology for aneuploidy screening is identification of cell-free fetal DNA (cfDNA) in the maternal circulation.
- cfDNA screening evaluates short segments of fetal DNA in maternal blood which can be used to screen for a variety of fetal conditions.
- Fetal fragments of cfDNA are released into the maternal circulation largely by placental cells that have undergone apoptosis or programmed cell death.
  - This makes up approximately 3–13% of the total cDNA in maternal blood (the remainder being maternal in origin). This amount increases throughout pregnancy and is cleared from the maternal circulation shortly after birth.
- Screening can be performed as early as 10 weeks and offers the highest screening detection rate for Down syndrome (>98%).
  - Detection rate is lower for trisomy 13 and 18.
  - Can be used to determine fetal sex, presence of Rh-positive fetus in Rh-negative mothers
- In addition to "no call" results that have been associated with an increased risk of aneuploidy, confined placental mosaicism, maternal mosaicism, and maternal malignancy have been associated with false-positive cfDNA screening. More information is needed to determine the implications of and appropriate counseling for a low fetal fraction or "no call" result. The most common reason for a "no call" result is maternal obesity.

Invasive/diagnostic testing
Indications

- Invasive or diagnostic testing should be made available to all patients. However, the following patients are at increased risk for genetic abnormalities:

- Older maternal age
- Older paternal age
- Parental carrier of chromosome rearrangement
- Parental aneuploidy or aneuploidy mosaicism
- Prior child with structural birth defect
- Parental carrier of genetic disorder
- Previous fetus or child with autosomal trisomy or sex chromosome aneuploidy
- Structural anomalies identified by ultrasonography
- Positive serum screening (either first or second trimester)
- Patients who conceive by in vitro fertilization

Preimplantation genetic diagnosis
- Preimplantation genetic diagnosis is the process that allows testing on an embryo for a particular genetic defect prior to implantation.
- It can be used to test for most genetic conditions in which a mutation has been identified in the family.
- Limitations
  - Though a biopsy of one or a few cells is obtained from an early embryo, confirmation of results with chorionic villus sampling (CVS) or amniocentesis is recommended.
  - This process requires in vitro fertilization and is, therefore, costly.

Chorionic villus sampling
- Placental villi are obtained under ultrasonographic guidance using a needle (transabdominal CVS or TA-CVS) or specialized catheter (transcervical CVS or TC-CVS) without entering the amniotic sac with chorionic villus sampling.
  - Negative pressure is created with a syringe and is then used to aspirate a small amount of placental villi.
- This procedure is performed between 10 weeks and 14 weeks of gestation, although the catheter used for TC-CVS is not FDA-approved for use after 12 weeks.
- Complications
  - The procedure-related loss is 0.22 to 2.6%
    - The large range in loss rates may be due to difficulties in accounting for background loss rate in the first trimester and therefore may be overestimated in some studies. However, a systematic review by the Cochrane Library in 2003 found similar rates of pregnancy loss with amniocentesis and transabdominal chorionic villus sampling.
  - Other complications include vaginal bleeding or spotting (as high as 32% after transcervical CVS).
  - The incidence of culture failure, amniotic fluid leakage or infection is less than 0.5% for chorionic villus sampling.
- One main advantage of CVS to amniocentesis is earlier diagnosis (though not earlier than 10 weeks due to increased risk of limb reduction defects).
- However, there are some disadvantages to chorionic villus sampling. DNA methylation patterns are not well-established in the first trimester, so for disorders where this is important (Fragile X), CVS may not be the best test. Additionally, in women who are Rh alloimmunized, there is theoretical risk that CVS may worsen the alloimmunization.

Amniocentesis
- Amniocentesis is the most common procedure performed worldwide to diagnose fetal aneuploidy and other genetic disorders.
- This procedure is performed after 15 1/2 weeks to 20 weeks (can be performed beyond this gestational age, though must consider risk of periviable preterm premature rupture of membranes and iatrogenic preterm birth, as well as the possibility that results from the test may not be available in a timeframe that

would allow for pregnancy termination, should a woman choose that option). Amniocentesis should not be performed prior to this gestational age due to concerns about talipes equinovarus (clubbed feet).
- The procedure is performed using sterile technique, using a 20- or 22-gauge spinal needle under ultrasonographic guidance.
  - 20–30 ml of amniotic fluid is obtained from a pocket free of fetal parts and umbilical cord.
  - Transplacental passage of the needle is avoided, if possible.
- Complications
  - The procedure-related loss is 0.06 to 1.0%.
    - The large range in procedure related loss may be due to preexisting abnormalities such as placental abruption, abnormal placental implantation, fetal anomalies, uterine anomalies, and infection.
    - The Tabor study in the 1980s is the only randomized trial to show a loss rate of 1%, however, this was done at a time before continuous ultrasound guidance was universal and ultrasound technology still crude at many centers.
  - Transient vaginal spotting or amniotic fluid leakage occurs in approximately 1–2% of all cases.

Reading list

Alfirevic Z, Sundberg K, Brigham S. Amniocentesis and chorionic villus sampling for prenatal diagnosis. *Cochrane Database Syst Rev* 2003(3):CD003252.

American College of Obstetricians and Gynecologists, Gynecologists' Committee on Practice Bulletins-Obstetrics, Committee on Genetics, Society for Maternal-Fetal Medicine. Practice bulletin no. 162: Prenatal diagnostic testing for genetic disorders. *Obstet Gynecol* 2016;127(5):e108-22.

Committee on Genetics. Committee opinion no. 691: Carrier screening for genetic conditions. *Obstet Gynecol* 2017;129(3):e41-e55.

Committee on Genetics. Committee opinion no. 693: Counseling about genetic testing and communication of genetic test results. *Obstet Gynecol* 2017;129(4):e96-e101.

Committee on Practice Bulletins—Obstetrics, Committee on Genetics, Society for Maternal-Fetal Medicine. Practice bulletin no. 163: Screening for fetal aneuploidy. *Obstet Gynecol* 2016;127(5):e123-37.

Committee opinion no. 640: Cell-free DNA screening for fetal aneuploidy. *Obstet Gynecol* 2015;126(3):e31-7.

Committee opinion no. 690: Carrier screening in the age of genomic medicine. *Obstet Gynecol* 2017;129(3):e35-e40.

Eddleman KA, Malone FD, Sullivan L, et al. Pregnancy loss rates after midtrimester amniocentesis. *Obstet Gynecol* 2006;108(5):1067-72.

Gregg AR, Gross SJ, Best RG, et al. ACMG statement on noninvasive prenatal screening for fetal aneuploidy. *Genet Med* 2013;15(5):395-8.

Grody WW, Thompson BH, Gregg AR, et al. ACMG position statement on prenatal/preconception expanded carrier screening. *Genet Med* 2013;15(6):482-3.

Tabor A, Philip J, Madsen M, et al. Randomised controlled trial of genetic amniocentesis in 4606 low-risk women. *Lancet* 1986;1(8493):1287-93.

Tabor A, Vestergaard CH, Lidegaard O. Fetal loss rate after chorionic villus sampling and amniocentesis: an 11-year national registry study. *Ultrasound Obstet Gynecol* 2009;34(1):19-24.

Suggested websites

American College of Obstetricians and Gynecologists. www.acog.org
American College of Medical Genetics and Genomics. www.acmg.net

Guidelines
National society guidelines

Title	Source	Date/full reference
Practice bulletin no. 162: Prenatal diagnostic testing for genetic disorders	American College of Obstetricians and Gynecologists, Gynecologists' Committee on Practice Bulletins-Obstetrics, Committee on Genetics, Society for Maternal-Fetal Medicine	*Obstet Gynecol* 2016;127(5):e108-22.

(Continued)

(*Continued*)

Title	Source	Date/full reference
Practice bulletin no. 163: Screening for fetal aneuploidy	Committee on Practice Bulletins—Obstetrics, Committee on Genetics, Society for Maternal-Fetal Medicine	*Obstet Gynecol* 2016;127(5):e123-37.
Committee opinion no. 640: Cell-free DNA screening for fetal aneuploidy	ACOG, Society for Maternal-Fetal Medicine	*Obstet Gynecol* 2015;126(3):e31-7.
Committee opinion no. 690: Carrier screening in the age of genomic medicine	ACOG Committee on Genetics	*Obstet Gynecol* 2017;129(3):e35-e40.
Committee opinion no. 691: Carrier screening for genetic conditions	ACOG Committee on Genetics	*Obstet Gynecol* 2017;129(3):e41-e55.
Committee opinion no. 693: Counseling about genetic testing and communication of genetic test results	ACOG Committee on Genetics	*Obstet Gynecol* 2017;129(4):e96-e101.

CHAPTER 9

Preterm Birth

Andrei Rebarber

Maternal Fetal Medicine Associates, New York, NY; Division of Maternal-Fetal Medicine – Department of Obstetrics, Gynecology and Reproductive Science, Icahn School of Medicine at Mount Sinai, New York, NY

OVERALL BOTTOM LINE

- Preterm birth occurs when an infant is born between 20 and 37 weeks of pregnancy.
- Complex multifactorial etiology prevents a singular universal treatment regimen to be applied but rather tailored approaches to various clinical scenarios can improve outcomes.
- Prematurity results in increased neonatal death and disability as well as being associated with increased maternal morbidity.

Background

- Premature birth is the leading cause of death of babies in the United States. Accurate identification of women truly in preterm labor allows appropriate application of interventions that can improve neonatal outcome such as antenatal corticosteroid therapy, group B streptococcal infection prophylaxis, magnesium sulfate for neuroprotection, and transfer to a facility with an appropriate level nursery (if necessary).

Disease classification

- Preterm is defined as babies born alive before 37 weeks of pregnancy are completed. There are subcategories of preterm birth, based on gestational age:
  - extremely preterm (<28 weeks)
  - very preterm (28 to <32 weeks)
  - moderate to late preterm (32 to <37 weeks).

Incidence/prevalence

- In 2016, preterm birth affected about 1 of every 10 infants born in the United States.
- Racial and ethnic disparities in preterm birth rates persist. In 2016, the rate of preterm birth among African American women (14%) was about 50% higher than the rate of preterm birth among white women (9%).

Economic impact

- A 2006 report from the Institute of Medicine estimated the annual cost of preterm birth in the United States to be $26.2 billion or more than $51 000 per premature infant. The breakdown was as follows:
  - $16.9 billion (65%) in medical and healthcare costs for the infant
  - $1.9 billion (7%) in labor and delivery cost for the mother
  - $611 million (2%) for early intervention services
  - $1.1 billion (4%) for special education services
  - $5.7 billion (22%) for lost household and labor market productivity

---

Mount Sinai Expert Guides: Obstetrics and Gynecology, First Edition. Edited by Rhoda Sperling.
© 2020 John Wiley & Sons Ltd. Published 2020 by John Wiley & Sons Ltd.
Companion Website: www.wiley.com/go/sperling/mountsinai/obstetricsandgynecology

Etiology

- Infants are born preterm after:
  - spontaneous labor with intact membranes
  - preterm premature rupture of the membranes (PPROM)
  - labor induction or caesarean delivery for maternal or fetal indications

Pathology/pathogenesis

- The pathophysiology of preterm labor involves five primary pathogenic processes that result in a final common pathway ending in spontaneous preterm labor and delivery:
  - Activation of the maternal or fetal hypothalamic-pituitary-adrenal axis associated with either maternal anxiety and depression or fetal stress
  - Infection
  - Decidual hemorrhage
  - Pathological uterine distention
  - Cervical insufficiency

Predictive/risk factors

Risk factors
No partner
Low socioeconomic level
Anxiety, stress
Depression, use of selective serotonin reuptake inhibitors
Life events (divorce, separation, death)
Abdominal surgery during pregnancy
Occupational issues (upright posture, use of industrial machines, physical exertion, mental or environmental stress related to work or working conditions)
Multiple gestation
Polyhydramnios
Uterine anomaly, including diethylstilbestrol-induced changes in uterus and leiomyomas
Preterm premature rupture of membranes
History of second-trimester abortion
History of cervical surgery
Premature cervical dilatation or effacement (short cervical length)
Sexually transmitted infections
Systemic infection, pyelonephritis, appendicitis, pneumonia
Bacteriuria
Periodontal disease
Placenta previa
Placental abruption
Vaginal bleeding, especially in more than one trimester

Risk factors
Previous preterm delivery
Substance abuse
Smoking
Maternal age (<18 or >40)
African American race
Poor nutrition and low body mass index
Inadequate prenatal care
Anemia (hemoglobin <10 g/dL)
Excessive uterine contractility
Low level of educational achievement
Maternal first-degree family history of spontaneous preterm birth, especially if the pregnant woman herself was born preterm
Fetal anomaly
Fetal growth restriction
Environmental factors (e.g. heat, air pollution)
Fetal demise
Positive fetal fibronectin test result in vaginal secretions
Genetic variants

Prevention

- Preconception GYN visit – to time pregnancies appropriately, identify modifiable risk factors noted previously, obtain baseline GYN examination/cultures, folic acid use beginning at least 3 months prior to conception (Frayne et al. 2016; Robbins et al. 2018)
- Smoking – smoking cessation programs, including use of nicotine replacement therapy (NRT) or bupropion supplementation (Bérard et al. 2016; Chamberlain et al. 2017; Cooper et al. 2014)
- Bacteriuria screening all pregnant women – Clean catch urine culture at 12–16 weeks or first prenatal visit (Nicolle et al. 2005)
- Periodontal disease – referral for dental care though impact on preterm birth is controversial (Michalowicz et al. 2013)
- Substance abuse – Comprehensive addiction programs including use of methadone maintenance (Jones et al. 2008; Sweeney et al. 2000)
- Low body mass index – Lifestyle, nutrition counseling (Jeric et al. 2013)
- Interpregnancy interval – Education and contraceptive counseling (Salihu et al. 2012)
- Anxiety/depressive disorders – medication for disease modification to be continued throughout pregnancy (Malm et al. 2015)
- Hx prior cervical surgery (LEEP/conization) – transvaginal cervical length evaluation at 18–22 weeks if short consider progesterone therapy (Romero et al. 2018)
- Uterine anomaly
  - One-transvaginal cervical length evaluation at 18–22 weeks if short consider progesterone therapy
  - Two-hysteroscopic metroplasty IF prior OB history indicates adverse outcomes
  (Daly et al. 1989; Romero et al. 2018)
- Higher order multiple gestation (≥3 fetuses) – multifetal pregnancy reduction (Stone et al. 2002)

- Short cervix in women WITHOUT a history of preterm birth (singleton/twin pregnancies) – transvaginal cervical screen performed between 18–22 weeks with cervical length ≤2.5 cm
  - progesterone and/or pessary
  (Goya et al. 2016; Romero et al. 2017, 2018)
- Women with ≥2 consecutive prior second-trimester losses* **or** ≥3 early (<34 weeks) preterm births – history indicated cerclage placement at 12–14 weeks and hydroxyprogesterone caproate 250 mg IM weekly from 16 to 36 weeks (Iams and Berghella 2010)
- Women with one prior second-trimester loss (16–24 weeks), **OR** one or two preterm births – hydroxyprogesterone caproate 250 mg IM weekly from 16 to 36 weeks and serial measurement of cervical length (q2 weeks) beginning at 14–16 weeks and ending at 24 weeks. IF cervical length ≤25 mm before 24 weeks, place transvaginal cerclage (Iams and Berghella 2010)
- Women with a history of early delivery because of preeclampsia – administration of low-dose aspirin (80–100 mg) starting at 10–12 weeks gestation (van Vliet et al. 2017)
- Women <24 weeks with minimal or no symptoms and physical examination reveals a dilated cervix – examination-indicated cerclage; consider amniocentesis to look for subclinical infection when the cervix is ≥2 cm dilated and on a case-by-case basis when ultrasound findings are consistent with inflammation (e.g. debris in the amniotic fluid ["sludge"] or when membranes are visible and exposed at the external os, as prolapsed membranes are associated with a poor perinatal prognosis) (Ehsanipoor et al. 2015)
- Women with prior history of a successful cerclage – placement of history-indicated cerclage OR serial measurement of cervical length 14–24 weeks, IF cervix ≤2.5 cm place ultrasound-indicated cerclage (Society for Maternal-Fetal Medicine 2012)

Primary prevention
- Although there are many risk factors for preterm delivery only some are modifiable; others are not. Identification of these before conception or early in pregnancy ideally would lead to interventions that could help prevent this complication as noted previously.
- Short cervical length on ultrasound examination between 16–24 weeks of gestation in the current pregnancy is a risk factor for preterm birth (PTB) and is the basis for screening for a short cervix in the midtrimester. Progesterone supplementation may prolong gestation.
- Singleton gestations are less likely to deliver preterm than multiple gestations. Prevention of multifetal gestations using single embryo transfers and controlled stimulation cycles in infertile couple can prevent preterm deliveries

Secondary prevention
- Prior PTB is the strongest risk factor and progesterone supplementation ± cerclage placement in certain circumstances has been shown to prevent recurrent disease

Diagnosis
- Although two-thirds of PTBs occur among women with no risk factors, the two biggest historical risk factors include multiple gestations and a prior history of preterm birth.
- We make the diagnosis of preterm labor based upon clinical criteria of regular painful uterine contractions accompanied by cervical change (dilation and/or effacement).
- Our initial evaluation of women with suspected preterm labor includes assessment of uterine contraction frequency, duration, and intensity; examination of the uterus to assess firmness and tenderness; maternal vital signs, digital and speculum examination of the cervix; ultrasound evaluation of the fetus for gestational age and estimated fetal weight.

Differential diagnosis

Differential diagnosis	Features
Urinary tract infection	Urinary symptoms including dysuria, frequency, urgency. Positive urinalysis for nitrates and/or leukocyte esterase. Focal suprapubic pain and/or costovertebral angle (CVA) tenderness
False labor	Contractions dissipate, no cervical change is documented over time, fetal fibronectin test is negative, cervical length using transvaginal imaging ≥2.5 cm.
Degenerating fibroid	History of fibroid uterus usually greater than 5–7 cm in size, focal rather than diffuse pain, no cervical change noted, often occurs in the second and early third trimesters.
Vaginal infection	Vaginal discharge is noted that is negative for rupture of membranes(using nitrazine paper, AmniSure testing, ferning on slide prep) or clinical exam dose not identify pooling of fluid in the posterior fornix. Vaginal discharge is consistent with infection by color or odor.
Dehydration	Often associated with gastrointestinal symptoms of nausea, vomiting, and/or diarrhea. Can be complication of severe hyperemesis gravidarum.

Typical presentation

- Prodromal signs and symptoms of preterm labor may be present for several hours before diagnostic criteria for true preterm labor (contractions with cervical change) are met. These include menstrual-like cramping; mild, irregular contractions; low back ache; pressure sensation in the vagina or pelvis; vaginal discharge of mucus, which may be clear, pink, or slightly bloody (i.e. mucus plug, bloody show); and finally spotting/light bleeding. Of note, mild irregular contractions are a normal finding at all stages of pregnancy, thereby adding to the challenge of distinguishing true labor from false labor. Additionally, increased vaginal discharge is also more common throughout gestation as is vaginal spotting from cervical ectropion, the latter particularly associated with a postcoital event.

Clinical diagnosis

History

- Review of the patient's past and present obstetrical, gynecologic, surgical, and medical history, including risk factors for preterm birth should be thoroughly evaluated. Recent activities including intercourse, travel, exercise, and/or trauma are important topics to discuss. Assessment of gestational age, based on the best estimate from the first ultrasound examination becomes of paramount importance in dictating management strategies.

Physical examination

- Obtain maternal vital signs (temperature, blood pressure, heart rate, respiratory rate)
- Heart and lung examination
- Evaluation for CVA tenderness
- Examination of the uterus to assess firmness, tenderness, fetal size, and fetal position
- *Speculum examination*
  - Estimate cervical dilation. Cervical dilation ≥3 cm supports the diagnosis of preterm labor
  - Assess the presence and amount of uterine bleeding.
  - Evaluate fetal membrane status (intact or ruptured) by standard methods
  - Obtain a fetal fibronectin (fFN) test ("Blind" sampling without a speculum is acceptable); some obtain fFN selectively, limiting its use to women with cervical length 20 to 30 mm

- *Digital cervical examination*
  - Cervical dilation and effacement are assessed by digital examination after speculum examination. Evaluate the cervix for its consistency and location – softening and movement to a more anterior position are more consistent with true labor features.

  NOTE: placenta previa and rupture of membranes should be excluded prior to examination

Useful clinical decision rules and calculators

Uterine contractions (≥4 every 20 minutes or ≥8 in 60 minutes) **AND**
- Cervical dilation ≥3 cm

  OR
- documented cervical change or cervical effacement ≥80% or cervical dilation >2 cm.
- IF transvaginal cervical length evaluation is available then consider
  - Cervical length <20 mm on transvaginal ultrasound **or**
  - Cervical length 20 to 30 mm on transvaginal ultrasound and positive fetal fibronectin

"The QUiPP app is a clinical decision-making tool to help calculate individualized percent risk scores of delivery within pre-specified time frames which may help determine management in the clinical setting" (Carter et al. 2020). It is designed for asymptomatic women at high risk for preterm birth as well for the management of women with symptoms of preterm labor.

Laboratory diagnosis

- No single test currently available is diagnostic of true preterm labor

List of diagnostic tests

- Uterine contraction monitoring (i.e. tocodynamometer) and fetal heart rate assessment
- Speculum examination with fFN testing in women <34 weeks of gestation with cervical dilation <3 cm and cervical length 20 to 30 mm on transvaginal ultrasound examination, AmniSure testing (i.e. evaluation for amniotic fluid leakage) in the setting of unclear clinical testing (e.g. nitrazine, pooling, ferning)
- Maternal blood testing including blood type and screen, complete blood count, complete chemistry panel only if clinical history indicates
- Rectovaginal group B streptococcal culture if not done within the previous 5 weeks; antibiotic prophylaxis depends on the results.
- Urine culture, because asymptomatic bacteriuria is associated with an increased risk of preterm labor and birth
- Drug testing in patients with risk factors for substance abuse, given the link between cocaine use and placental abruption.
- Testing for sexually transmitted infections (e.g. chlamydia, gonorrhea) depends on the patient's risk factors for these infections

List of imaging techniques

- Transabdominal ultrasound assessment of the fetal weight, placental location, and amniotic fluid volume should be performed in all cases
- Transvaginal ultrasound (TVU) measurement of cervical length – a short cervix ≤2.5 cm prior to 34 weeks of gestation is predictive of preterm birth in all populations, whereas a long cervix has a high negative predictive value for preterm birth. A meta-analysis of individual patient data reported that clinician knowledge of cervical length in women with threatened preterm labor reduced the rate of preterm birth compared with absence of this information (22 versus 35%; relative risk [RR] 0.64. 95% confidence

interval [CI] 0.44–0.94; three trials; n = 287 participants), but other outcomes were not significantly different (Berghella et al. 2016)

Note: The 34th week of gestation is the threshold at which perinatal morbidity and mortality are too low to justify the potential maternal and fetal complications and costs associated with inhibition of preterm labor, which results in only short-term delay in delivery. The American College of Obstetricians and Gynecologists states administration of betamethasone is recommended for women with a singleton pregnancy at 34 + 0 to 36 + 6 weeks of gestation at imminent risk of preterm birth within 7 days, with the following caveats: (a) antenatal corticosteroid administration should not be administered to women with chorioamnionitis; (b) tocolysis should not be used to delay delivery in women with symptoms of preterm labor to allow administration of antenatal corticosteroids, and medically/obstetrically indicated preterm delivery should not be postponed for steroid administration; (c) antenatal corticosteroids should not be administered if the patient has already received a course antenatal corticosteroids; and (d) newborns should be monitored for hypoglycemia. Recent data also suggest that betamethasone can be beneficial in pregnant women at high risk of late preterm birth, between 34 0/7 weeks and 36 6/7 weeks of gestation who have not received a prior course of antenatal corticosteroids (Committee on Obstetric Practice 2017; Lockwood 2018). See Algorithm 9.1.

Potential pitfalls/common errors made regarding diagnosis of disease

- Only 13% of women presenting at <34 weeks of gestation who meet explicit contraction criteria for preterm labor deliver within 1 week.
- In symptomatic women the positive predictive value of a positive qualitative fetal fibronectin test (set at 50 ng/mL as positive) to delivery in 14 days is only 20% in one prospective trial; and to delivery <34 weeks it is only 32% positive predictive value.
- Symptomatic women with cervical length <20 mm are at high risk (>25%) of delivery within 7 days; the addition of fFN testing does not significantly improve the predictive value of cervical length measurement alone.
- Symptomatic women with cervical length ≥30 mm are at low risk (<5%) of delivery within 7 days, regardless of fFN result; the addition of fFN testing does not significantly improve the predictive value of cervical length measurement alone.
- Recent intercourse and vaginal bleeding can lead to false-positive fetal fibronectin results.
- In general observation period of at least 4 to 6 hours should be an adequate time period in symptomatic women to determine true preterm labor. Those without progressive cervical dilation and effacement in this time period and no other obvious clinical obstetrical complication with fetal well-being reassured often can be safely discharged.

Treatment
Treatment rationale
- Although an inexact process, attempts at accurate identification of women in true preterm labor allows appropriate interventions that can improve neonatal outcome such as antenatal corticosteroid therapy, group B streptococcal infection prophylaxis, magnesium sulfate for neuroprotection, and transfer to a facility with an appropriate level nursery (if necessary). On the contrary, accurate triage of women in false preterm labor can avoid unnecessary interventions and associated costs for the ≥50% of patients with suspected preterm labor who will go on to deliver at term without treatment.

When to hospitalize
- We hospitalize women diagnosed with preterm labor between 20 and <37 weeks of gestation if we believe they are at high risk for imminent delivery or when we are in the process of considering other diagnosis that require hospitalization (e.g. pyelonephritis, degenerating fibroids requiring pain management).

Algorithm 9.1 Suggested approach to management of suspected preterm labor

Patient with preterm uterine contractions, intact membranes, reassuring maternal and fetal status, no placenta previa or abruption

Gestational age <34 weeks of gestation

Gestational age ≥34 weeks of gestation

Cervix dilated ≥3 cm

Cervix dilated <3 cm

No tocolysis or antenatal corticosteroids. Admit for delivery if labor progresses; discharge home if contractions cease.

Obtain specimen for fetal fibronectin testing. Hold until results of ultrasound measurement of cervical length are available.

Transvaginal ultrasound measurement of cervical length

Cervical length <20 mm

Cervical length 20 to 30 mm

Cervical length <30 mm

Perform fetal fibronectin test

Preterm labor unlikely. Observe for 4 to 6 hours. Women without progressive cervical dilation and effacement are discharged to home. Follow up in 1 to 2 weeks. Patient should call if she experiences signs or symptoms of preterm labor.

Fetal fibronectin (+)

Fetal fibronectin (−)

Preterm labor likely

Preterm labor unlikely. Observe for 6 to 12 hours. Women without progressive cervical dilation and effacement are discharged to home. Follow up in 1 to 2 weeks. Patient should call if she experiences signs or symptoms of preterm labor.

• Tocolysis
• Antibiotics for GBS prophylaxis
• Magnesium sulfate for neuroprotection if 24 to 32 weeks
• Antenatal corticosteroids if 23 to 34 weeks and delivery is not imminent

GBS: group B streptococcus.

Table of treatment

Treatment	Comments
Antenatal corticosteroids One repeat "rescue" course may be administered as long as they have not had a course of antenatal corticosteroids at least 14 days previously and at ≤34 weeks of gestation.	**Betamethasone suspension** 12 mg intramuscularly every 24 hours for two doses **or** four doses of 6 mg **Dexamethasone** intramuscularly 12 hours apart 1-Transient maternal hyperglycemia; the steroid effect begins approximately 12 hours after the first dose and may last for 5 days. 2-Transient fetal heart rate (FHR) and behavioral changes that typically return to baseline by 4 to 7 days after treatment: most consistent FHR finding is a decrease in variability on days 2 and 3 after administration, reduced fetal breathing and body movements have also been reported.
Tocolytic drugs for up to 48 hours to delay delivery so that betamethasone given to the mother can achieve its maximum fetal effect.	**Indomethicin** 50 to 100 mg loading dose (orally or per rectum), followed by 25 mg orally every 4 to 6 hours. Maternal effects: nausea, esophageal reflux, gastritis, and emesis Fetal effects: oligohydramnios, fetal ductus arteriosus closure **Nifedipine** (calcium channel blocker) initial loading dose of 20 to 30 mg orally, followed by an additional 10 to 20 mg orally every 3 to 8 hours for up to 48 hours, with a maximum dose of 180 mg/day. Maternal effects: nausea, flushing, headache, dizziness, and palpitations **Terbutaline** (Beta-2 agonist) 0.25 mg can be administered subcutaneously every 20 to 30 minutes for up to four doses or until tocolysis is achieved. Once labor is inhibited, 0.25 mg can be administered subcutaneously every 3 to 4 hours until the uterus is quiescent for 24 hours. Maternal effects: tachycardia, palpitations, and lower blood pressure. Hypokalemia, hyperglycemia, and lipolysis. Fetal effects: hyperinsulinemia, hypoglycemia
Antibiotics for Group B streptococcus chemoprophylaxis. Intrapartum antibiotic prophylaxis is most effective if administered at least 4 hours before delivery.	**Penicillin G** 5 million units intravenously initial dose, then 2.5 to 3 million units intravenously every 4 hours until delivery **Ampicillin** 2 g intravenously initial dose, then 1 g intravenously every 4 hours until delivery **Patients with penicillin allergy** Low risk: Cefazolin 2 g intravenously initial dose, then 1 g every 8 hours until delivery High risk: Clindamycin 900 mg intravenously every 8 hours until delivery OR Vancomycin 2 g intravenously initially and then 1 g every 12 hours thereafter until delivery
Magnesium sulfate for pregnancies at 24–32 weeks of gestation who will likely deliver within 24 hours. In utero exposure to magnesium sulfate provides neuroprotection against cerebral palsy and other types of severe motor dysfunction in offspring born preterm. We limit the magnesium sulfate infusion to a maximum of 24 hours, even if delivery has not occurred. Retreatment of the full dose of magnesium sulfate if delivery was again considered imminent may be performed and the pregnancy is still <32 weeks gestation, and the initial magnesium infusion had been discontinued for more than 6 hours.	4 g loading of **magnesium sulfate** over 20 minutes and a maintenance dose of 1 g/hour. Fetal effects: Decrease in baseline fetal heart rate (generally remains within the normal range) and a decrease in fetal heart rate variability, which may be absent or minimal Maternal effects: diaphoresis, flushing, warmth, drop in blood pressure, nausea, vomiting, headache, muscle weakness, visual disturbances, and palpitations. Dyspnea or chest pain may be symptoms of pulmonary edema, which is a rare side effect.

Prevention/management of complications

The primary fetal concerns with use of indomethacin and other COX inhibitors (e.g. sulindac, nimesulide) are constriction of the ductus arteriosus and oligohydramnios. Several cases of premature ductal constriction have been reported in pregnancies in which the duration of indomethacin exposure exceeded 48 hours and is most common after 31 to 32 weeks. Therefore, indomethacin is **not** recommended after 32 weeks of gestation. Between 24–32 weeks, fetal echocardiographic evaluation is useful for monitoring ductal effects if the duration of therapy exceeds 48 hours. Sonographic signs of ductal narrowing include tricuspid regurgitation, right ventricular dysfunction, and pulsatility index less than 1.9.

Calcium-channel blockers are contraindicated in women with known hypersensitivity to the drugs, hypotension, or preload-dependent cardiac lesions and should be used with caution in women with left ventricular dysfunction or congestive heart failure. The concomitant use of a calcium-channel blocker and magnesium sulfate could act synergistically to suppress muscular contractility, which could result in respiratory depression.

Pulmonary edema is an uncommon side effect of beta-agonist therapy, occurring in 0.3% of patients. Pulmonary edema probably results from several additive factors including fluid overload from excessive intravenous crystalloid infusion, decreased time for diastolic filling time due to increased heart rate and the increased plasma volume of pregnancy. Alternatively, pulmonary edema may be unrelated to the beta-agonist therapy and instead may be due to increased vascular permeability related to infection, inflammation, or preeclampsia. Therefore, careful attention to fluid management and signs of infection and fluid overload are warranted if this drug is used. Myocardial ischemia is a rare complication. In the United States, the Food and Drug Administration (FDA) has warned that injectable terbutaline should not be used in pregnant women for prolonged (beyond 48 to 72 hours) treatment of preterm labor or prevention of recurrent preterm labor because of the potential for serious maternal heart problems and death. The FDA also opined that oral terbutaline should not be used for prevention or any treatment of preterm labor because it has not been shown to be effective and has similar safety concerns.

(US FDA 2011)

Prognosis

- In women with an acute episode of preterm labor, bedrest, hydration, sedatives, antibiotics, and progesterone supplementation are ineffective for preventing preterm birth.
- Tocolytic drugs for inhibition of acute preterm labor has limited benefit of prolonging gestation. A 2009 meta-analysis of randomized trials found that these drugs were more effective than placebo/control for delaying delivery for 48 hours (75 to 93% versus 53% for placebo/control) and for 7 days (61 to 78% versus 39% for placebo/control) but not for delaying delivery to 37 weeks (Haas et al. 2009).
- The goal of treatment of preterm labor is to
  - delay delivery so that antenatal corticosteroids can be completed
  - allow safe transport of the mother to a facility that can provide an appropriate level of neonatal care if the patient delivers preterm
  - prolong pregnancy when self-limited causes of pathologic labor, such as abdominal surgery, are unlikely to cause recurrent events

Natural history of untreated disease

- The preterm labor syndrome is associated with multiple mechanisms of disease resulting in an often unstoppable course of early delivery with significant neonatal mortality and morbidity.

Prognosis for treated patients

- Infants delivered prematurely who have received optimal treatment appear to have improved short-term and long-term morbidity and decreased neonatal mortality. Implementation of evidence-based practice improves outcome. This was illustrated in a prospective multinational European study that reported implementation of four evidence-based practices reduced in-hospital mortality (RR 0.72, 95% confidence interval [CI] 0.60–0.87), and the risk of the composite outcome of in-hospital mortality or severe morbidity (defined as intraventricular hemorrhage [IVH] grade III or IV, cystic periventricular leukomalacia [PVL], retinopathy of prematurity [ROP] stages III to V, and severe necrotizing enterocolitis [NEC]), or both (RR 0.82, 95% CI 0.73–0.92). The four evidence-based practices included delivery in a maternity unit with appropriate level of neonatal care, administration of antenatal corticosteroids, prevention of hypothermia (temperature on admission to neonatal unit ≥36 °C), surfactant used within 2 hours of birth, or early nasal continuous positive airway pressure (nCPAP). (Zeitlin et al. 2016)

Follow-up tests and monitoring

- Evaluation of the uterine cavity may be performed in the postpartum period between pregnancies to determine the normality of the uterine cavity in the setting of an initial spontaneous preterm birth.
- Progesterone supplementation in women with a prior history of spontaneous preterm birth has been shown to decrease recurrence in most publications. We suggest hydroxyprogesterone caproate 250 mg weekly (also known as 17-alpha-hydroxyprogesterone caproate or 17OHPC) administered intramuscularly for women with a history of spontaneous preterm birth. However, a recent publication has called into questions the efficacy of this approach and individualized management may be appropriate based on risks of recurrence and other cofactors (Blackwell et al. 2019). Some clinicians have switched to use of natural progesterone vaginally in patient with a history of preterm birth based upon a comparative analysis of 17OHP vs vaginal progesterone suggesting improved effects (Saccone et al. 2017). Proper patient counseling and shared decision-making models must be applied during follow up discussions.

Reading list

American College of Obstetricians and Gynecologists. Prevention of group B streptococcal early-onset disease in newborns. ACOG committee opinion no. 782. *Obstet Gynecol* 2019;134:e19-40.

Bérard A, Zhao JP, Sheehy O. Success of smoking cessation interventions during pregnancy. *Am J Obstet Gynecol* 2016;215(5):611.e1.

Berghella V, Saccone G. Fetal fibronectin testing for prevention of preterm birth in singleton pregnancies with threatened preterm labor: a systematic review and metaanalysis of randomized controlled trials. *Am J Obstet Gynecol* 2016 Oct;215(4):431-8.

Berghella V, Palacio M, Ness A, et al. Cervical length screening for prevention of preterm birth in singleton pregnancy with threatened preterm labor: systematic review and meta-analysis of randomized controlled trials using individual patient-level data. *Ultrasound Obstet Gynecol* 2017;49:322. Epub 2017 Feb 8.

Blackwell SC, Gyamfi-Bannerman C, Biggio JR Jr, et al. 17-OHPC to prevent recurrent preterm birth in singleton gestations (PROLONG study): a multicenter, international, randomized double-blind trial. *Am J Perinatol* 2020; 37(2):127. Epub 2019 Oct 25.

Carter J, Seed PT, Watson HA, et al. Development and validation of prediction models for QUiPP App v.2: tool for predicting preterm birth in women with symptoms of threatened preterm labor. *Ultrasound Obstet Gynecol* 2020; 55:357-67.

Chamberlain C, O'Mara-Eves A, Porter J, et al. Psychosocial interventions for supporting women to stop smoking in pregnancy. *Cochrane Database Syst Rev* 2017;2:CD001055. Epub 2017 Feb 14.

Chawanpaiboon S, Vogel JP, Moller AB, et al. Global, regional and national estimates of levels of preterm birth in 2014: a systematic review and modelling analysis. *Lancet Global Health* 2019;7:e37-46.

Committee on Obstetric Practice. Committee opinion no. 713: Antenatal corticosteroid therapy for fetal maturation. *Obstet Gynecol* 2017;130(2):e102.

Cooper S, Taggar J, Lewis S. Effect of nicotine patches in pregnancy on infant and maternal outcomes at 2 years: Follow-up from the randomised, double-blind, placebo-controlled SNAP trial. Smoking, Nicotine and Pregnancy (SNAP) Trial Team. *Lancet Respir Med* 2014;2(9):728. Epub 2014 Aug 10.

Daly DC, Maier D, Soto-Albors C. Hysteroscopic metroplasty: six years' experience. *Obstet Gynecol* 1989;73(2):201.

Ehsanipoor RM, Seligman NS, Saccone G, et al. Physical examination-indicated cerclage: A systematic review and meta-analysis. *Obstet Gynecol* 2015;126(1):125.

Frayne DJ, Verbiest S, Chelmow D, et al. Health care system measures to advance preconception wellness: Consensus recommendations of the Clinical Workgroup of the National Preconception Health and Health Care Initiative. *Obstet Gynecol* 2016 May;127(5):863-72.

Goya M, de la Calle M, Pratcorona L, et al., PECEP-Twins Trial Group. Cervical pessary to prevent preterm birth in women with twin gestation and sonographic short cervix: a multicenter randomized controlled trial (PECEP-Twins). *Am J Obstet Gynecol* 2016;214(2):145. Epub 2015 Nov 25.

Gyamfi-Bannerman C, Thom EA, Blackwell SC, et al. Antenatal betamethasone for women at risk for late preterm delivery. *N Engl J Med* 2016;374:1311-20.

Haas DM, Imperiale TF, Kirkpatrick PR, et al. Tocolytic therapy: a meta-analysis and decision analysis. *Obstet Gynecol* 2009;113(3):585.

Iams JD, Berghella V. Care for women with prior preterm birth. *Am J Obstet Gynecol* 2010;203:89.

Jeric M, Roje D, Medic N, et al. Maternal pre-pregnancy underweight and fetal growth in relation to institute of medicine recommendations for gestational weight gain. *Early Hum Dev* 2013;89(5):277. Epub 2012 Nov 8.

Jones HE, O'Grady KE, Malfi D, et al. Methadone maintenance vs. methadone taper during pregnancy: maternal and neonatal outcomes. *Am J Addict* 2008;17(5):372.

Lockwood CJ. Preterm labor: Clinical findings, diagnostic evaluation, and initial treatment. Uptodate Chapter – Algorithm, last updated 27 June 2018.

Malm H, Sourander A, Gissler M, et al. Pregnancy complications following prenatal exposure to SSRIs or maternal psychiatric disorders: Results from population-based national register data. *Am J Psychiatry* 2015;172(12):1224.

Michalowicz BS, Gustafsson A, Thumbigere-Math V, et al. The effects of periodontal treatment on pregnancy outcomes. *J Clin Periodontol* 2013 Apr;40 Suppl 14:S195-208.

Nicolle LE, Bradley S, Colgan R, et al. Infectious Diseases Society of America guidelines for the diagnosis and treatment of asymptomatic bacteriuria in adults. Infectious Diseases Society of America, American Society of Nephrology, American Geriatric Society. *Clin Infect Dis* 2005;40(5):643.

Robbins C, Boulet SL, Morgan I, et al. Disparities in preconception health indicators. Behavioral Risk Factor Surveillance System, 2013–2015, and Pregnancy Risk Assessment Monitoring System, 2013–2014. *MMWR Surveill Summ* 2018;67(1):1. Epub 2018 Jan 19.

Romero R, Conde-Agudelo A, El-Refaie W, et al. Vaginal progesterone decreases preterm birth and neonatal morbidity and mortality in women with a twin gestation and a short cervix: an updated meta-analysis of individual patient data. *Ultrasound Obstet Gynecol* 2017;49(3):303.

Romero R, Conde-Agudelo A, Da Fonseca E, et al. Vaginal progesterone for preventing preterm birth and adverse perinatal outcomes in singleton gestations with a short cervix: a meta-analysis of individual patient data. *Am J Obstet Gynecol* 2018;218(2):161. Epub 2017 Nov 17.

Saccone G, Khalifeh A, Elimian A, et al. Vaginal progesterone vs intramuscular 17α-hydroxyprogesterone caproate for prevention of recurrent spontaneous preterm birth in singleton gestations: systematic review and meta-analysis of randomized controlled trials. *Ultrasound Obstet Gynecol* 2017 Mar;49(3):315-21.

Salihu HM, August EM, Mbah AK, et al. The impact of birth spacing on subsequent feto-infant outcomes among community enrollees of a federal healthy start project. *J Community Health* 2012 Feb;37(1):137-42.

Society for Maternal-Fetal Medicine Publications Committee, with assistance of Vincenzo Berghella. Progesterone and preterm birth prevention: translating clinical trials data into clinical practice. *Am J Obstet Gynecol* 2012;206(5):376.

Stone J, Eddleman K, Lynch L, et al. A single center experience with 1000 consecutive cases of multifetal pregnancy reduction. *Am J Obstet Gynecol* 2002;187(5):1163.

Sweeney PJ, Schwartz RM, Mattis NG, et al. The effect of integrating substance abuse treatment with prenatal care on birth outcome. *J Perinatol* 2000 Jun;20(4):219-24.

US Food and Drug Administration. FDA Drug Safety Communication: *New warnings against use of terbutaline to treat preterm labor.* 2011 (updated 2017). Available from: http://www.fda.gov/Drugs/DrugSafety/ucm243539.htm#ds.

van Vliet EO, Askie LA, Mol BW, et al. Antiplatelet agents and the prevention of spontaneous preterm birth: A systematic review and meta-analysis. *Obstet Gynecol* 2017 Feb;129(2):327-336.

Zeitlin J, Manktelow BN, Piedvache A, et al. EPICE Research Group. Use of evidence based practices to improve survival without severe morbidity for very preterm infants: results from the EPICE population based cohort. *BMJ* 2016;354:i2976. Epub 2016 Jul 5.

Zhang Ge, Feenstra B, Bacelis J, et al. Genetic associations with gestational duration and spontaneous preterm birth. *N Engl J Med* 2017;377:1156-67.

Suggested websites

American College of Obstetricians and Gynecologists. www.acog.org (Practice Bulletins and Committee Opinions available at this website)

March of Dimes Prematurity Collaborative. http://www.marchofdimes.org/professionals/prematurity-collaborative.aspx

Antenatal Corticosteroids (ANCS Toolkit) – Ohio Perinatal Quality Collaborative. http://www.opqc.net/projects/OB-ANCS

Maternal and Infant Health. http://www.cdc.gov/reproductivehealth/maternalinfanthealth

Society for Maternal-Fetal Medicine toolkit with practice algorithms and other materials to better implement clinical screening and interventions to prevent PTB. http://www.smfm.org/publications/231-smfm-preterm-birth-toolkit

World Health Organization recommendations on interventions to improve preterm birth outcomes. http://www.who.int/reproductivehealth/publications/maternal_perinatal_health/preterm-birth-highlights/en/

The Quipp app. https://quipp.org/

Guidelines
National society guidelines

Title	Source	Date/full reference
Prediction and prevention of preterm birth (Practice Bulletin)	ACOG (Committee on Practice Bulletins – Obstetrics) Reaffirmed 2018	American College of Obstetricians and Gynecologists. Prediction and prevention of preterm birth. Practice bulletin no. 130. *Obstet Gynecol* 2012;120:964–73.
Magnesium sulfate before anticipated preterm birth for neuroprotection (Committee Opinion)	ACOG (Committee on Obstetric Practice) Reaffirmed 2018	American College of Obstetricians and Gynecologists. Magnesium sulfate before anticipated preterm birth for neuroprotection. Committee opinion no. 455. *Obstet Gynecol* 2010;115:669–71.
Cerclage for the management of cervical insufficiency (Practice Bulletin)	ACOG (Committee on Practice Bulletins – Obstetrics) Reaffirmed 2019	American College of Obstetricians and Gynecologists. Cerclage for the management of cervical insufficiency. Practice bulletin no. 142. *Obstet Gynecol* 2014;123:372–9.
Management of preterm labor (Practice Bulletin)	ACOG (Committee on Practice Bulletins – Obstetrics) Reaffirmed 2018	American College of Obstetricians and Gynecologists. Management of preterm labor. Practice bulletin no. 171. *Obstet Gynecol* 2016;128:e155–64.
Antenatal corticosteroid therapy for fetal maturation	ACOG (Committee on Obstetric Practice) Reaffirmed 2018	American College of Obstetricians and Gynecologists. Antenatal corticosteroid therapy for fetal maturation. Committee opinion no. 713. *Obstet Gynecol* 2017;130:e102–9.

CHAPTER 10

Abnormal Labor

Dyese Taylor[1], Lois Brustman[2], and Frederick Friedman Jr.[1]

[1] Department of Obstetrics, Gynecology and Reproductive Science, Icahn School of Medicine at Mount Sinai, New York, NY
[2] Division of Maternal-Fetal Medicine, Department of Obstetrics, Gynecology and Reproductive Science, Icahn School of Medicine at Mount Sinai, New York, NY

OVERALL BOTTOM LINE

- Abnormal labor is labor that does not fall within the 95th percentile of labor progress. Although the precise definition of "normal labor" is disputed, there are guidelines for anticipated progress of labor; any deviation from these may be considered "abnormal."
- Abnormal labor is divided into protracted disorders or arrest disorders. A protracted labor is one that is slower than expected but progresses. Arrest of labor is defined as complete cessation of progress.
- The exact cause of an abnormal labor is not always apparent but may be categorized as disorders of either contractile forces or relative disproportion of the maternal pelvic size and the baby's size.
- Labor is divided into three stages. The first stage starts from the onset of labor until the cervix is completely dilated. The first stage is separated into latent and active phases. The second stage begins after the first stage and continues until the infant is delivered. The third stage of labor begins after the baby delivers and ends when the placenta delivers.
- There are no highly effective treatments for abnormal labor. When appropriate, augmentation of labor and operative vaginal deliveries can lower the rate of cesarean delivery.

Background

Definition of disease

- Labor may be defined as the act of regular painful uterine contractions that leads to serial dilatation and effacement of the cervix with eventual descent and expulsion of the baby.
- Abnormal or difficult labors ("dystocias") are those that deviate from the progress seen in the majority of parturients and may be divided into protraction ("slow progress") or arrest ("lack of progress") disorders.

Disease classification

- Abnormal labor is divided into protracted labor or arrest of labor.
- Historically, the definition of abnormal labor was based on the Friedman curve, which was published in 1955. However, an updated curve was created based on two retrospective analyses of the data from the National Collaborative Perinatal Project Cohort and the Safe Labor Consortium published by Zhang et al., in 2010 and 2013, respectively. This labor curve is felt to be more representative of current labor practices inclusive of the increased use of oxytocin, regional anesthetics, and a population of women with increased body mass index.

Incidence/prevalence

- Abnormal labor occurs in 21% of live births in the United States. Given that there are a little under 4 million births in the United States, this occurs in about 840 000 live births.
- The incidence of abnormal labor is highest in term nulliparas.

Mount Sinai Expert Guides: Obstetrics and Gynecology, First Edition. Edited by Rhoda Sperling.
© 2020 John Wiley & Sons Ltd. Published 2020 by John Wiley & Sons Ltd.
Companion Website: www.wiley.com/go/sperling/mountsinai/obstetricsandgynecology

- Abnormal or arrest of progress of labor is the most common indication for primary cesarean delivery in term gestations.

Economic impact

- The exact economic impact of abnormal labors is difficult to quantify – one would have to consider costs of augmentation (and the cost of complications thereof), the costs of cesarean deliveries if augmentation efforts are unsuccessful, lawsuits that might arise from maternal and/or fetal complications of prolonged labors (whether perceived or actually due to these efforts), and compare those to the costs of elective cesarean deliveries and direct or indirect costs of complications from those.
- Abnormal labors result in greater lengths of hospital stays, more involvement (time, effort, and materials) from the healthcare team, and more frequent neonatal intensive care unit admissions.

Etiology

- Although the exact cause of abnormal labors may not always be apparent the underlying etiology may be categorized as disorders of either contractile forces or relative disproportion of the maternal pelvic size and the fetus. These etiologies of abnormal labor are commonly referred to as the three Ps: power, passenger, and passage.
- Abnormal presentations – persistent occiput posterior, brow, face, or marked asynclitism often result in abnormal labors and may necessitate cesarean delivery.
- A small pelvis, whether the inlet, midpelvis, or outlet, will often result in an abnormal labor. Although rare, a contracted pelvis (any diameter less than 8 cm) will necessitate cesarean delivery.
- Certain complications increase the likelihood of dystocias likely due to interference with uterine contractile forces: infection (e.g. chorioamnionitis or endomyometritis) and uterine overdistension (e.g. multiple gestations or polyhydramnios) have been cited for this.

Pathology/pathogenesis

- Abnormal labor is caused by dysfunction in any of the previously described causes.

Predictive/risk factors

- There is no strong evidence but the following are believed to be risk factors for labor dystocia.

Risk factor	Odds ratio
Obesity	N/A
Increasing maternal age	N/A
Increased interpregnancy interval	N/A
Abnormal fetal presentation	N/A

Prevention

> **BOTTOM LINE/CLINICAL PEARLS**
> - No interventions have strong evidence to prevent abnormal labor. Some interventions that are still being studied are active management of labor, hydration and glucose intake during labor, laboring down, and amniotomy.

Screening

- Screening for cephalopelvic disproportion with clinical pelvimetry or X-ray evaluations of the maternal pelvis have poor predictive value in determining if labor will end in a spontaneous vaginal delivery (Maharaj 2010).

Primary prevention

- There are no effective primary interventions for abnormal labor. However, active management of labor may prevent the occurrence of labor abnormalities.

Diagnosis

> **BOTTOM LINE/CLINICAL PEARLS**
> - Prolonged latent phase is diagnosed when ≥ 20 hours in nulliparous women or ≥ 14 hours in multiparous have passed and the patient has not dilated beyond 4 cm.
> - In primigravida patients, labor is protracted if it takes more than 6 hours to progress from 4–5 cm, 3 hours to progress from 5–6 cm, 2 hours to progress from 6–7 cm, and 1 cm every 2 hours after until the patient is fully dilated.
> - In multiparous patients, labor is protracted if it takes more than 7 hours to progress from 4–5 cm, 3 hours to progress from 5–6 cm, 2 hours to progress from 6–7 cm, and 1 cm per hour after until the patient is fully dilated.
> - Arrest of dilation is diagnosed if the patient is ≥ 6 cm with ruptured membranes and has any of the following: adequate contractions with no cervical change for ≥ 4 hours or inadequate contractions with no cervical change for ≥ 6 hours.
> - In nulliparous patients, second stage should not be longer than 3 hours. In multiparous patients, 2 hours. However, in the face of neuraxial anesthesia an additional hour is acceptable if descent of the fetal head is progressive.

Differential diagnosis

Differential diagnosis	Features
False labor or prodromal contractions	It is hard to tell the difference between false labor and the latent phase of labor. False labor usually decreases in frequency and intensity over time with no cervical dilation.

Typical presentation

- There is no typical presentation of abnormal labor. It is suspected once the diagnostic criteria are reached (see Algorithm 10.1).

Clinical diagnosis

History

- A patient with a history of known fetal anomalies that can obstruct labor is someone that can present with abnormal labor.

Physical examination

- Cervical exam and contraction frequency and strength are used to diagnose abnormal labor. Contractions can be palpated and their strength and frequency assessed. In active labor, contractions should occur approximately every 2–3 minutes lasting 60 seconds.
- Clinical pelvimetry will be helpful in assessing the adequacy or the pelvis.
- Estimated fetal weight can be determined by Leopold maneuver (Abnormal Labor, in Cunningham et al. 2013).

Algorithm 10.1 Algorithm for diagnosis of arrest of labor

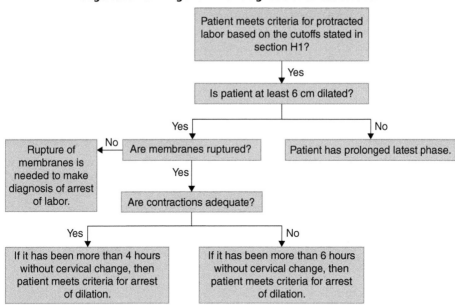

Laboratory diagnosis
List of diagnostic tests
- External tocometer can be used to assess frequency and duration of contractions.
- Internal pressure catheter (IUPC) can be used to assess strength, frequency, and duration of contractions. Strength of contractions is reported by Montevideo units with between ≥ 200 MVU and ≤ 300 MVU in a 10-minute window as a measurement of adequacy.
- Sonography can be used to assess fetal weight and position if there is uncertainty during pushing.

List of imaging techniques
- Historically, it was thought that X-ray assessment of the pelvis could predict if abnormal labor would occur; however, this has been proven to be a poor predictor.
- Ultrasound evaluation of the uterus and fetus can detect structural or positional abnormalities when abnormal labor is suspected.
- Magnetic resonance imaging is rarely used for assessing pelvic adequacy but is an alternative to traditional X-ray pelvimetry.

Potential pitfalls/common errors made regarding diagnosis of disease
- Abnormal labor is not exact. Women who go on to have spontaneous vaginal deliveries can have labor patterns outside the 95th percentile. It should be used as a guide to facilitate further management along with clinical judgment.

Treatment
Treatment rationale
- In cases of abnormal labor where uterine contractions are not adequate in frequency and strength, oxytocin, amniotomy, or a combination of both may be effective in shortening the length of labor. Importantly, neither of these interventions separately or together decreases the rate of cesarean or operative delivery.

Table of treatment

Treatment	Comments
Conservative	Expectant management or amniotomy to stimulate contractions.
Medical (nested list of all drugs or drug combinations) together with dose	Pitocin to stimulate uterine contractions. Pitocin should be titrated to prevent uterine tachysystole, which is defined as more than five contractions in 10 minutes averaged over a 30 minute window.
Surgical (list techniques)	Cesarean delivery if patient meets criteria for arrest of labor.
Radiological	Not applicable.
Psychological (includes cognitive, behavioral, etc., therapies)	Not applicable.
Complementary	Not applicable.
Other	Not applicable.

Prevention/management of complications
- Cesarean delivery
- Chorioamnionitis

CLINICAL PEARLS
- If the etiology of abnormal labor is believed to be a hypocontractile uterus, start Pitocin or perform amniotomy.
- An ultrasound should be performed to assess fetal position.
- There is no highly effective intervention in treating abnormal labor to ensure a vaginal delivery.
- See Algorithm 10.2.

Algorithm 10.2 Algorithm for management of abnormal labor

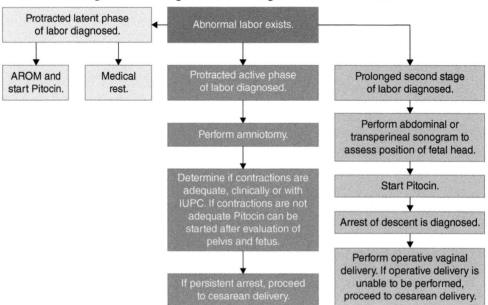

Prognosis

> **BOTTOM LINE/CLINICAL PEARLS**
> * If the cause of abnormal labor was due to an etiology that does not change between pregnancies (i.e. maternal pelvis) then the chance of having abnormal labor in subsequent pregnancies is high.
> * Most patients who have protracted labor will end up with a vaginal delivery if given more time.

Reading list

Cahill AG, Tuuli MG. Labor in 2013: the new frontier. *Am J Obstet Gynecol* 2013;209:531-4.

Cunningham F, Leveno KJ, Bloom SL, et al. Chapter 20. Abnormal Labor. In: Cunningham F, Leveno KJ, Bloom SL, et al., eds. *Williams obstetrics*. 23rd ed. New York, NY: McGraw-Hill; 2010.

Ehsanipoor, R, Satin, A. Diaphragmatic pacing. In: Post, TW, ed. *UpToDate*. Waltham, MA: UpToDate; 2016.

Friedman EA. Primigravid labor: a graphicostatistical analysis. *Obstet Gynecol* 1955;6:567-89.

Laughon SK, Branch DW, Beaver J, et al. Changes in labor patterns over 50 years. *Am J Obstet Gynecol* 2012;206:419. e1-9.

Maharaj D. Assessing cephalopelvic disproportion: back to the basics. *Obstet Gynecol Surv* 2010;65:387.

Safe prevention of the primary cesarean delivery. Obstetric care consensus no. 1. American College of Obstetricians and Gynecologists. *Obstet Gynecol* 2014;123:693-711.

Spong CY, Berghella V, Wenstrom KD, et al. Preventing the first cesarean delivery: Summary of a Joint *Eunice Kennedy Shriver* National Institute of Child Health and Human Development, Society for Maternal-Fetal Medicine, and American College of Obstetricians and Gynecologists Workshop. *Obstet Gynecol* 2012;120(5):1181-93.

Zhang J, Troendle JF, Yancey MK. Reassessing the labor curve in nulliparous women. *Am J Obstet Gynecol* 2002;187: 824–8.

Zhang J, Landy HJ, Branch DW, et al. Contemporary patterns of spontaneous labor with normal neonatal outcomes. *Obstet Gynecol* 2010;116(6):1281-87. doi:10.1097/AOG.0b013e3181fdef6e.

Guidelines
National society guidelines

Title	Source	Date/URL
The American College of Obstetricians and Gynecologists (ACOG) Consensus for the Safe Prevention of the Primary Cesarean Delivery	ACOG Comment: gives an overview of the diagnosis and management of abnormal labor.	2014 – reaffirmed 2019 http://www.acog.org/Resources-And-Publications/Obstetric-Care-Consensus-Series/Safe-Prevention-of-the-Primary-Cesarean-Delivery

Evidence

Type of evidence	Title and comment	Date/full reference
Systematic review	Preventing the first cesarean delivery Comment: This summary reviews the most current literature on the indications for primary cesarean deliveries and recommends strategies to reduce the rate of first cesarean delivery. It also reviews the diagnosis and management of abnormal labor and options for treatment before cesarean delivery is performed.	Spong CY, Berghella V, Wenstrom KD, et al. Preventing the first cesarean delivery: Summary of a Joint Eunice Kennedy Shriver National Institute of Child Health and Human Development, Society for Maternal-Fetal Medicine, and American College of Obstetricians and Gynecologists Workshop. *Obstet Gynecol* 2012;120(5):1181-93.

(Continued)

(Continued)

Type of evidence	Title and comment	Date/full reference
Retrospective, cross-sectional study	Contemporary patterns of spontaneous labor with normal neonatal outcomes Comment: This retrospective study questioned the definition of active labor and the duration of labor based on parity that was established by Friedman et al. in the 1950s. It established 6 cm as the cutoff of active labor in comparison to Friedman's cutoff of 4 cm and recommended more time to allow for the progression of normal labor.	Zhang J, Landy HJ, Branch DW, et al. Contemporary patterns of spontaneous labor with normal neonatal outcomes. *Obstet Gynecol* 2010;116(6):1281-87. doi:10.1097/AOG.0b013e3181fdef6e.
Retrospective, cross-sectional study	Primigravid labor: a graphicostatistical analysis Comment: This seminal paper was the original retrospective study in the 1950s that determined the normal pattern of labor in women who would go on to have a spontaneous vaginal delivery. This was accepted as doctrine in obstetrics until the time frame of normal labor in the study was questioned by Zhang et al.	Friedman EA. Primigravid labor: a graphicostatistical analysis. *Obstet Gynecol* 1955;6:567-89.

Additional material for this chapter can be found online at:
www.wiley.com/go/sperling/mountsinai/obstetricsandgynecology

This includes a case study, multiple choice questions, advice for patients, and ICD codes.

CHAPTER 11

Cesarean Delivery and Operative Vaginal Delivery

Francesco Callipari, Anna Kremer, Fahimeh Sasan, and Jian Jenny Tang
Department of Obstetrics, Gynecology and Reproductive Science, Icahn School of Medicine at Mount Sinai, New York, NY

OVERALL BOTTOM LINE
- Cesarean delivery is safe and has significantly reduced both fetal and maternal morbidity and mortality.
- Compared to vaginal delivery, women undergoing cesarean delivery are at higher risk for short-term and long-term health consequences.
- The short-term risks of cesarean delivery include hemorrhage, infection, and prolonged healing time.
- Antibiotic prophylaxis has significantly reduced the incidence of postoperative fever, endomyometritis, wound infections, and other serious maternal infectious complications.
- The long-term risks of cesarean delivery include the high likelihood of a repeat cesarean delivery and the risk of placental abnormalities such as placenta previa and placenta accreta.
- In the appropriately selected patient, operative vaginal delivery (either forceps or vacuum-assisted delivery) can expedite a safe vaginal delivery and avoid the need for cesarean delivery.

Background
- Childbirth, regardless of route of delivery, carries risks for both the mother and the baby.
- Cesarean delivery (CD) is the method of delivering a baby through a surgical incision in the abdomen and then through the uterus.
- Although cesarean deliveries are safe and are often the preferred route of delivery for many obstetrical and fetal complications, cesarean delivery poses a greater risk of maternal morbidity and mortality than vaginal delivery.
- Compared to vaginal delivery, the short-term risks of cesarean delivery include hemorrhage, infection, prolonged healing time, and increased cost.
- Compared to vaginal delivery, the long-term risks of cesarean delivery include the need for repeat cesarean delivery and the risk of placental abnormalities such as placenta accrete and placenta previa.
- CD is categorized as either primary or repeat.
- The rates of primary and total cesarean deliveries increased rapidly from 1996 to 2011 reaching a high of 32.9% of all US births in 2009.
- Approximately 60% of cesarean deliveries in the United States are primary cesarean deliveries.
- There is concern among the obstetrical and public health community that primary cesarean delivery is overused and efforts are underway to reduce the rates of primary cesarean delivery.
- Appropriate labor management can reduce the need for primary cesarean delivery and also reduce complications of cesarean delivery.
- In the appropriately selected patient, operative vaginal delivery (either forceps or vacuum-assisted delivery) can expedite a safe vaginal delivery and avoid the need for cesarean delivery.

Mount Sinai Expert Guides: Obstetrics and Gynecology, First Edition. Edited by Rhoda Sperling.
Companion Website: www.wiley.com/go/sperling/mountsinai/obstetricsandgynecology

Incidence/prevalence
- More than 30% of births in the United States occur by CD.
- Selected factors are responsible for increased CD rates. (Figure 11.1).
- Prevalence of operative vaginal delivery decreased from 9% in 1990 to 3.4% in 2012. Forceps have been used for less than 1% of all births in the United States since 2005.

Barber et al. 2011; Hamilton et al. 2015; Martin et al. 2015; Menacker and Hamilton 2010

Economic impact
- 1.3 million cesarean deliveries are performed in the United States every year and about 20 million are done worldwide.

Selected factors responsible for increased cesarean delivery (CD) rate

Obstetrical factors

    Increased primary CD rate

    Failed induction, increased use of induction

    Decreased use of operative vaginal delivery

    Increased macrosomia, CD for macrosomia

    Decline in vaginal breech delivery

    Increased repeat CD rate

    Decreased use of vaginal birth after CD

Maternal factors

    Increased proportion of women > 35 yr

    Increased proportion of nulliparous women

    Increased primary CDs on maternal request

    Obesity

Physician factors:

    Malpractice litigation concerns

Gabbe et al. 2016; Chapter 19 Cesarean Delivery, p. 426

Prevention
- Given the morbidity associated with cesarean deliveries, the American College of Obstetrics and Gynecologists and Society for Maternal-Fetal Medicine recently published a consensus statement in attempting to reduce the incidence of primary cesarean delivery (ACOG 2014; Safe prevention 2014). Recommendations are classified as either strong (Grade 1) or weak (Grade 2), and quality of evidence is classified as high (Grade A), moderate (Grade B), and low (Grade C).

First stage of labor
- A prolonged latent phase (>20 hr in nulliparous [NP] women and > 14 hr in multiparous [MP] women) should not be an indication for CD. (Grade 1B)
- Slow but progressive labor in the first stage rarely should be an indication for CD. (Grade 1B)
- As long as fetal and maternal status are reassuring, cervical dilation of 6 cm should be considered the threshold for the active phase in most laboring women. Thus before 6 cm of dilation is achieved, standards of active-phase progress should not be applied. (Grade 1B)

- CD for active-phase arrest in the first stage of labor should be reserved for women at or beyond 6 cm of dilation with ruptured membranes who fail to progress despite 4 hr of adequate uterine activity or at least 6 hr of oxytocin administration with inadequate uterine activity and no cervical change. (Grade 1B)

Second stage of labor

- A specific absolute maximum length of the second stage of labor above which all women should be delivered operatively has not been identified. (Grade 1C)
- Before diagnosing arrest of labor in the second stage, if the maternal and fetal conditions permit, allow for the following:
  - At least 2 hr of pushing in MP women (Grade 1B)
  - At least 3 hr of pushing in NP women (Grade 1B)
  Longer durations may be appropriate on an individualized basis (e.g. with the use of epidural analgesia or with fetal malposition) as long as progress is being documented. (Grade 1B)
- Operative vaginal delivery in the second stage of labor should be considered an acceptable alternative to CD. Training in, and ongoing maintenance of, practical skills related to operative vaginal delivery should be encouraged. (Grade 1B)
- Manual rotation of the fetal occiput in the setting of fetal malposition in the second stage of labor is a reasonable alternative to operative vaginal delivery or CD. To safely prevent CD in the setting of malposition, it is important to assess fetal position throughout the second stage of labor. (Grade 1B)

Fetal heart rate monitoring

- Amnioinfusion for repetitive variable fetal heart rate decelerations may safely reduce the CD rate. (Grade 1A)
- Scalp stimulation can be used as a means of assessing fetal acid-base status when abnormal or indeterminate (*nonreassuring*) fetal heart patterns (e.g. minimal variability) are present, and it is a safe alternative to CD in this setting. (Grade 1C)

Induction of labor

- Induction of labor should generally be performed based on maternal and fetal medical indications and after obtaining and documenting informed consent. Inductions at 41 0/7 weeks of gestation and beyond should be performed to reduce the risk of CD and the risk of perinatal morbidity and mortality. (Grade 1A)
- Cervical ripening methods should be used when labor is induced in women with an unfavorable cervix. (Grade 1B)
- If the maternal and fetal status allow, CDs for failed induction of labor in the latent phase can be avoided by allowing longer durations of the latent phase (up to 24 hr or longer) and requiring that oxytocin be administered for at least 18 hr after membrane rupture before deeming the induction a failure. (Grade 1B)

Fetal malpresentation

- Fetal presentation should be assessed and documented beginning at 36 0/7 weeks of gestation to allow for external cephalic version to be offered. (Grade 1C)

Suspected fetal macrosomia

- CD to avoid potential birth trauma should be limited to estimated fetal weights of at least 5000 g in women without diabetes and at least 4500 g in women with diabetes. The prevalence of birth weight of 5000 g or more is rare, and patients should be counseled that estimates of fetal weight, particularly late in gestation, are imprecise. (Grade 2C)

• Women should be counseled about the Institute of Medicine maternal weight guidelines in an attempt to avoid excessive weight gain. (Grade 1B)

Twin gestations

• Perinatal outcomes for twin gestations in which the first twin is in cephalic presentation are not improved by CD. Thus women with either cephalic/cephalic-presenting twins or cephalic/noncephalic-presenting twins should be counseled to attempt vaginal delivery. (Grade 1B)

Other

• Individuals, organizations, and governing bodies should work to ensure that research is conducted to provide a better knowledge base to guide decisions regarding CD and to encourage policy changes that safely lower the rate of primary CD. (Grade 1C)

Modified from American College of Obstetricians and Gynecologists (ACOG), Society for Maternal-Fetal Medicine (SMFM) et al. 2014

Diagnosis

Indications for primary cesarean delivery

• Approximately 60% of cesarean deliveries in the United States are primary. The most common indications for primary CD in the United States account for 80% of these deliveries:
  • Failure to progress during labor (34%)
  • Nonreassuring fetal status (23%)
  • Fetal malpresentation (17%)
  • Multiple gestation (7%)
  • Abnormal placentation (i.e. placenta previa, vasa previa)
  • Suspected macrosomia (4%)

Timing

• Planned term cesarean delivery should be scheduled for ≥ 39 weeks of gestation (Barber et al. 2011; Martin et al. 2013; Safe prevention 2014).

Precesarean antibiotics

• Prophylactic antibiotics, usually a single intravenous dose of narrow-spectrum antibiotics, such as cefazolin, should be given approximately 30 to 60 minutes before the skin incision to allow for adequate tissue concentrations (Mackeen et al. 2014). For women who have anaphylactic reaction to penicillin, either metronidazole or clindamycin and gentamicin can be used.

Laboratory testing

• Complete blood count
• Blood type and screen

Technique

• Pfannenstiel skin incision with scalpel, which is associated with less postoperative pain, greater wound strength, and better cosmetic appearance than the vertical midline incision
• Use fingers to bluntly open the peritoneum to minimize injury to other organs
• Bladder flap to protect the bladder
• Low transverse uterine hysterotomy for entry into the uterine cavity
• Spontaneous, rather than manual extractions of the placenta
• Two-layer uterine closure for primary cesarean delivery

- Closure of peritoneum to reduce future adhesions
- For women with subcutaneous tissue depth ≥ 2 cm, we recommend closure of the subcutaneous tissue layer with sutures, which decreases the risk of subsequent wound disruption.
- Reapproximation of the skin with subcuticular suture rather than staples

Anesthesia
- Regional or neuraxial anesthesia is used for 95% of cesarean deliveries.
- Patient is awake for the birth.
- Minimizes risk for aspiration pneumonia or airway instrumentation
- Minimizes systemic medication and transfer to the fetus
- Allows administration of postoperative analgesia with long-term opioids

Thromboembolism prophylaxis
- Mechanical thromboprophylaxis
- Pharmacologic thromboprophylaxis in high-risk patient with obesity, increased risk of deep vein thrombosis

Skin preparation
- Chlorhexidine-based antiseptic agents

Hair removal
- Hair removal is unnecessary, but if it is, use hair clippers the morning of the surgery.

Operative vaginal delivery
Forceps delivery
- The indications for forceps maybe maternal or fetal. Maternal indications include maternal exhaustion, failure to progress, or bleeding. Fetal indications include signs of nonreassuring fetal status and malposition (Committee on Practice Bulletins 2015).
- The prerequisites for forceps delivery are of vital importance and should be emphasized.
  - Cervix must be fully dilated and retracted.
  - Membranes ruptured
  - Fetal head must be engaged in the + 2 to + 3 station.
  - Exact position of the head should be determined.
  - The type of pelvis should be known.
  - Appropriate anesthesia should be in effect.
  - Operator should have knowledge of the instruments.
  - Know gestational age and size
  - Bladder is empty.
  - Operator is knowledgeable.
  - Informed consent obtained

Operative vaginal delivery classification
Outlet
- Scalp is visible at the introitus without separating the labia.
- Fetal skull has reached the pelvic floor.
- Sagittal suture is in the AP diameter or left/right occiput anterior (LOA/ROA) or left/right occiput posterior (LOP/ROP) position.
- Fetal head is at or on the perineum.
- Rotation does not exceed 45 degrees.

Low forceps

- Leading point of the fetal skull is at + 2 cm or greater and not on the pelvic floor.
- Rotation is 45 degrees or less from LOA/ROA to OA or LOP/ROP to OP, or rotation is 45 degrees or more.

Vacuum-assisted vaginal delivery (VAVD)

- The same prerequisites for forceps apply to VAVD. The mushroom-shaped cups are a hybrid of the stainless steel and plastic devices. Example is Omnicup (Kiwi). This is most commonly used at our institution.
- The vacuum cup must be placed on the bony surface of the fetal scalp and avoid the fontanelles.
- Leading point of the head is the ideal position for vacuum cup placement, which is labeled as the flexion point, or pivot point and is located on the sagittal suture 2 to 3 cm below the posterior for the OA position and 2 to 3 cm above the posterior fontanel for the OP position.
- Maximum number of pop-offs should be limited to three.
- No use of both forceps and vacuum.

Vacuum extraction devices

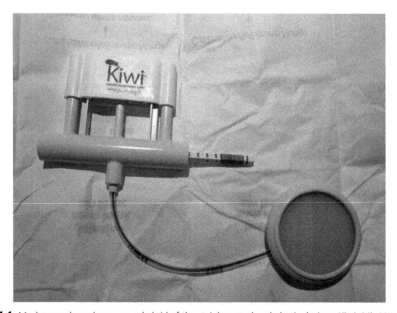

Figure 11.1 Mushroom-shaped cups are a hybrid of the stainless steel and plastic devices: Kiwi, MityVac, CMI.

Reading list

American College of Obstetricians and Gynecologists. Safe prevention of the primary cesarean delivery. Obstetric care. Consensus no. 1. *Obstet Gynecol* 2014;123:693-711.

American College of Obstetricians and Gynecologists, Society for Maternal-Fetal Medicine, Caughey AB, Cahill AG, Guise JM, et al. Safe prevention of the primary cesarean delivery. *Am J Obstet Gynecol* 2014;210(3):179-93.

Barber EL, Lundberg L. Belanger K, et al. Contributing indications to the rising cesarean delivery rate. *Obstet Gynecol* 2011;118:29-38.

Bucklin BA, Hawkins JL, Anderson JR, et al. Obstetric anesthesia workforce survey: twenty-year update. *Anesthesiology* 2005;103(3):645-53.

Committee on Practice Bulletins – Obstetrics. ACOG practice bulletin no. 154. Summary: operative vaginal delivery. *Obstet Gynecol* 2015;126:1118.

Gabbe S, Niebyl J, Simpson J, et al. *Obstetrics: normal and problem pregnancies.* 7th ed. Amsterdam: Elsevier; 2016.

Hamilton BE, Martin JA, Osterman MJ, et al. Births: Final data for 2014. *National Vital Stat Report* 2015;64:1-64.

Mackeen AD, Packard RE, Ota E, et al. Timing of intravenous prophylactic antibiotics for preventing postpartum infection morbidity in women undergoing cesarean delivery. *Cochrane Database Syst Rev* 2014;(2): CD 009516.

Martin JA, Hamilton BE, Osterman MJ, et al. Births: Final data for 2013. *National Vital Stat Report* 2015;64:1-65.

Menacker F, Hamilton BE. *Recent trends in Cesarean delivery in the United States*. NCHS data brief 2010;(35):1-8.

Osterman MJK, Martin JA. Primary cesarean delivery rates by state. Results from the revised birth certificate, 2006-2012. *Natl Vital Stat Rep* 2014 Jan;63(1):1-11.

Small FM, Grivell RM. Antibiotic prophylaxis versus no prophylaxis for preventing infection after cesarean section. *Cochrane Database Syst Rev* 2014;CD 007482.

Tsakiridis I, Giouleka S, Mamopoulos A, et al. Operative vaginal delivery: a review of four national guidelines. *Perinat Med* 2020 Jan 11. pii: /j/jpme.ahead-of-print/jpm-2019-0433/jpm-2019-0433.xml. doi: 10.1515/jpm-2019-0433. [Epub ahead of print]

Suggested website

American College of Obstetricians and Gynecologists. www.acog.org

Guidelines
National society guidelines

Title	Source	Date/full reference or URL
Safe prevention of the primary cesarean delivery: Obstetric care consensus no. 1	ACOG and SMFM	2014 (reaffirmed 2019) https://www.acog.org/Clinical-Guidance-and-Publications/Obstetric-Care-Consensus-Series/Safe-Prevention-of-the-Primary-Cesarean-Delivery
Operative vaginal delivery: ACOG practice bulletin #154	ACOG	Committee on Practice Bulletins–Obstetrics. ACOG Practice Bulletin No. 154: operative vaginal delivery. *Obstet Gynecol* 2015;126:e56–65.

International society guidelines

Title	Source	Date/full reference
Operative vaginal delivery: a review of four national guidelines	A descriptive review of guidelines from the Royal College of Obstetricians and Gynaecologists (RCOG), the Royal Australian and New Zealand College of Obstetricians and Gynaecologists (RANZCOG), the Society of Obstetricians and Gynaecologists of Canada (SOGC) and the American College of Obstetricians and Gynecologists (ACOG) on instrumental vaginal birth was conducted.	*J Perinat Med* 2020 Jan 11. pii: /j/jpme.ahead-of-print/jpm-2019-0433/jpm-2019-0433.xml. doi: 10.1515/jpm-2019-0433. [Epub ahead of print]

CHAPTER 12

Intrapartum and Postpartum Hemorrhage

Faith J. Frieden
Department of Obstetrics, Gynecology and Reproductive Science, Icahn School of Medicine at Mount Sinai, New York, NY

OVERALL BOTTOM LINE
- Obstetrical hemorrhage is the single most significant cause of maternal death and morbidity worldwide.
- The most common causes are uterine atony, trauma, and coagulation defects.
- Anticipation, preparation, and prompt recognition are key to the management of obstetrical hemorrhage, which may require a multidisciplinary team approach.

Background
Definition of disease
- Intrapartum/postpartum hemorrhage refers to excessive blood loss during or after delivery, generally defined as *cumulative* blood loss greater than or equal to 1000 mL or blood loss accompanied by signs or symptoms of hypovolemia within 24 hours after the birth process, including intrapartum blood loss, regardless of the route of delivery. Note that this is in contrast to the traditional definitions: more than 500 mL for a vaginal delivery and more than 1000 mL for a cesarean delivery.

Disease classification
- Primary – occurs within 24 hours of delivery
- Secondary – occurs between 24 hours and 6–12 weeks postpartum

Incidence/prevalence
- Hemorrhage is estimated to occur in 4–6% of pregnancies.
- It is a leading cause of maternal morbidity and mortality, accounting for 140 000 maternal deaths per year worldwide, or 1 death every 4 minutes.

Etiology
- Uterine atony is responsible for at least 80% of postpartum hemorrhage.
- Hemorrhage can be related to trauma, such as lacerations, incisions, or uterine rupture.
- Coagulopathy may be both a cause and a result of hemorrhage, because persistent heavy bleeding leads to consumption of clotting factors.

Pathology/pathogenesis
- The uterus at full term receives 600 mL of blood per minute, which places the woman at risk for massive amounts of blood loss in a short time. Normally, hemostasis occurs by a combination of mechanisms: contraction of the myometrium, which causes mechanical compression of the blood vessels, and local

---

Mount Sinai Expert Guides: Obstetrics and Gynecology, First Edition. Edited by Rhoda Sperling.
© 2020 John Wiley & Sons Ltd. Published 2020 by John Wiley & Sons Ltd.
Companion Website: www.wiley.com/go/sperling/mountsinai/obstetricsandgynecology

and systemic coagulation factors that promote clotting. When either of these mechanisms is disturbed or overwhelmed, massive bleeding will result.

Predictive/risk factors

Risk factor
Abnormal placentation (previa, accreta, abruption)
Prior uterine surgery
Overdistended uterus (multiple gestation, polyhydramnios, large for gestational age [LGA] fetus, myomata)

Prevention

> **BOTTOM LINE/CLINICAL PEARLS**
> - In an effort to prevent uterine atony and the associated bleeding, it is routine to administer oxytocin immediately after delivery of the baby/placenta.

Screening
- According to the Safe Motherhood Initiative (SMI), all patients should be screened for risk factors during their prenatal course, upon admission for delivery, and during the course of labor, in order to identify those at highest risk and prepare for potential hemorrhage.

Primary prevention
- The best prevention is anticipation/preparation, which may involve interdisciplinary team huddles for high-risk patients and, when indicated, transfer to an appropriate level of care for delivery.
- For patients with prior uterine surgery, placental location should be documented prior to delivery, with imaging to evaluate risk for accreta.
- Upon admission, patients at medium risk (prior cesarean, multiple gestation, >4 prior births, prior post-partum hemorrhage, myomata, obesity, hematocrit <30) should have a type and screen.
- Patients at high risk (placenta previa/accreta, thrombocytopenia, active bleeding, coagulopathy, two or more medium risk factors) should have type and cross.
- During the course of labor, additional risk factors may develop that would increase the risk for hemorrhage (e.g. chorioamnionitis, prolonged labor, the use of magnesium sulfate), which is the rationale for ongoing evaluation.

Diagnosis

> **BOTTOM LINE/CLINICAL PEARLS**
> - The key to managing obstetrical hemorrhage is prompt diagnosis, based on estimated or quantitative assessment of blood loss of greater than or equal to 1000 mL.
> - In addition to assessing blood loss, which is often underestimated, attention must be paid to any changes in vital signs and urine output.
> - Laboratory evaluations, such as complete blood count (CBC) and coagulation studies, are helpful in diagnosis and management; however, treatment should not be delayed while awaiting lab results.

Differential diagnosis

Differential diagnosis	Features
Intra-abdominal bleeding	There may be a change in vital signs, with minimal visible bleeding, due to internal bleeding or an enlarging hematoma.
Vasovagal reaction or vasodilatation due to neuraxial anesthesia	Lightheadedness, tachycardia, hypotension with abrupt onset immediately following administration of an anesthetic or drug known to cause hypotension.

Typical presentation
- Obstetrical hemorrhage typically presents with bleeding that is greater than expected and causes signs/symptoms of hypovolemia, such as lightheadedness, palpitations, hypotension, tachycardia, oliguria, and decreased oxygen saturation.

Clinical diagnosis
History
- History should include a search for potential risk factors for increased bleeding, such as prior postpartum hemorrhage, prior uterine surgery, any reason to anticipate a morbidly adherent placenta, clinically significant bleeding disorder, more than four prior births, and history of myomata.
- The clinician should ascertain whether or not the patient would be willing to accept blood products.

Physical examination
- The physical evaluation should include a measurement of blood loss and assessment of vital signs, as this will inform the response to the hemorrhage.
- Next, there is a search for etiology, starting with a bimanual pelvic exam to determine if the uterus is soft and poorly contracted, since uterine atony is the leading cause of hemorrhage.
- If bleeding persists, the clinician should inspect the lower genital tract for cervical or vaginal lacerations.
- Ultrasound evaluation of the uterus can also be performed to look for evidence of retained placental fragments, prior to manual or instrumental exploration.

Disease severity classification
SMI Classification
- Stage I: Blood loss >1000 mL after delivery with normal vital signs and lab values; vaginal delivery with 500–999 mL should be treated as Stage I.
- Stage II: Continued bleeding (estimated blood loss up to 1500 mL OR >2 uterotonics) with normal vital signs and lab values
- Stage III: Continued bleeding (>1500 mL OR >2 units red blood cells given OR patient at risk for occult bleeding/coagulopathy OR abnormal vital signs/labs/oliguria)
- Stage IV: Cardiovascular collapse (massive hemorrhage, profound hypovolemic shock, or amniotic fluid embolism)

Laboratory diagnosis
List of diagnostic tests
- When intrapartum or postpartum hemorrhage is suspected, the provider should immediately send blood for type and crossmatch, hemoglobin and hematocrit, platelet count, prothrombin time/partial thromboplastin time (PT/PTT), international normalized ratio (INR), and fibrinogen.
- If bleeding continues, send follow-up hematocrit, platelets, and coagulation studies to help guide transfusion requirements; however, transfusion should not be delayed while awaiting lab results.

- In women with bleeding many weeks after delivery, a quantitative pregnancy test is useful for evaluating for choriocarcinoma.

List of imaging techniques
- Ultrasound evaluation of the uterus may be helpful to look for retained products of conception; for delayed postpartum bleeding, it may also help detect choriocarcinoma.

Potential pitfalls/common errors made regarding diagnosis of disease
- The most common pitfall in diagnosis is underestimation of the extent of the blood loss, especially because otherwise healthy young women can maintain their vital signs until large amounts of blood are lost.

Treatment
Treatment rationale
- Treatment almost always starts with uterotonics, because atony is the leading cause of postpartum hemorrhage, with prompt escalation to other interventions as needed.
- Generally, less-invasive methods should be tried initially, with advancing to more aggressive surgical management if necessary, as dictated by the etiology of the bleeding and the extent of the blood loss.

Table of treatment

Treatment	Comments
Conservative	For patients with Stage I hemorrhage: ensure large-bore IV access; increase IV crystalloid fluids; insert indwelling urinary catheter; perform fundal massage; draw labs; notify blood bank and operating room Physical exam to determine etiology: • Tone (atony, uterine inversion) • Trauma (laceration, rupture) • Tissue (retained products, accreta) • Thrombin (coagulation dysfunction)
Medical (nested list of all drugs or drug combinations) together with dose	• Oxytocin 10–40 units per 500–1000 mL solution or 10 units IM • Methylergonovine 0.2 mg IM (avoid with hypertension) every 2–4 hrs • 15-methyl PGF2alpha 250 mcg IM every 15 minutes up to 8 doses (avoid with asthma, hypertension) • Misoprostol 800–1000 mcg PR once • Tranexamic acid 1 gram IV over 10 minutes; may be repeated once after 30 minutes • Initiate massive transfusion protocol
Surgical (list techniques)	• Bakri balloon • Uterine packing • Curettage • Exploratory laparotomy • Compression/B-Lynch suture • Uterine artery ligation • Hysterectomy
Radiological	Uterine artery embolization

CLINICAL PEARLS
- Management of obstetrical hemorrhage should employ a *multidisciplinary*, multifaceted, stepwise approach that involves maintaining hemodynamic stability while simultaneously identifying and treating the cause of the blood loss.

Reading list

Alexander JM, Wortman AC. Intrapartum hemorrhage. *Obstet Gynecol Clin N Am* 2013;40:15-26.

American College of Obstetricians and Gynecologists. Practice Bulletin 183: postpartum hemorrhage. *Obstet Gynecol* 2017 Oct;130(4):e168-e186.

American College of Obstetricians and Gynecologists District II, *Safe motherhood initiative, Maternal Safety Bundle for Obstetric Hemorrhage*, November 2015, revised June 2019.

American College of Obstetricians and Gynecologists, Society for Maternal-Fetal Medicine. Obstetric care consensus no. 7: placenta accreta spectrum. *Obstet Gynecol* 2018 Dec;132(6):e259-e275.

Belfort MA. Overview of postpartum hemorrhage. *UpToDate* 2017 Mar.

Suggested websites

California Maternal Quality Care Collaborative. www.cmqcc.org

Council on Patient Safety in Women's Health Care. safehealthcareforeverywoman.org

Guidelines
National society guidelines

Title	Source	Date/full reference or URL
Maternal safety bundle for obstetric hemorrhage: obstetric hemorrhage checklist	ACOG District II – Safe Motherhood Initiative	2019 https://www.acog.org/-/media/Districts/District-II/Public/SMI/v2/SMIHemorrhageChecklistREVISEDJUNE2019
Practice guidelines for obstetric anesthesia	American Society of Anesthesiologists, Society for Obstetric Anesthesia and Perinatology	Practice guidelines for obstetric anesthesia: an updated report by the American Society of Anesthesiologists Task Force on Obstetric Anesthesia and the Society for Obstetric Anesthesia and Perinatology. *Anesthesiology* 2007 Apr;106(4):843-63.

International society guidelines

Title	Source	Date/URL
WHO recommendations for the prevention and treatment of postpartum hemorrhage (PPH)	World Health Organization Comment: provides evidence based guidelines for PPH care particularly in underresourced settings	https://apps.who.int/iris/bitstream/handle/10665/75411/9789241548502_eng.pdf;jsessionid=2EDC38C7B511933CFAF410028A91FC0E?sequence=1

CHAPTER 13

Intraamniotic Infection

Andrew Ditchik
Department of Obstetrics and Gynecology, Elmhurst Hospital Center, Queens, NY; Department of Obstetrics, Gynecology and Reproductive Science, Icahn School of Medicine at Mount Sinai, New York, NY

OVERALL BOTTOM LINE

Intraamniotic infection (IAI) is a poorly defined heterogeneous condition including both clinical and subclinical histologic diagnoses.

- Recently developed tiered classification system may assist in guiding standardized approach to diagnosis and treatment.
- Incidence of IAI is inversely proportional to the gestational age at delivery.
- Preventive measures include:
  - Screening and treating patients for group B strep colonization
  - Antibiotic treatment for patients with preterm premature rupture of membranes
- Treatment consists of broad-spectrum antibiotics and delivery; cesarean delivery should be reserved for usual indications.

Background
Definition of disease
- IAI is defined as an active infection or inflammation in the amniotic sac resulting in inflammatory changes in the mother and/or fetus.
- May include subclinical histologic evidence of chorioamnionitis or funisitis

Incidence/prevalence
- Clinical IAI: 1–4% term births; 5–10% preterm births
- Histologic IAI: 20% term births; 50% preterm births

Economic impact
- Difficult to quantify although direct costs include neonatal care for preterm infants as well as long-term costs for children born with disabilities due to prematurity and/or neonatal sepsis.

Etiology
- Most commonly ascending infection from lower genital tract (e.g. group B strep, mycoplasma, ureaplasma)
- Hematogenous spread from gastrointestinal tract (e.g. listeria monocytogenes), oral, urinary, or respiratory tract
- Invasive procedure such as amniocentesis
- Inflammatory processes without bacterial contamination may result in similar clinical features and sequelae.

Mount Sinai Expert Guides: Obstetrics and Gynecology, First Edition. Edited by Rhoda Sperling.
© 2020 John Wiley & Sons Ltd. Published 2020 by John Wiley & Sons Ltd.
Companion Website: www.wiley.com/go/sperling/mountsinai/obstetricsandgynecology

Pathology/pathogenesis

- Often includes low virulent organisms resulting in chronic or subacute condition.
- Infection or inflammation results in maternal inflammatory response (SIRS) as well as fetal inflammatory response (FIRS).
- Inflammatory mediators responsible for much of fetal damage regardless of bacterial invasion.
- Maternal complications include preterm premature rupture of membranes, preterm labor, dysfunctional labor, increased risk of cesarean delivery, postpartum hemorrhage, postpartum infection (endometritis, wound infection), sepsis, adult respiratory distress syndrome, death.
- Fetal complications include sepsis, pneumonia, respiratory distress, asphyxia, necrotizing enterocolitis, intraventricular hemorrhage, periventricular leukomalacia, cerebral palsy, long-term neuro developmental delay, death.

Predictive/risk factors

Risk factor
Prolonged labor
Prolonged rupture of membranes
Multiple digital exams
Intrauterine monitoring
Group B strep colonization
Bacterial vaginosis
Other genital tract infection
Meconium stained amniotic fluid
Tobacco use
Alcohol use
History of intraamniotic infection in prior pregnancy

Prevention

> **BOTTOM LINE/CLINICAL PEARLS**
> - Screening for group B strep colonization and prophylactic treatment in labor has been shown to decrease the risk of early onset neonatal sepsis due to this organism without subsequent increase in sepsis due to other organisms.
> - Induction of labor for patients with preterm premature rupture of membranes > 34 weeks gestation is currently recommended, although this is an area of active research.
> - Antibiotics have been shown to prolong latency and improve clinical outcome for patients with preterm premature rupture of membranes but not for preterm labor with intact membranes or rupture of membranes at term.

Screening

- All pregnant women should be screened for group B strep colonization unless they have a prior pregnancy complicated by group B strep neonatal infection.

Primary prevention
- Patients with a positive group B strep screen, positive urine culture for group B strep, or prior pregnancy complicated by group B strep neonatal infection should be treated prophylactically in labor.
- Induction of labor for patients with preterm premature rupture of membranes after 34 weeks gestation has been shown to reduce the incidence of maternal infection and need for neonatal intensive care admission and is currently recommended, although this is an area of active investigation.
- Antibiotics have been shown to prolong latency and improve clinical outcome for patients with preterm premature rupture of membranes but not for preterm labor with intact membranes or rupture of membranes at term. Multiple regimens have been used effectively; amoxicillin/clavulonic acid should be avoided due to increased risk of neonatal necrotizing enterocolitis.
- Although poor dental hygiene is associated with preterm premature rupture of membranes and preterm labor, treatment during labor has not been shown to be effective.
- There is mixed evidence whether treatment of bacterial vaginosis in high-risk populations results in reduced incidence of preterm premature rupture of membranes or preterm labor.

Secondary prevention
- Women with prior pregnancy complicated by neonatal group B strep infection should be prophylactically treated in labor.

Diagnosis

> **BOTTOM LINE/CLINICAL PEARLS**
> - Diagnosis of IAI should be suspected for patients presenting with preterm premature rupture of membranes or preterm labor.
> - Fever is hallmark of the disease. Additional findings may include maternal or fetal tachycardia, uterine tenderness, or purulent cervical discharge.
> - Maternal leukocytosis supports the diagnosis; fluid obtained by amniocentesis may also be examined for evidence of infection or inflammation.

Differential diagnosis

Differential diagnosis	Features
Epidural in labor	Fever after epidural placement. Differential diagnosis may be complicated by uterine tenderness, maternal tachycardia, and leukocytosis commonly seen during labor.
Placental abruption	Usually presents with bleeding and/or tetanic uterine contractions without fever
Other infections (urinary tract infection, influenza, appendicitis, pneumonia)	Signs and symptoms specific to that disease may be present (e.g. cough, dysuria) as well as laboratory tests specific to that disease state (e.g. urine analysis, influenza rapid assay).
Thrombophlebitis	Evidence of thrombophlebitis may include swollen, tender extremity.
Colitis	Gastrointestinal symptoms

Typical presentation
- IAI usually presents with fever in the setting of labor or ruptured membranes. It may be accompanied by maternal or fetal tachycardia, uterine tenderness, or purulent cervical discharge. Subclinical IAI should be suspected in the setting of preterm labor and/or preterm premature rupture of membranes in asymptomatic patients.

Clinical diagnosis

History

- Clinicians should focus on evidence of maternal fever, leakage of fluid or preterm labor as well as prior pregnancy complicated by preterm labor, preterm premature rupture of membranes, or evidence of IAI.
- Additional history should be obtained to assist in differential diagnosis as described previously.

Physical examination

- Physical exam should include evaluation of maternal vital signs (temperature, blood pressure, pulse, respiratory rate, and oxygen saturation) as well as fetal heart rate, palpation of the uterus for the presence of contractions and/or fundal tenderness, vaginal exam to examine for evidence of rupture of membranes and/or labor, as well as general evaluation of the patient to exclude other diagnoses.

Disease severity classification

- IAI can be divided into histologic or clinical disease.
  - Histologic IAI represents subclinical infection or inflammation resulting in characteristic changes in the placenta and/or umbilical cord (Figure 13.1).
- Current evidence supports tiered classification of clinical IAI:
  - Isolated maternal fever: Maternal oral temperature 38 °C < 39 °C on two separate occasions 30 minutes apart.
  - Suspected IAI: Fever as defined above plus fetal tachycardia ≥ 160 bpm for ≥ 10 minutes, leukocytosis ≥ 15 000 per mm^3, or purulent cervical discharge; OR maternal oral temperature ≥ 39 °C.
    - NOTE: maternal oral temp ≥ 39 °C without additional clinical criteria was reclassified from isolated maternal fever to suspected IAI in Committee Opinion No. 712: Intrapartum Management of Intraamniotic Infection.
  - Confirmed intraamniotic infection: All of the above plus amniocentesis proven infection (positive gram stain, glucose < 15 mg/dL, white blood cell [WBC] count > 30 cells/mm^3, leukocyte esterase activity or positive amniotic fluid culture); OR placental pathology with histologic evidence of infection
- See Algorithm 13.1.

Algorithm 13.1 Stepwise approach to diagnosing intraamniotic infection

Fever 38 °C < 39 °C on two separate occasions 30 minutes apart → fetal tachycardia ≥ 160 bpm for ≥ 10 min and/or leukocytosis ≥ 15 000 per mm^3 and/or purulent cervical discharge
OR
Fever ≥ 39 °C →

Amniocentesis evidence of infection (positive gram stain, glucose < 15 mg/dL, WBC count > 30 cells/mm^3, leucocyte esterase activity, positive bacterial culture); OR
placental pathology with histologic evidence of infection

Laboratory diagnosis

List of diagnostic tests

- Complete blood count (CBC) and lactate should be drawn for all febrile patients; blood and urine cultures should be strongly considered prior to starting antibiotics.
- Urinalysis should be drawn to evaluate for urinary tract infection.
- Evaluation of renal and/or liver function may be appropriate for select cases.
- Amniocentesis may be considered for patients with questionable diagnosis such as patients with preterm labor and intact membranes or prior to rescue cerclage.

- Current evidence supports the following laboratory studies (positive values suggestive of IAI shown later)
  - Gram stain (presence of bacteria)
  - Glucose (<15 mg/dL)
  - WBC cell count (>30 cells/mm^3)
  - Leukocyte esterase activity (trace or greater on dipstick)
  - Bacterial culture
- Markers for inflammation such as interleukin-6 and proteomic biomarkers are actively being studied but should be considered investigatory at this time.
- Pathologic evaluation of the placenta should be sent for all patients with suspected IAI.

List of imaging techniques
- Ultrasound should be performed to evaluate status of the fetus and amniotic fluid volume.
- Chest X-ray is appropriate for patients presenting with respiratory signs or symptoms.
- Abdominal imaging with ultrasound or magnetic resonance imaging (MRI) should be considered if appendicitis or other inflammatory bowel disease is suspected.

Potential pitfalls/common errors made regarding diagnosis of disease
- Overdiagnosis continues to be problematic for patients who present with single low-grade isolated fever in labor.

Treatment
Treatment rationale
- Prompt initiation of broad-spectrum antibiotics reduces the incidence of neonatal sepsis by 80%.
- Prolongation of pregnancy for patients with documented IAI has been shown to worsen fetal as well as maternal outcome; therefore, delivery is indicated in all such cases.
- Antipyretics should be used to treat maternal fever, which is an independent risk factor for the development of neonatal encephalopathy.
- There is no evidence that patients receiving appropriate treatment benefit from immediate cesarean delivery.

When to hospitalize
- All patients with suspected IAI should be hospitalized.

Managing the hospitalized patient
- For patients with suspected IAI, broad-spectrum antibiotic should be administered covering the most common pathogens.
- Coverage should include common commensal organisms including mycoplasma and ureaplasma.
  - First-line treatment: ampicillin (2 g IV every 6 hours) PLUS gentamicin (5 mg/kg IV every 24 hours or 2 mg/kg IV load followed by 1.5 mg/kg every 8 hours)
    - Prior to cesarean delivery consider addition of clindamycin (900 mg IV) or metronidazole (500 mg IV).
  - Penicillin-allergic patients with mild allergic reactions may receive cefazolin (2 g IV every 8 hours) PLUS gentamicin as described previously.
  - Penicillin-allergic patients with severe allergic reactions may receive vancomycin (1 g every 12 hours) or clindamycin (900 mg IV every 8 hours) PLUS gentamicin as described previously.
  - Other regimens include ampicillin-sulbactam (3 g IV every 6 hours), piperacillin-tazobactam (3.375 g IV every 6 hours or 4.5 g every 8 hours), cefotetan (2 g IV every 12 hours), cefoxitin (2 g IV every 8 hours), or ertapenem (1 g IV every 24 hours).

- Induction of labor should be initiated for all patients with suspected IAI not already in labor. Current evidence does not support any particular method of induction.
- There are not enough data to support or refute the practice of continuing antibiotics after delivery. Studies do suggest that a single dose of antibiotics after cesarean delivery is more effective than discontinuing antibiotics and as effective as continuing antibiotics until the patient has remained afebrile for 24 hours.

Table of treatment

Treatment	Comments
Medical	
Antibiotics Antipyretics	Antibiotic can be used as a preventative measure (such as with preterm premature rupture of membranes or group B strep colonization) and also as a primary treatment for IAI. Antipyretic agents such as acetaminophen should be used to reduce maternal temperature. There is evidence that maternal temperature is an independent risk factor for neonatal encephalopathy.
Other	Delivery is indicated for all cases of suspected IAI. Cesarean delivery should be reserved for the usual obstetrical indications.

Prevention/management of complications
- Aminoglycoside and vancomycin levels should be checked for patients receiving weight-based dosing regimens to reduce likelihood of renal toxicity.

CLINICAL PEARLS
- Patients with suspected IAI should be started on broad-spectrum antibiotics and, if not in labor, induction of labor is indicated.
- Prompt initiation of antibiotics reduces the risk of neonatal sepsis by 80%.
- There is no evidence that immediate cesarean delivery provides benefit; cesarean delivery should be reserved for the usual indications.
- See Algorithm 13.2.

Algorithm 13.2 Treatment of intra-amniotic infection
Prompt initiation of broad-spectrum antibiotics and antipyretics

Delivery (cesarean should be limited to the usual obstetrical indications)

Prognosis

BOTTOM LINE/CLINICAL PEARLS
- Prompt initiation of antibiotics and induction of labor greatly reduces risk to both mother and neonate.

Natural history of untreated disease
- Untreated IAI increases the risk of neonatal sepsis and multiorgan failure. It also increases maternal morbidity including sepsis and wound infections.

Prognosis for treated patients

- Prompt utilization of antibiotics can reduce the incidence of neonatal sepsis by 80% and reduces the incidence of maternal complications.

Follow-up tests and monitoring

- Monitoring of vital signs, physical exam, and labwork (CBC, lactate, cultures) should be continued as needed. Renal function should be checked for patients receiving aminoglycosides or vancomycin.

Reading list

Chapman E, Reveiz L, Illanes E, et al. Antibiotic regimens for management of intra-amniotic infection. *Cochrane Database Syst Rev* 2014;12:1-85.

Goldenberg RL, Hauth JA, Andrews WW. Intrauterine infection and preterm delivery. *N Engl J Med* 2000;342: 1500-07.

Higgins RD, Saade G, Polin RA, et al. Evalution and management of women and newborns with a maternal diagnosis of chorioamnionitis: summary of a workshop. *Obstet Gynecol* 2016;127(3):426-36.

Johnson CT, Farzin A, Burd I. Current management and long-term outcomes following chorioamnionitis. *Obstet Gynecol Clin North Am* 2014;41(4):646-69.

Kenyon S, Boulvain M, Neilson JP. Antibiotics for preterm rupture of membranes. *Cochrane Database Syst Rev* 2013;12:1-97.

Kenyon SL, Taylor DF, Tarnow-Mordi W. Broad-spectrum antibiotics for preterm, prelabour rupture of fetal membranes: the ORACLE 1 randomised trial. *Lancet* 2001;357:979-88.

Mendz GL, Kaakoush NO, Quinlivan JA. Bacterial aetological agents of intra-amniotic infections and preterm birth in pregnant women. *Front Cell Infect Microbiol* 2013;3(58):1-7.

Mercer BM, Miodovnik M, Thurnau GR, et al. Antibiotic therapy for reduction of infant morbidity after preterm premature rupture of the membranes. *JAMA* 1997;278(12):989-95.

Tita ATN, Andrews WW. Diagnosis and management of clinical chorioamnionitis. *Clin Pernatol* 2010;37(2):339-54.

Wojcieszek AM, Stock OM, Flenady V. Antibiotics for prelabour rupture of membranes at or near term. *Cochrane Database Syst Rev* 2014;10:1-66.

Guidelines
National society guidelines

Title	Source	Date/URL
ACOG practice bulletin no. 188: Prelabor rupture of membranes	American College of Obstetricians and Gynecologists (ACOG)	January 2018 https://www.acog.org/Clinical-Guidance-and-Publications/Practice-Bulletins/Committee-on-Practice-Bulletins-Obstetrics/Prelabor-Rupture-of-Membranes
ACOG committee opinion no. 485: Prevention of early onset group B streptococcal disease in newborns	ACOG	April 2011 https://www.acog.org/Clinical-Guidance-and-Publications/Committee-Opinions/Committee-on-Obstetric-Practice/Prevention-of-Early-Onset-Group-B-Streptococcal-Disease-in-Newborns
ACOG committee opinion no. 712: intrapartum management of intraamniotic infection	ACOG	August 2017 https://www.acog.org/Clinical-Guidance-and-Publications/Committee-Opinions/Committee-on-Obstetric-Practice/Intrapartum-Management-of-Intraamniotic-Infection

Evidence

Type of evidence	Title and comment	Date/full reference
Randomized controlled trial	Broad-spectrum antibiotics for preterm, prelabour rupture of fetal membranes Comment: Comparison of antibiotic regimens for treatment of preterm premature rupture of membranes showed efficacy of erythromycin and discouraged use of amoxicillin/clavulonic acid in this population due to increased incidence of necrotizing enterocolitis.	Kenyon SL, Taylor DF, Tarnow-Mordi W. Broad-spectrum antibiotics for preterm, prelabour rupture of fetal membranes: the ORACLE 1 randomised trial. *Lancet* 2001;357:979-88.
Randomized controlled trial	Antibiotic therapy for reduction of infant morbidity after preterm premature rupture of the membranes Comment: Comparison of antibiotics vs placebo for patients with preterm premature rupture of membranes. Showed effectiveness of IV ampicillin and erythromycin for 2 days followed by 5 days of oral amoxicillin and erythromycin in reducing neonatal morbidity.	Mercer BM, Miodovnik M, Thurnau GR, et al. Antibiotic therapy for reduction of infant morbidity after preterm premature rupture of the membranes. *JAMA* 1997;278(12):989-95.
Meta-analysis	Antibiotic regimens for management of intra-amniotic infection Comment: Compared various antibiotic regimens for the treatment of intraamniotic infections in labor. Results showed that there is limited evidence guiding both the choice of antibiotics and the duration of treatment.	Chapman E, Reveiz L, Illanes E, Bonfill Cosp X. Antibiotic regimens for management of intra-amniotic infection. *Cochrane Database Syst Rev* 2014;12:1-85.
Meta-analysis	Antibiotics for prelabour rupture of membranes at or near term Comment: Evaluated various antibiotic regimens for term rupture of membranes. Results showed no benefit to prophylactic treatment and suggested antibiotics should be avoided due to potential adverse effects and the development of resistant organisms	Wojcieszek AM, Stock OM, Flenady V. Antibiotics for prelabour rupture of membranes at or near term. *Cochrane Database Syst Rev* 2014;10:1-66.

Images

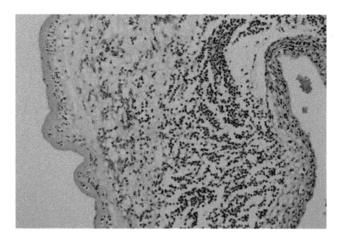

Figure 13.1 Acute chorioamnionitis showing inflammation. Source: https://upload.wikimedia.org/wikipedia/commons/9/94/Chorioamnionitis_-_low_mag.jpg. Licensed under CC BY SA 3.0. See color version on website.

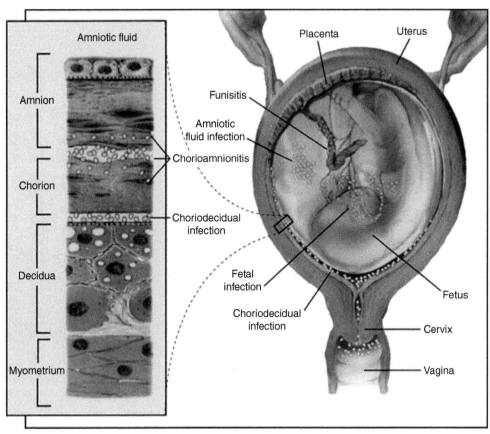

Figure 13.2 Potential sites of bacterial infection within the uterus. From: https://clinicalgate.com/infections-of-the-neonatal-infant/ Original source: Goldenberg RL, Hauth JA, Andrews WW: Intrauterine infection and preterm delivery. *N Engl J Med* 2000;342:1500–1507. Copyright 2000, Massachusetts Medical Society. See color version on website.

Additional material for this chapter can be found online at:
www.wiley.com/go/sperling/mountsinai/obstetricsandgynecology

This includes a case study, multiple choice questions, a video clip, advice for patients, and ICD codes. The following images are available in color: Figure 13.1 and Figure 13.2.

CHAPTER 14

Liver Disease and Pregnancy

Tatyana Kushner[1] and Rhoda Sperling[2]

[1] Department of Medicine – Division of Liver Diseases, Icahn School of Medicine at Mount Sinai, New York, NY

[2] Department of Obstetrics, Gynecology and Reproductive Science – Department of Medicine, Division of Infectious Diseases, Icahn School of Medicine at Mount Sinai, New York, NY

OVERALL BOTTOM LINE
- Physiologic changes during pregnancy can lead to fluctuations in liver tests during pregnancy.
- Certain liver diseases such as intrahepatic cholestasis of pregnancy, hemolysis elevated liver enzymes and low platelets (HELLP) syndrome, and acute fatty liver of pregnancy are unique to pregnancy.
- Coincident liver disease with pregnancy is liver disease that may be more common and more severe during pregnancy, such as Budd-Chiari disease or gallstone disease.
- In chronic liver diseases such as hepatitis B and hepatitis C, management during pregnancy as well as minimization of mother to child transmission during pregnancy should be prioritized; in liver diseases such as hepatitis E and autoimmune hepatitis, attention should be given to minimizing maternal complications with appropriate disease management.

Background
Definition of disease
- Liver diseases unique to pregnancy occur only in association with pregnancy and typically resolve with delivery.
- Coincident liver disease with pregnancy is liver disease that is not unique to pregnancy but whose disease course may be affected by pregnancy.

Disease classification
- Liver diseases unique to pregnancy are classified based on trimester during which they occur, with hyperemesis gravidarum occurring in the first 20 weeks, intrahepatic cholestasis of pregnancy occurring in the second and/or third trimesters, preeclampsia/eclampsia/HELLP after 20 weeks gestation, and acute fatty liver of pregnancy predominantly occurring in the third trimester.
- Coincident liver disease is classified based on serologic evaluation for presence of viral hepatitis (i.e. hepatitis B surface antigen, hepatitis C antibody, hepatitis E antibody), autoimmune liver disease (i.e. positive antinuclear antibody and antismooth muscle antibody), or imaging findings of thrombus (blood clot) or gallstones in the gallbladder.

Incidence/prevalence
- Intrahepatic cholestasis of pregnancy is the most common disease of pregnancy, with prevalence ranging from 0.3–5.6%.
- About 2% of all pregnancies are affected by severe preeclampsia/eclampsia.
- Acute fatty liver of pregnancy is very rare, with an estimated 5 per 100 000 maternities affected.
- The rates of hepatitis B and hepatitis C during pregnancy are estimated to be 105 per 100 000 and 210 per 100 000 deliveries, and are becoming more prevalent over time.

Mount Sinai Expert Guides: Obstetrics and Gynecology, First Edition. Edited by Rhoda Sperling.

© 2020 John Wiley & Sons Ltd. Published 2020 by John Wiley & Sons Ltd.

Companion Website: www.wiley.com/go/sperling/mountsinai/obstetricsandgynecology

Etiology

- Although the cause of liver diseases unique to pregnancy is unknown, risk factors for hyperemesis gravidarum (HG) include molar pregnancy, multiple pregnancies, trophoblastic disease, prior HG, and fetal abnormalities (triploidy, trisomy 21, and hydrops fetalis).
- Risk factors for intrahepatic cholestasis of pregnancy (IHCP) include advanced maternal age, a history of cholestasis secondary to oral contraceptives, and a personal or family history of IHCP.
- The cause of acute fatty liver of pregnancy (AFLP) is thought to be related to fetal deficiency of LCHAD enzyme, which leads to spilling of unmetabolized long-chain fatty acids into the maternal circulation, leading to maternal hepatotoxicity.
- Risk factors for preeclampsia, eclampsia, and HELLP include advanced maternal age, nulliparity, and multiparity.
- The etiology of viral hepatitis during pregnancy is the hepatitis B and hepatitis C viruses that are blood-borne pathogens transmitted from those who are infected to those who are not immune; etiology of autoimmune hepatitis is unknown.

Pathology/pathogenesis

- HG presents with persistent vomiting with loss of 5% or more prepregnancy body weight, dehydration, and ketosis; 50–60% of hospitalized women with this condition will have a mild elevation in aminotransferase levels.
- IHCP presents with persistent pruritus, which involves the entire body including the palms and soles and elevated bile acid levels. Elevated aminotransferase levels and jaundice can also occur.
- Preeclampsia and eclampsia are manifested with new onset hypertension (blood pressure > 140/90) and proteinuria. Severe preeclampsia is characterized by organ dysfunction, including hepatomegaly and hepatocellular injury. Eclampsia is present when grand mal seizures occur.
- HELLP syndrome is characterized by hemolytic anemia, increased liver enzymes, and low platelets.
- Acute fatty liver disease of pregnancy is characterized by microvesicular fatty infiltration of the liver leading to liver failure.
- Chronic liver diseases such as autoimmune hepatitis and hepatitis B can present with liver disease flare characterized by elevated liver enzymes and hepatic failure, especially in the postpartum period.

Predictive/risk factors

Liver disease	Risk factor
Hyperemesis gravidarum	1. Molar pregnancy 2. Multiple pregnancies 3. Trophoblastic disease 4. Prior hyperemesis gravidarum 5. Fetal abnormalities (triploidy, trisomy 21, and hydrops fetalis)
Intrahepatic cholestasis of pregnancy	1. Advanced maternal age 2. History of cholestasis secondary to oral contraceptives 3. Personal or family history of IHCP
Preeclampsia/eclampsia/HELLP	1. Advanced maternal age 2. Nulliparity 3. Multiparity
Acute fatty liver disease of pregnancy	1. Twin pregnancy 2. Low body mass index
Hepatitis B flare	1. Antiviral therapy discontinuation 2. HBeAg positive status

Prevention

> **BOTTOM LINE/CLINICAL PEARLS**
> - No interventions have been demonstrated to prevent the development of liver disease unique to pregnancy.
> - For chronic liver disease, it is imperative to have disease control during pregnancy in order to prevent disease flare or pregnancy complications.

Screening
- There is no screening recommended for liver diseases unique to pregnancy.
- All women are screened for hepatitis B when they present for pregnancy care by checking hepatitis B surface antigen.
- Risk-based screening for hepatitis C is recommended during pregnancy in women with a history of injection drug use, incarceration, HIV, and/or blood transfusion before 1992. Universal screening for hepatitis C is now recommended by the American Association for the Study of Liver Diseases (AASLD), the Infectious Diseases Society of America, the United States Preventative Task Force (USPSTF), and the Centers for Disease Control and Prevention (CDC).

Primary prevention
- Hepatitis B vaccine is universally recommended for all infants born in the US and provides lifelong immunity against hepatitis B.

Secondary prevention
- Active–passive immunoprophylaxis with hepatitis B immunoglobulin and the hepatitis B virus (HBV) vaccination series should be administered to all infants born to HBV-infected mothers to prevent perinatal transmission; treatment of hepatitis B in the mother (if they are not already on treatment) with antiviral therapy during third trimester is indicated in women with high viral loads (>200 000 IU/mL).
- All women with AFLP and their children should have molecular testing for long-chain 3-hydroxyacyl-CoA dehydrogenase.
- There are no interventions that have been shown to prevent reoccurrence of liver diseases unique to pregnancy, including IHCP, HELLP, or hyperemesis gravidarum.

Diagnosis

> **BOTTOM LINE/CLINICAL PEARLS**
> - A careful clinical history should identify if the patient has a prior history of liver disease during prior pregnancies and in general, when the current symptoms began (i.e. during which trimester of pregnancy), medication history, what the symptoms are (pruritus, jaundice, and/or evidence of hepatic decompensation are key symptoms to elicit).
> - A physical exam should involve a careful skin exam to evaluate for jaundice and evidence of excoriations, a neurologic exam (to evaluate for hepatic encephalopathy as manifested by asterixis), a cardiovascular exam including assessment for lower extremity edema, and a gastrointestinal exam including evaluation for hepatosplenomegaly.
> - Laboratory testing should include testing of liver enzymes. If the patient presents with symptoms of pruritus, bile acids should be tested as well.
> - A pregnant patient with abnormal liver enzymes should undergo standard workup as with any nonpregnant individual (see the following chart).
> - An ultrasound of the liver is safe during pregnancy and can evaluate for presence of chronic liver disease, cirrhosis, and/or other etiologies such as liver masses or thrombus in the liver.

Differential diagnosis

Differential diagnosis of abnormal liver tests during pregnancy	Features
Viral Hepatitis	Test with acute viral serologies including hepatitis A IgM, hepatitis B surface antigen and core IgM, hepatitis C antibody, hepatitis E virus IgM
Autoimmune Liver Disease	Can present in women with a history of autoimmune disease/ rheumatologic disorders; laboratory evaluation would include positive antinuclear antibody, antismooth antibody, and serum IgG
Wilson's Disease	Can present with changes in mental status and evidence of Kayser-Fleischer rings on ophthalmologic exam; laboratory evaluation would include low serum ceruloplasmin (<20 mg/dL) and high urinary copper excretion
Budd-Chiari Syndrome	Typically presents with new ascites and abdominal swelling; ultrasound with Doppler would demonstrate thrombus in the hepatic vein
Drug-Induced Liver Injury	Elevated liver enzymes in the setting of ingestion of Tylenol or other new medication or herb.

Typical presentation

- Liver disease in pregnancy presents in different ways depending on etiology. During the first trimester, hyperemesis gravidarum presents with persistent vomiting that may prompt laboratory testing that reveals elevated liver enzymes. During second and third trimester, a patient who presents with significant pruritus, and/or a prior history of IHCP should prompt evaluation for IHCP. Preeclampsia and HELLP present in the late second and third trimesters, and occasionally postpartum, with elevated blood pressures, organ dysfunction, and proteinuria, with the latter occasionally presenting with markedly elevated aspartate transaminase and alanine transaminase (AST and ALT) in the 1000s. AFLP also typically presents in the third trimester with nonspecific symptoms such as nausea, vomiting, and abdominal pain, but with striking aminotransferase elevations and hyperbilirubinemia, as well as evidence of hepatic dysfunction, including encephalopathy, coagulopathy, and hypoglycemia. Chronic liver disease such as autoimmune hepatitis and hepatitis B can present with disease flare, most typically postpartum.

Clinical diagnosis

History

- The clinician should ask the patient about prior history of liver disease, medication use, liver disease that occurred during prior pregnancies, and family history of liver disease during pregnancy and otherwise. A detailed history of symptoms, including timing of onset, development of symptoms since onset, and any medications used for symptom management should be evaluated. Targeted questions about signs of hepatic decompensation, including jaundice, signs of encephalopathy, coagulopathy (i.e. bleeding history), new ascites, and hypoglycemia should be elicited, especially if there is concern for HELLP or AFLP.

Physical examination

- A careful head-to-toe examination should be performed. Neurologic exam, including exam for asterixis should be performed. Eye exam should look for scleral icterus. Skin exam should evaluate for jaundice and/or excoriations related to pruritus. Heart and lung exam should be performed, to evaluate for signs of end-organ dysfunction, and for evidence of volume overload such as lower extremity edema and pulmonary crackles. Abdominal exam should include evaluation for fluid wave if ascites is suspected and for hepatosplenomegaly.

Useful clinical decision rules and calculators
- The Swansea criteria for diagnosis of acute fatty liver of pregnancy require the presence of six or more of the following criteria in the absence of another cause in order to diagnose AFLP:

Vomiting	
Abdominal pain	
Polydypsia/polyuria	
Encephalopathy	
Elevated bilirubin	>14 mmol/l
Hypoglycemia	<4 mmol/l
Elevated urea	>340 mmol/l
Leucocytosis	>11 x 10^6 cells/l
Ascites or bright liver on ultrasound scan	
Elevated transaminases (AST or ALT)	>42 IU/l
Elevated ammonia	>47 mmol/l
Renal impairment; creatinine	>150 mmol/l
Coagulopathy; prothrombin time	>14s or activated partial thromboplastin time (aPTT)>34s
Microvesicular steatosis on liver biopsy	

- The Tennessee System Criteria has been used to diagnose and grade the severity of HELLP
  - Tennessee System
    - AST > 70 IU/L
    - lactate dehydrogenase (LDH) >600 IU/L
    - Platelets < 100x10^9/L

Disease severity classification
- Mississippi Protocol for HELLP states that class 1 requires severe thrombocytopenia (platelets ≤ 50 000/μl), evidence of hepatic dysfunction (AST and/or ALT ≥ 70 IU/l), and evidence suggestive of hemolysis (total serum LDH ≥ 600 IU/l); class 2 requires similar criteria except thrombocytopenia is moderate (>50 000 to ≤ 100 000/μl); and class 3 includes patients with mild thrombocytopenia (platelets > 100 000 but ≤ 150 000/μl), mild hepatic dysfunction (AST and/or ALT ≥ 40 IU/l), and hemolysis (total serum LDH ≥ 600 IU/L).

Laboratory diagnosis
List of diagnostic tests
- Patients with suspected liver disease should have their liver tests checked (see Algorithm 14.1).
- Women with elevated liver tests should undergo workup as with any nonpregnant individual, including laboratory testing to rule out viral hepatitis with anti-hepatitis A virus (HAV) IgM, HBsAg, hepatitis E IgM, and herpes simplex virus polymerase chain reaction (HSV PCR).
- All pregnant women should be screened for hepatitis B with hepatitis B surface antigen. If positive, a hepatitis B DNA level should be checked prior to third trimester.
- All pregnant women should be screened for hepatitis C with hepatitis C antibody screening and reflex hepatitis C RNA (hepatitis C viral load).

Algorithm 14.1 Workup of abnormal liver test in pregnant woman

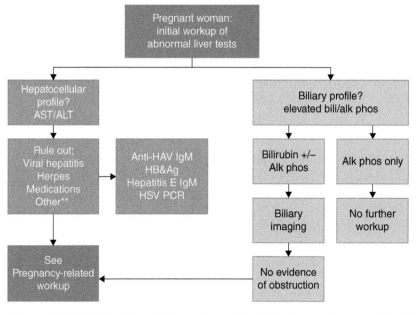

Taken from Tran et al. 2016. **Other differential diagnosis to consider if clinically appropriate: AIH, Wilson disease.

- Bile acid concentration should be checked if suspicion for IHCP.
- Complete blood count should be checked if HELLP is suspected to evaluate for thrombocytopenia.

List of imaging techniques
- Ultrasound is safe and the preferred imaging modality to assess patients with abnormal liver tests suggestive of biliary tract disease.
- Magnetic resonance imaging with gadolinium can be used in the second and third trimesters.
- Computed tomography scans carry a higher risk of teratogenesis but may be used if necessary with minimized radiation protocols.
- Upper endoscopy is safe but should be deferred until the second trimester if possible, with use of meperidine and propofol for sedation.

Potential pitfalls/common errors made regarding diagnosis of disease
- HG can lead to elevated liver enzymes.
- IHCP can present with elevated liver enzymes before elevated bile acids and can be confused for HELLP/AFLP.
- Do not assume it is liver disease unique to pregnancy – it can be liver disease unrelated to pregnancy (i.e. chronic liver disease) that is coincident with pregnancy.

Treatment
Treatment rationale
- Intrahepatic cholestasis of pregnancy: first-line therapy is ursodeoxycholic acid (UDCA) at 10–15 mg/kg maternal body weight; early delivery at 37 weeks
- Eclampsia: expectant management and delivery if possible
- HELLP: emergent delivery; possible liver transplantation for hepatic decompensation
- AFLP: prompt delivery and supportive care

When to hospitalize

- First trimester
  - Severe hyperemesis gravidarum with evidence of dehydration
- Second trimester/third trimester
  - Severe preeclampsia
  - Eclampsia
  - HELLP
- All trimesters: Elevated liver enzymes of unknown etiology with evidence of jaundice or hepatic decompensation (ascites, variceal bleed, hepatic encephalopathy)

Managing the hospitalized patient

- Supportive care
- Workup for elevated liver enzymes
- Prompt delivery if indicated
- Evaluation for liver transplantation if evidence of hepatic decompensation
- See Algorithm 14.2

Table of treatment

Treatment	Comments
Conservative	Supportive care in patients with preeclampsia, eclampsia

Medical
  UDCA
  Tenofovir
	Safe during pregnancy

Surgical (list techniques) Liver transplantation	Liver transplantation can be considered after delivery if indicated
Other	

Prevention/management of complications

- Tenofovir has been associated with renal insufficiency with prolonged exposure, although short duration treatment during pregnancy would likely not lead to this.

Algorithm 14.2 Management/treatment of elevated liver enzymes

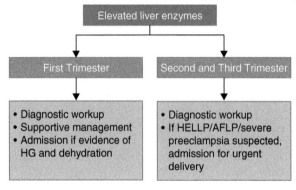

CLINICAL PEARLS
- Although hyperemesis gravidarum does not progress to fulminant liver failure, supportive care is crucial to decrease risk of adverse outcomes such as low birth weight and prematurity.
- Intrahepatic cholestasis of pregnancy should be treated with UDCA and serum bile acids monitored weekly to evaluate treatment response; it has a 40–60% rate of recurrence so should be suspected in subsequent pregnancies.
- Early recognition and prompt delivery should be performed in patients with AFLP and HELLP.

Prognosis

BOTTOM LINE/CLINICAL PEARLS
- Hyperemesis gravidarum is not associated with any permanent liver damage.
- Intrahepatic cholestasis of pregnancy is associated with an increased risk of fetal complications, particularly if bile acids are over 100 umol/L and spontaneous preterm delivery if bile acids are over 40 umol/L; typically improves within 6 weeks post delivery; is associated with the development of hepatobiliary disease later in life.
- Preeclampsia/eclampsia/HELLP, associated with up to 15% mortality
  - When associated with hepatic rupture, is associated with a 56–76% maternal mortality and 62–77% fetal mortality
- AFLP – with appropriate treatment, is associated with <10% maternal mortality, 23% fetal mortality.
- Liver diseases unique to pregnancy, including cholestasis of pregnancy and preeclampsia/HELLP, are associated with increased risk of recurrence in future pregnancies.

Natural history of untreated disease
- If left untreated, AFLP and HELLP are associated with poor pregnancy outcome and high mortality.

Prognosis for treated patients
- When treated and urgent delivery achieve, prognosis is significantly improved.

Follow-up tests and monitoring
- Liver enzymes should be rechecked within 6 weeks post delivery to confirm resolution.
- Patients with pregnancy-specific liver diseases should be monitored in future pregnancies due to risk of recurrence.

Reading list
Ma K, Berger D, Reau N. Liver diseases during pregnancy. *Clin Liver Dis* 2019;23(2):345-61.
Orekondy N, Cafardi J, Kushner T, et al. HCV in women and pregnancy. *Hepatology* 2019;70(5):1836-40.
Tran T, Ahn J, Reau N. ACG clinical guideline: liver disease and pregnancy. *Am J Gastroenterol* 2016 Feb;111(2): 176-94.

Guidelines
National society guidelines

Title	Source	Date/URL
HCV in pregnancy	American Association for the Study of Liver Diseases, Infectious Diseases Society of America	April 2018 https://www.hcvguidelines.org/unique-populations/pregnancy
Screening for hepatitis C virus infection in adolescents and adults	US Preventive Services Task Force	March 2020 https://jamanetwork.com/journals/jama/fullarticle/2762186

(Continued)

(Continued)

Title	Source	Date/URL
Hepatitis B in pregnancy screening, treatment and prevention of vertical transmission	Society for Maternal-Fetal Medicine (SMFM)	January 2016 https://www.sciencedirect.com/science/article/pii/S0002937815012144
Liver disease and pregnancy	American College of Gastroenterology	February 2016 https://journals.lww.com/ajg/Fulltext/2016/02000/ACG_Clinical_Guideline__Liver_Disease_and.15.aspx

Additional material for this chapter can be found online at:
www.wiley.com/go/sperling/mountsinai/obstetricsandgynecology

This includes advice for patients.

CHAPTER 15

Thyroid Disease and Pregnancy

Carol Levy[1], Danielle Brooks[1], and Keerti Murari[2]

[1] Department of Medicine – Division of Endocrinology, Diabetes, and Metabolism, Icahn School of Medicine at Mount Sinai, New York, NY
[2] Department of Medicine – Division of Endocrinology and Metabolism, Yale School of Medicine, New Haven, CT

OVERALL BOTTOM LINE

- Thyroid disease is the second most common endocrine disorder affecting women of reproductive age.
- Symptoms of thyroid dysfunction can mimic the symptoms of pregnancy resulting in difficulty identifying the disease in pregnant women.
- Untreated thyroid disease results in increased risk of miscarriage, placental abruption, hypertensive disorders, and fetal growth restriction.
- In women with hypothyroidism, levothyroxine is administered to achieve a serum thyroid stimulating hormone (TSH) <2.5 during the first trimester and < 3 during the second and third trimester. For women with hyperthyroidism, antithyroid medications are used with a goal of maintaining serum-free thyroxine level in the upper third of normal range.
- Postpartum thyroiditis is the most common form of postpartum thyroid dysfunction and may present as hyper- or hypothyroidism.

Background

Definition of disease

- Overt hypothyroidism is defined as an elevated TSH and decreased serum-free thyroxine (FT_4) concentration outside the trimester specific ranges.
- Hyperthyroidism is defined as elevated FT_4 and suppressed TSH.

Incidence/prevalence

- 2–3% of healthy, nonpregnant women of childbearing age have an elevated TSH with higher prevalences observed in iodine deficient regions.
- Incidence of diagnosis during pregnancy:
  - Overt hypothyroidism 0.3–0.5%
  - Subclinical hypothyroidism 2–3%
  - Postpartum thyroiditis 1.1–21.1%
  - Hyperthyroidism 0.2%
- Prevalence of Graves disease ranges from 0.1 to 1%.

Economic impact

- Worldwide, cretinism and infant mental retardation resulting from maternal hypothyroidism and iodine deficiency can lead to devastating effects on families with significant costs on health systems.

Mount Sinai Expert Guides: Obstetrics and Gynecology, First Edition. Edited by Rhoda Sperling.
© 2020 John Wiley & Sons Ltd. Published 2020 by John Wiley & Sons Ltd.
Companion Website: www.wiley.com/go/sperling/mountsinai/obstetricsandgynecology

Etiology
- Causes of hypothyroidism in pregnancy or postpartum:
  - Hashimoto's thyroiditis
  - Postpartum thyroiditis
  - Iodine deficiency
  - Iatrogenic hypothyroidism
  - *Other uncommon causes:* Central hypothyroidism, thyroid resistance, isolated hypothyroxinemia
- Causes of hyperthyroidism in pregnancy:
  - Graves disease
  - Gestational transient thyrotoxicosis
  - *Other uncommon causes:* hydatidiform mole, multinodular toxic goiter, toxic adenoma, subacute thyroiditis, struma ovarii

Pathology/pathogenesis
- **Hashimoto's thyroiditis:** Autoimmune mediated destruction of the thyroid gland resulting in a low thyroid state that is the most frequent cause of hypothyroidism in iodine sufficient regions.
- **Postpartum thyroiditis:** A destructive thyroiditis induced by an autoimmune mechanism involving inflammatory autoimmune destruction of the thyroid gland within 1 year after parturition after the relative immunosuppressed state of pregnancy. This can result in transient hyperthyroidism, hypothyroidism, or both followed by recovery.
- **Iodine deficiency:** Iodine deficiency results in reduction of thyroid hormone production as it is an essential substrate.
- **Central hypothyroidism:** Insufficient stimulation of a normal gland due to disease affecting the hypothalamic pituitary axis or defect in the TSH structure.
- **Thyroid resistance:** Reduced activity of thyroid hormone at tissue level despite normal or increased levels of production. Usually results from rare anomalies of thyroid hormone metabolism and nuclear signaling.
- **Graves disease:** An autoimmune condition against the thyroid-stimulating hormone receptor (TSHR). TSHR antibodies (TRAb) bind to the TSH receptor, leading to overstimulation of thyrocytes with increased production of thyroid hormone.
- **Gestational transient thyrotoxicosis:** High concentrations of human chorionic gonadotropin (hCG) stimulate TSH receptor due to similar structure between hCG and TSH.

Prevention

> **BOTTOM LINE/CLINICAL PEARLS**
> - Iodine supplementation is critical in preventing maternal hypothyroidism in iodine insufficient regions.
> - Women who are at high risk for thyroid disease should be screened at their initial prenatal visit and further testing depends on their risk factors.
> - Women with hypothyroidism prior to pregnancy should have their levothyroxine increased by 25–30% as soon as pregnancy is suspected.

Screening
- There is an increased thyroid hormone requirement to maintain a euthyroid state in pregnancy. During pregnancy, the production of FT_4 increases by 40–50% to maintain a euthyroid state. The increased requirement for FT_4 occurs early as 4–6 weeks during the first trimester, gradually increasing until 20 weeks gestation.
- The thyroid gland increases in size by 18% and is thought to be due to thyrotropic effect of β-HCG.

Table 15.1 **Trimester-specific reference ranges for common thyroid tests.**

Test	Nonpregnant	First trimester	Second trimester	Third trimester
Thyroid stimulating hormone (mIU per L)	0.3 to 4.3	0.1 to 2.5	0.2 to 3.0	0.3 to 3.0
Thyroxine-binding globulin (mg per dL)	1.3 to 3.0	1.8 to 3.2	2.8 to 4.0	2.6 to 4.2
Thyroxine, free (ng per dL)	0.8 to 1.7	0.8 to 1.2	0.6 to 1.0	0.5 to 0.8
Thyroxine, total (mcg per dL)	5.4 to 11.7	6.5 to 10.1	7.5 to 10.3	6.3 to 9.7
Triiodothyronine, free (pg per mL)	2.4 to 4.2	4.1 to 4.4	4.0 to 4.2	Not reported
Triiodothyronine, total (ng per dL)	77 to 135	97 to 149	117 to 169	123 to 162

- In pregnant women, reference ranges for TSH are lower due to cross-reactivity of the alpha subunit of hCG with the TSH receptor (Table 15.1).
- Screening is recommended at the initial prenatal visit or once pregnancy is confirmed for women at high risk of thyroid disease.
- Risk factors:
  - History of thyroid disease and/or current thyroid therapy
  - History of hemithyroidectomy, radioactive iodine, amiodarone, or lithium use
  - Personal history of autoimmune disorder such as type 1 diabetes mellitus (DM), high dose neck radiation, or postpartum thyroid dysfunction
  - History of infertility, preterm delivery, pregnancy loss, or previous delivery of infant with thyroid disease
  - Presence of goiter or known thyroid antibody positivity
  - Family history of autoimmune thyroid disease or goiter
  - Age > 30 years
  - Morbid obesity (body mass index $\geq 40 \, kg/m^2$)
  - Residing in iodine deficient region (Alexander et al. 2017)
- Women who are euthyroid but thyroid peroxidase antibody (TPO) Ab positive, post-hemithyroidectomy, or treated previously with radioactive iodine should be monitored with serum TSH every 4 weeks until midgestation and at least once near 30 weeks gestation.
- Women with type 1 DM with thyroglobulin or TPO-Ab are at increased risk of postpartum thyroiditis and should be screened at 3 and 6 months postpartum using TSH even when asymptomatic.

Primary prevention
- Adequate iodine supplementation is critical in preventing maternal hypothyroidism. Maternal iodine deficiency remains problematic in developing nations and is the leading cause of hypothyroidism worldwide.

Secondary prevention
- Euthyroid women who are taking stable dose of levothyroxine should increase their medication by two additional doses per week (25–30%) after a missed menstrual cycle or positive home pregnancy test.
- Thyroid function monitoring during pregnancy should occur at the first prenatal visit and every 4–8 weeks thereafter.
- Increased doses of thyroid hormone are needed in 50–80% of women, with some requiring dose increases of 50%.
- Radioactive iodine treatment at least 6 months prior to conception can reduce the risk of maternal hyperthyroidism and prevent fetal adverse outcomes such as radiation exposure and cretinism. Treatment does not prevent the transfer of maternal thyroid antibodies and it should not cause infertility.

Table 15.2 Changes in thyroid function tests during normal pregnancy and in pregnant women with thyroid disease.

Maternal condition	Thyroid stimulating hormone	Free thyroxine	Total thyroxine	Triiodothyronine
Normal Pregnancy	Decrease	No change	Increase	Increase
Hypothyroidism	Increase	Decrease	Decrease	Decrease or no change
Hyperthyroidism	Decrease	Increase	Increase	Increase or no change

Diagnosis

> **BOTTOM LINE/CLINICAL PEARLS**
> - A complete medical history including screening for risk factors and symptoms of thyroid disease.
> - A thorough physical exam should be conducted and the thyroid should be evaluated for nodularity or increased size.
> - To confirm the diagnosis obtain a serum TSH and free T_4.
> - See Table 15.2.

Differential diagnosis

Differential diagnosis for hypothyroidism	Features
Hashimoto's thyroiditis	• Autoimmune disease that may or may not be associated with a goiter. • Serum TPO-Ab (thyroid peroxidase antibodies) are usually present with an elevated TSH and most commonly a low FT_4.
Postpartum thyroiditis	• Abnormal TSH level within the first 12 months postpartum in previously euthyroid patients. No associated toxic thyroid nodules or thyrotoxin receptor antibodies. • Presents as symptoms of fatigue, which is common after delivery. • The clinical course varies greatly and is typically transient with 25% of patients presenting with symptoms of hyperthyroidism followed by hypothyroidism, 43% with isolated hypothyroidism, and 32% with isolated hyperthyroidism. • Radioactive iodine uptake scan, to help distinguish postpartum thyroiditis from Graves disease, is contraindicated in breastfeeding women.
Iatrogenic hypothyroidism	• Physical exam for thyroidectomy scar or history of Graves disease treated with radioactive iodine can help distinguish this etiology.
Iodine deficiency	• History of dietary intake and without thyroid antibodies can help distinguish this condition.
Central hypothyroidism	• Labs notable for inappropriately low TSH and low FT_4 and total T_4
Thyroid resistance	• Labs notable for elevated TSH, free, and total T_4 without clinical features of hyperthyroidism

Differential diagnosis for hyperthyroidism	Features
Graves disease	• Often diagnosed before pregnancy • May see goiter or ophthalmopathy • Not associated with hyperemesis • Often have positive TSH-receptor antibodies

Differential diagnosis for hyperthyroidism	Features
Gestational transient thyrotoxicosis	• Associated with hyperemesis • No goiter or ophthalmopathy • Negative TSH-receptor and TPO antibodies
Hydatidiform mole	• May present with hyperemesis gravidarum with clinical hyperthyroid signs later in pregnancy • Very elevated hCG levels
Subclinical hyperthyroidism	• Low TSH with normal serum FT_4 and T_3 • Often artificial effect due to hCG-induced suppression of TSH • Usually no symptoms or signs of hyperthyroidism

Typical presentation
- Women with thyroid disease may present with symptoms that are common in pregnancy.
- Thyroid disease can have manifestations in almost every organ system. Symptoms are driven by the degree of hormone deficiency or excess and are independent of the underlying etiology.

Clinical diagnosis
History
- Patients should be screened for risk factors for thyroid disease (See section on Screening)
- Providers should conduct a complete review of systems inquiring about changes in exercise tolerance, fatigue, weight changes, mood changes, palpitations, angina, shortness of breath, visual changes, lower extremity swelling, muscle weakness, hair or skin changes, appetite changes, constipation or diarrhea, hyperemesis, tremors, and altered temperature sensitivity.

Physical examination

Physical examination	Hypothyroidism	Hyperthyroidism
Constitutional	Weight gain Slowed speech	Weight loss Diaphoresis Fatigue
HEENT	Loss of lateral third of eyebrow Enlargement and/or nodular thyroid	Goiter Stare, lid lag Infiltrative ophthalmopathy (specific to Graves disease: includes periorbital edema, injected conjunctiva, exophthalmos)
Cardiovascular	Bradycardia Narrowed pulse pressure Weak distal pulses	Tachycardia Hypertension
Respiratory	Tachypnea, particularly with exertion Hypoventilation	Dyspnea
Gastrointestinal	Abdominal distention Ascites, in rare cases	Abdominal pain

(Continued)

(*Continued*)

Physical examination	Hypothyroidism	Hyperthyroidism
Neurologic	Memory impairment Lethargy and somnolence Reduced hearing and visual acuity Slow body movements Ataxia Slow reflexes with delayed relaxation phase	Tremors Brisk reflexes
Psychiatric	Paranoia Depression	Depression Anxiety Restlessness Inattention Emotional lability
Musculoskeletal	Reduced muscle mass	Proximal muscle weakness
Skin	Boggy, nonpitting edema of skin along face, hands, feet, supraclavicular fossa, and pretibial area Pale, cool, dry and coarse skin; poor wound healing Easy bruising Dry and brittle head and body hair Loss of skin pigmentation	Pretibial myxedema (violaceous indurated skin) Warm, moist skin Friable hair

Laboratory diagnosis
List of diagnostic tests
- TSH, free T_4 and T_3: Population and trimester specific reference ranges for serum TSH, free T_4 and T_3 during pregnancy should be used when diagnosing thyroid disease. Current guideline reference ranges are defined for healthy TPO-Ab negative pregnant women without iodine deficiency (see Tables 15.1 and 15.2).
- Thyroid peroxidase antibody (TPO-Ab): Greater risk of adverse events is associated with TPO-Ab positive status. Presence of TPO-Ab is associated with a high risk of developing hypothyroidism.
- TRab testing: Indications include patients with untreated or treated hyperthyroidism in pregnancy, history of Graves disease treated with radioiodine or thyroidectomy, or delivery of an infant with hyperthyroidism. Serum TRAb levels three times the upper limit of normal is an indication for close monitoring to prevent fetal loss or fetal hyperthyroidism.

List of imaging techniques
- Radionuclide scintigraphy and radioiodine uptake testing are **contraindicated** in pregnancy.
- Ultrasound can be used to evaluate thyroid nodules. Fine-needle aspiration is used if suspicious features are present or if > 1 cm.

Potential pitfalls/common errors made regarding diagnosis of disease
- Laboratory diagnosis of thyroid disease can be difficult if pregnancy-specific reference ranges are not listed.
- Healthy pregnant women may also have elevated FT_4 levels.

Treatment
Treatment rationale
Hypothyroidism
- Pregnant women with overt hypothyroidism should receive levothyroxine treatment; TPO-Ab positive women with subclinical hypothyroidism should also receive treatment.

- Isolated hypothyroxinemia and subclinical hypothyroidism with negative TPO-Ab do not routinely require treatment.
- Levothyroxine (synthetic FT_4) is the mainstay of treatment with incremental dose adjustments based on the TSH elevation. Avoid synthetic T_3, which does not cross the placenta.
- Serum TSH should be measured every 4–6 weeks until 20 weeks gestation or until patient is on a stable dose; remeasure again at 24–28 weeks' and 32–34 weeks' gestation.
- Levothyroxine dose should be adjusted to maintain TSH < 2.5 during the first trimester and < 3.0 during second and third trimesters.

Hyperthyroidism
- Propylthiouracil is recommended during the first trimester to minimize risk of teratogenicity. Methimazole is recommended after the first trimester to reduce the risk of maternal hepatotoxicity.
- The goal of treatment is a FT_4 in the upper one third of normal range for nonpregnant women using the lowest doses possible of antithyroid medication.
- Monitor serum TSH/FT_4 every 2–4 weeks until a stable dose is reached, then monitor levels every 4–6 weeks.

When to hospitalize
- **Myxedema coma** is a severe hypothyroid state associated with a high mortality rate is extremely rare with only a few case reports in pregnant women.
- **Thyroid storm** is a rare, life-threatening condition of decompensated thyrotoxicosis. Symptoms include fever, altered mental status, tachyarrhythmias, heart failure, nausea, vomiting, diarrhea, and hepatotoxicity.

Managing the hospitalized patient
- Oral levothyroxine can be administered intravenously at half the oral dose for dose equivalency (i.e. PO to IV, 2:1) for hospitalized patients unable to take PO.
- **Myxedema coma**
  - Treatment consists of stress dose steroids followed by high dose IV T_4 and IV T_3.
  - Supportive care measures include intravenous fluid resuscitation, correction of hypothermia with passive rewarming.
- **Management of thyroid storm**
  - Supportive care, IV fluids
  - PO or IV propranolol or IV esmolol for tachyarrhythmias
  - Higher dose antithyroid drugs +/- high dose hydrocortisone or dexamethasone
  - PO potassium iodide 1 hour *after* antithyroid drugs are initiated **rarely** considered if the risks to the mother outweighed the risks of iodine to the fetus.

Table of treatment
Treatment of hypothyroidism

Treatment	Comments
Medical	
Levothyroxine (synthetic free T_4) • 1.7mcg/kg/day (range 100–125 mcg daily)	Common adverse reactions: headache, insomnia, irritability, hyperhidrosis, palpitations, increased appetite, weight loss Goal TSH: • First Trimester: <2.5 • Second and Third Trimester < 3.0

Treatment of hyperthyroidism

Treatment	Comments
Medical:	
1. **Propylthiouracil** (PTU): preferred agent in first trimester (50–100 mg administered BID or TID) 2. **Methimazole** (MMI): preferred agent after first trimester (5–30 mg/day) 3. **Propranolol**: to reduce symptoms (20–40 mg q8h) 4. **Metoprolol**: to reduce symptoms (100 mg daily or BID)	Common adverse reactions for both PTU and MMI include rash, GI upset, and fever. **Propylthiouracil** is associated with hepatotoxicity. **Methimazole** is associated with dose-related agranulocytosis. Routine monitoring of complete blood count is not recommended. Reports of teratogenicity including aplasia cutis congenita, choanal atresia, tracheoesophageal fistula, omphalocele, and developmental delay. β-**blocking agents** may be associated with neonatal bradycardia and hypoglycemia, small for gestational age infants.
Surgical	
- **Total or subtotal thyroidectomy**	**Indications include** antithyroid medication allergy, lack of response to recommended doses, medication noncompliance or intolerance, goiter with compressive symptoms. Preferred in second trimester.

Prevention/management of complications

- Overly aggressive treatment with levothyroxine can lead to a suppressed TSH. Care should be taken to not overtreat hypothyroidism with routine monitoring of serum TSH levels and for clinical symptoms of hyperthyroidism.
- Obtain baseline liver function tests (LFTs) in patients starting propylthiouracil. Patients developing symptoms of jaundice, abdominal pain, nausea, dark urine, or light stools require LFTs. Discontinue PTU if transaminases are 3x upper limit of reference range, monitor LFTs weekly.

> **CLINICAL PEARLS**
> - Levothyroxine is the mainstay of treatment for hypothyroidism in pregnancy and should be adjusted for a goal TSH is < 2.5 during the first trimester and < 3.0 during the second and third trimester.
> - Patients on levothyroxine should be monitored clinically for signs of hyperthyroidism.
> - In hyperthyroid patients, use propylthiouracil in the first trimester, methimazole after the first trimester, and beta-blockers for symptom control.

Prognosis

> **BOTTOM LINE/CLINICAL PEARLS**
> - There is a reduced risk of adverse pregnancy outcomes when high-risk patients are screened and treated for thyroid disease.
> - Overt maternal hypothyroidism is associated with premature birth, low birth weight, pregnancy loss, gestational hypertension, and lower IQ in offspring.
> - Poorly controlled hyperthyroidism is associated with pregnancy loss, premature birth, stillbirth, low birth weight, preeclampsia, hypertension, thyroid storm, and maternal heart failure.

Prognosis for treated patients

- No evidence suggests that treated overt and subclinical hypothyroidism during pregnancy is associated with obstetrical complications.
- Women with thyroid disease are at increased risk of developing gestational hypertension.
- Pregnant women with subclinical hypothyroidism in the first trimester treated with levothyroxine had decreased rates of miscarriage and premature delivery.

- Isolated hypothyroxinemia in the first trimester of pregnancy is associated with reduced IQ among off-spring.
- Women with untreated overt hypothyroidism during pregnancy have a 60% risk of fetal loss. This risk increases proportionally with TSH elevation.
- TPO-Ab positive women with subclinical hypothyroidism have an increased risk of preterm delivery and pregnancy loss.

Follow-up tests and monitoring
- After delivery, levothyroxine should be decreased to the prepregnancy dosage over a 4-week period. Repeat TSH levels 4–6 weeks postpartum.
- Women with a history of postpartum thyroiditis are at increased risk of permanent hypothyroidism and should be screened annually. Women with a history of Graves disease in pregnancy should have TSH and FT_4 checked 6 weeks postpartum. Monitor every 4 months if thyroid function tests (TFTs) are normal, more frequently if abnormal.

Reading list
Amino N, Tanizawa O, Mori H, et al. Aggravation of thyrotoxicosis in early pregnancy and after delivery in Graves' disease. *J Clin Endocrinol Metab* 1982;55(1):108-12.

Carney LA, Quinlan JD, West JM. Thyroid disease in pregnancy. *Am Fam Physician* 2014;89(4):273-78.

Cooper DS, Laurberg P. Hyperthyroidism in pregnancy. *Lancet Diabetes Endocrinol* 2013;1(3):238-49.

Davies TF, Laurberg P, Bahn RS. Hyperthyroid disorders. In: *Williams textbook of endocrinology*. 13th ed. Philadelphia: Elsevier; 2016:369-415.

Hershman JM. Physiological and pathological aspects of the effect of human chorionic gonadotropin on the thyroid. *Best Pract Res Clin Endocrinol Metab* 2004;18(2):249-65.

Krassas G, Karras SN, Pontikides N. Thyroid disease during pregnancy: a number of important issues. *Hormones* 2015;14(1):59-69.

Latif R, Morsed SA, Zaidi M, et al. The thyroid-stimulating hormone receptor: impact of thyroid-stimulating hormone and thyroid-stimulating hormone receptor antibodies on multimerization, cleavage, and signaling. *Endocrinol Metab Clin N Am* 2009;38 (2):319-41.

Mestman, JH. Hyperthyroidism in pregnancy. *Clin Obstet Gynecol* 1997;40(1):45-64.

Patil-Sisodia K, Mestman JH. Graves hyperthyroidism and pregnancy: a clinical update. *Curr Opin Endocrinol Diabetes Obes* 2010;19(5):394-401.

Ross DS, Burch HB, Cooper DS, et al. 2016 American Thyroid Association guidelines for diagnosis and management of hyperthyroidism and other causes of thyrotoxicosis. *Thyroid* 2016;26(10):1343-1421.

Sisson JC, et al. American Thyroid Association Taskforce on Radioiodine Safety. Radiation safety in the treatment of patients with thyroid diseases by radioiodine 131I: Practice Recommendations of the American Thyroid Association. *Thyroid* 2011;21(4):335-46

Suggested website
Thyroid Disease in Pregnancy. https://www.thyroid.org/thyroid-disease-pregnancy

Guidelines
National society guidelines

Title	Source	Date /full reference
Management of thyroid dysfunction during pregnancy and post-partum: an Endocrine Society clinical practice guideline.	Endocrine Society	De Groot L, et al. Management of thyroid dysfunction during pregnancy and postpartum: an Endocrine Society clinical practice guideline. *J Clin Endocrinol Metab* 2012;7(8): 2543-65.
2017 Guidelines of the American Thyroid Association for the diagnosis and management of thyroid disease during pregnancy and the postpartum	American Thyroid Association	Alexander EK, et al. 2017 Guidelines of the American Thyroid Association for the diagnosis and management of thyroid disease during pregnancy and the postpartum. *Thyroid* 2017;27(3):315-89.

Evidence

Type of evidence	Title and comment	Date/URL
Systematic review	Interventions for clinical and subclinical hypothyroidism in pregnancy. Comment: Systematic review that intended to identify interventions used in the management of hypothyroidism and subclinical hypothyroidism in pregnancy and to ascertain the impact of these interventions on important maternal, fetal, neonatal and childhood outcomes.	2010 https://www.ncbi.nlm.nih.gov/pubmed/20614463
Randomized controlled trial	Universal screening versus case finding for detection and treatment of thyroid hormonal dysfunction during pregnancy. Comment: 4562 pregnant women were randomized to universal screening versus case-finding in Italy. No significant differences in adverse pregnancy outcomes were found between the groups. This study suggests that universal screening for thyroid disease is not necessary to reduce negative pregnancy outcomes.	2010 https://doi.org/10.1210/jc.2009-2009
Cohort study	Outcomes of pregnancy complicated with hyperthyroidism: a cohort study. . Comment: This study looked at outcomes of 203 pregnant women with hyperthyroidism. They demonstrated that hyperthyroidism is associated with an increased risk of gestational hypertension, fetal growth restriction, and preterm birth.	2011 https://www.ncbi.nlm.nih.gov/pubmed/20087627
Retrospective review	Increased need for thyroxine during pregnancy in women with primary hypothyroidism. Comment: This retrospective review of 12 women with hypothyroidism on levothyroxine demonstrated the need for thyroxine increases during pregnancy. This study also reaffirms the need for TFT monitoring throughout gestation and after delivery with adjustment of thyroxine to maintain a euthyroid state.	2001 http://www.nejm.org/doi/full/10.1056/NEJM200106073442302#t=article

---

Additional material for this chapter can be found online at:
www.wiley.com/go/sperling/mountsinai/obstetricsandgynecology

This includes a case study, advice for patients, and ICD codes.

CHAPTER 16

Perinatal Mood and Anxiety Disorders

Matthew Dominguez[1], Laudy Burgos[2], and Veerle Bergink[3]

[1] Department of Psychiatry, Icahn School of Medicine at Mount Sinai, New York, NY
[2] Department of Social Work Services – MSH, NERA-Undergraduate Behavioral Health Fellowship Program, Icahn School of Medicine at Mount Sinai, New York, NY
[3] Department of Psychiatry and Department of Obstetrics, Gynecology and Reproductive Science, Icahn School of Medicine at Mount Sinai, New York, NY

> **OVERALL BOTTOM LINE**
> - Perinatal mood and anxiety disorders (PMADs) are highly prevalent during pregnancy and the postpartum period.
> - There is evidence that screening for PMADs alone can have clinical benefits, although initiation of treatment or referral to mental healthcare providers offers maximum benefit.
> - Both behavioral and pharmacologic interventions are effective treatment options.

Background

Definition of disease
- Depressive disorders are characterized by abnormal low mood.
- Bipolar disorder is a severe mood disorder characterized by periods of depression and periods of abnormally elevated mood.
- Anxiety disorders include generalized anxiety disorder, panic disorder, and social anxiety disorder.

Disease classification
- Any mental health disorder with symptoms specifically during pregnancy or during the first year postpartum may be referred to with one of the following specifiers:
  - with peripartum onset
  - with peripartum exacerbation

Incidence/prevalence
- Depressive and anxiety disorders affect 10–20% of patients. Mood and anxiety disorders frequently co-occur and may be complicated by substance use or psychotic symptoms.
- Bipolar disorders have a prevalence of 2–5%. These women are at extremely high risk for postpartum depression and postpartum psychosis.

Economic impact
- There is an approximate cost to society of $32 000 per mother with PMAD over a 6-year time frame with about 60% attributed to maternal outcomes and the remaining 40% to child outcomes.

Etiology
- PMADs are defined by symptom clusters in the *Diagnostic and Statistical Manual of Mental Disorders*, 5th edition (DSM-5) but cannot be classified by pathogenesis.

Mount Sinai Expert Guides: Obstetrics and Gynecology, First Edition. Edited by Rhoda Sperling.
© 2020 John Wiley & Sons Ltd. Published 2020 by John Wiley & Sons Ltd.
Companion Website: www.wiley.com/go/sperling/mountsinai/obstetricsandgynecology

Pathology/pathogenesis
- Familial aggregations suggest a genetic susceptibility.
- Poor sleep during the peripartum period can prompt onset or exacerbation of PMAD symptoms.
- Estrogen and progesterone fluctuations affect cognitive function, circadian rhythms, and mood, which might increase the risk for development of PMADs.
- Immune dysregulation has been linked to the acute onset of mood episodes postpartum.
- Conditions such as autoimmune thyroiditis, anemia, and infection can mimic PMADs and exacerbate their symptoms.

Predictive/risk factors

Risk factor
A personal history of mood or anxiety disorder
Family psychiatric history
Obstetric complications
Early life trauma (maltreatment, abuse)
Personality factors
Unplanned pregnancy
Lack of social support from partner or family
Substance abuse
Financial problems, unemployment
Teen pregnancy
Congenital malformations/neonatal complications

Prevention

> **BOTTOM LINE/CLINICAL PEARLS**
> - The US Preventive Services Task Force issued a statement in 2019 endorsing the benefits of psychotherapy in the prevention of perinatal mood and anxiety disorders.

Screening
- The Edinburgh Postnatal Depression Scale (EPDS) has been validated for screening during both pregnancy and the postpartum period. http://perinatology.com/calculators/Edinburgh%20Depression%20Scale.htm
- Patient Health Questionnaire (PHQ2 and PHQ9) have been validated for general screening of depressive and anxiety symptoms. https://www.hiv.uw.edu/page/mental-health-screening/phq-2

Primary prevention
- Standardized preconception counseling or counseling at the first pregnancy visit can be performed, including review of psychiatric history, alterations in mental health symptoms, and significant life changes.
- There is evidence that screening for PMAD during pregnancy and the postpartum period can have clinical benefits.

- Resource assessment and optimization can be provided via social worker referral to aid with issues such as insurance coverage, housing/financial instability, and interventions for substance use or domestic/intimate partner violence.

Secondary prevention
- Treatment guidelines do not provide guidance about continuation of antidepressant medication (AD) due to lack of evidence regarding risk of peripartum relapse.
- Risks and benefits of ADs, as well as the risks of untreated PMADs should be thoroughly discussed with patients so that they may make informed and individualized decisions.
- If patients decide to continue antidepressant medication, guidelines advise against switching to another antidepressant.
- For patients who decide to discontinue antidepressants, psychotherapy can be offered as an effective alternative treatment option.
- Patients with a history of bipolar disorder or postpartum psychosis should be referred to a psychiatrist. Initiate pharmacologic prophylaxis, preferably with lithium or antipsychotics, immediately after delivery for relapse prevention.

Diagnosis

> **BOTTOM LINE/CLINICAL PEARLS**
> - Diagnosis of perinatal mood and anxiety disorders are established by psychiatric evaluation, using DSM-5 criteria as guideline.
> - On exam, providers should briefly screen for mental health symptoms such as depressed mood or excessive worrying, with observation of concerning signs like poor self-care, lack of engagement, sad/anxious affect, or significant alterations in behavior.
> - Medical causes of mood and anxiety disorders such as medication side effects, anemia, metabolic derangement, thyroid dysfunction, and infection should be ruled out before diagnosing a PMAD.
> - Symptoms of mania or psychosis or concern for risk of harm to self or others should prompt acute referral to a psychiatrist.

Differential diagnosis

Differential diagnosis	Features
Postpartum blues	Mild and transient mood/anxiety symptoms in the first days of postpartum period.
Postpartum psychosis	Acute symptoms of mania or psychosis with an onset < 6 weeks postpartum.
Medical condition	Medication side effects, anemia, metabolic derangement, thyroid dysfunction, or infection, which may be mimicking symptoms of PMADs.

Typical presentation
- Patients with PMADs will typically present with emotional symptoms (sadness, mood swings, crying bouts, excessive worry about the baby) or somatic complaints (fatigue, headaches, poor sleep, low energy, appetite changes). They may express concerns with the life changes brought about by pregnancy and parenthood or state that they feel overwhelmed by their current social stressors.

Clinical diagnosis

History
- Depression: Ask patients if they have experienced the two main symptoms of depression (depressed mood or anhedonia). If one or both are present, screening for additional symptoms of depression is indicated: change in appetite, decreased concentration, decreased energy levels, feelings of guilt/worthlessness/hopelessness, psychomotor retardation/agitation, recurrent thoughts of death.
- Mania: Elevated/irritable mood or increased energy/goal-directed behavior for a period of at least 1 week. If present, screening for other symptoms is indicated: inflated self-esteem, decreased need for sleep, rapid speech, racing thoughts, distractibility, and impulsivity.
- Anxiety: Excessive anxiety/worrying that the patient finds difficult to control. Accompanying symptoms include edginess or restlessness, more fatigued than usual, impaired concentration, irritability, increased muscle aches or soreness, difficulty sleeping, hypervigilance, panic attacks.

Physical examination
- Observe the patient for signs such as poor eye contact, slowed or rapid speech or movements, lack of engagement with provider or the baby, and absence of response when the baby cries.

Useful clinical decision rules
- Women with scores above 10 during pregnancy and above 12 postpartum on the EPDS should be referred to a mental health practitioner for follow-up.
- Manic symptoms, psychotic symptoms, or thoughts of harm to self or others are reasons for acute referral to a psychiatrist.

Laboratory diagnosis
- Patients presenting with symptoms of PMADs should have routine lab work to rule out other medical causes and substance abuse (complete blood count, basic metabolic panel, thyroid panel, urine toxicology).

Potential pitfalls
- Providers often fail to rule out medical mimics of PMADs that, when resolved, may alleviate symptoms.

Treatment

Treatment rationale
- Psychotherapy and/or counseling are indicated for the new onset of mild to moderate symptoms of depression and anxiety. There is most evidence for cognitive behavior therapy, but there is also evidence for other interventions.
- Guidelines advise to start antidepressant medication for severe depressive episodes. Zoloft/Sertraline is first line due to low levels in breast milk/infant serum. Paxil/Paroxetine is not a preferred treatment option.

When to hospitalize
- Severe depression
- Mania
- Psychosis
- Concern for harm to self or others

Table of treatment

Treatment	Comments
Conservative	Psychosocial interventions including counseling, support, and groups are appropriate for patients with mild mood and anxiety symptoms.
Medical	Antidepressants: e.g. Sertraline (50–200 mg PO daily).
Surgical	Electroconvulsive therapy (ECT) for very severe cases of depression, mixed states or mania.
Psychological	Psychotherapy including cognitive behavioral therapy (CBT) and interpersonal psychotherapy (IPT) are appropriate as sole treatment for mild/moderate PMAD and adjuncts to ADs.

CLINICAL PEARLS
- Treatment guidelines do not provide guidance whether or not to continue treatment with antidepressant medication.
- Psychotherapy is the preferred treatment option for mild to moderate episodes of anxiety or depression.
- There is an indication to start with antidepressant medication if the episode is considered severe.
- Emergency symptoms such as thoughts of self-harm or violence require referral to an ED for immediate psychiatric evaluation.

Prognosis

BOTTOM LINE/CLINICAL PEARLS
- Perinatal mood and anxiety disorders have a good prognosis when timely diagnosed and adequately treated.

Natural history of untreated disease
- Untreated PMADs lead to increased risk of negative mental and physical health outcomes, including suicide.
- Untreated PMADs are associated with adverse neonatal outcomes including low birth weight, premature birth, poor cognitive and social development, language problems, adiposity, and psychopathology in adolescence.
- Untreated postpartum psychosis is associated with increased risk of suicide and infanticide.

Reading list
Bergink V, Rasgon N, Wisner KL. Postpartum psychosis: madness, mania and melancholia in motherhood. A review. *Am J Psychiatry* 2016 Dec 1;173(12):1179-88.

Johansen SL, Robakis TK, Williams KE, et al. Management of perinatal depression with non-drug interventions. *BMJ* 2019 Feb 25;364:l322.

Kendig, S, Keats J, Hoffman C, et al. Consensus bundle on maternal mental health. *Obstet Gynecol* 2017 March;129(3):422-30.

Meltzer-Brody S, Howard LM, Bergink V, et al. Postpartum psychiatric disorders. *Nat Rev Dis Primers* 2018 Apr 26;4:18022.

Molenaar N, Kamperman A, Boyce P, et al. Guidelines on treatment of perinatal depression with antidepressants: an international review. *Aust N Z J Psychiatry* 2018 Apr;52(4):320-27.

US Preventive Services Task Force Recommendation Statement. Interventions to prevent perinatal depression. *JAMA* 2019;321(6):580-87.

Guidelines
National society guidelines

Title	Source	Date/URL
Screening for perinatal depression	American College of Obstetricians and Gynecologists	2018 https://www.acog.org/Clinical-Guidance-and-Publications/Committee-Opinions/Committee-on-Obstetric-Practice/Screening-for-Perinatal-Depression
Perinatal Depression: Resource Overview	American College of Obstetricians and Gynecologists	2019 https://www.acog.org/Womens-Health/Depression-and-Postpartum-Depression?IsMobileSet=false

Additional material for this chapter can be found online at:
www.wiley.com/go/sperling/mountsinai/obstetricsandgynecology

This includes advice for patients.

PART 2

Gynecology

CHAPTER 17

Surgical Site Infections

V. Ord Sarabanchong
Department of Obstetrics, Gynecology and Reproductive Science, Icahn School of Medicine at Mount Sinai, New York, NY

OVERALL BOTTOM LINE
- Surgical site infections (SSIs) are associated with increased morbidity and mortality, prolonged hospital stay, and increased cost.
- Antibiotic prophylaxis and attention to surgical risk factors can help prevent SSIs.
- Appropriate treatment can help reduce morbidity and mortality.

Background

Definition of disease
- Centers for Disease Control and Prevention (CDC) define surgical site infections as infections that occur at or near the surgical incision within 30 days after surgery.

Disease classification
- SSIs are classified as superficial incisional (skin or subcutaneous tissue), deep incisional (fascial and muscle layers), and involving the organ/space (tissue deeper than the muscle/fascial layer that was opened/manipulated during surgery).

Incidence/prevalence
- Approximately 2–5% of all surgical procedures in the US are complicated by SSI.
- 2–4% of cesarean deliveries and 2% of hysterectomies in the US are complicated by SSI.
- Two-thirds of gynecologic SSIs are superficial incisional infections.

Economic impact
- An SSI can add $10 000 in excess hospital cost and prolong hospitalization by more than 4 days.

Etiology
- Microbial contamination of the surgical site is the precursor to SSI.
- SSIs related to abdominal Gyn surgery are most often infected with aerobic gram-positive cocci (*Staphylococcus aureus*, *Staphylococcus epidermidis*); incisions around the groin or perineum can also involve anaerobic bacteria and gram-negative aerobes (*Enterococcus* species, *E. coli*); incisions in the vagina may be polymicrobial, involving aerobes and anaerobes (*Enterococcus* species, aerobic gram-negative bacilli, *Bacteroides* species).
- SSIs related to cesarean delivery are polymicrobial: *Ureaplasma* species, coagulase-negative staphylococci, *Enterococcus faecalis*, anaerobes, gram-negative rods, *Staphyloccocus aureus*, and group B Streptococcus.

Mount Sinai Expert Guides: Obstetrics and Gynecology, First Edition. Edited by Rhoda Sperling.
© 2020 John Wiley & Sons Ltd. Published 2020 by John Wiley & Sons Ltd.
Companion Website: www.wiley.com/go/sperling/mountsinai/obstetricsandgynecology

Pathology/pathogenesis
- Incision of the skin exposes tissue to endogenous flora.
- Increased microbial concentrations and altered host defenses affect the risk of SSI.

Predictive/risk factors

Risk factor	Odds ratio
Host risk factors:	
Obesity (body mass index ≥ 40)	2.23–2.65
Diabetes	1.4–2.5
Preoperative anemia (Hematocrit < 36%)	1.72
Tobacco use	1.99–5.32
Corticosteroid use	3.11
Bacterial vaginosis	3.2
Colonization with methicillin-resistant *Staphylococcus aureus* (MRSA)	12.4–25.3
American Society of Anesthesiologists class ≥ 3	1.8–5.3
Obstetrical risk factors:	
Labor	1.3–4.01
Rupture of membranes	1.3–2.61
Vaginal exams	2.19
Chorioamnionitis	5.62–10.6
Nonelective vs elective cesarean	1.3–2.5
Surgical risk factors:	
Duration of surgery (>75th percentile)	1.84–2.4
Abdominal skin preparation with chlorhexidine vs povidone-iodine	0.55–0.59
Intravaginal cleansing before cesarean	0.45
Antibiotic prophylaxis	0.4
Manual removal of placenta	1.64
Subcutaneous tissue closure	0.68
Hyperglycemia	1.4–9.4
Preoperative disinfection	0.36
Normothermia	0.36
Preoperative hair shaving vs clipping	2.09
Abdominal hysterectomy vs laparoscopic/vaginal	2.0–3.74

Prevention

BOTTOM LINE/CLINICAL PEARLS
- Prevention of SSIs focuses on addressing modifiable risk factors.
- Antibiotic prophylaxis, management of comorbid conditions, appropriate operative technique, and surgical site preparation can help prevent SSIs.

Primary prevention

* Remote infection such as skin or urinary tract infection should be treated before elective surgery, or surgery should be postponed until the infection has resolved.
* Consider preoperative screening for bacterial vaginosis before hysterectomy.
* Advise patients to shower or bathe with soap (preferably chlorhexidine) on at least the night before surgery.
* Do not shave the incision site; when hair removal is necessary, clippers rather than a razor should be used immediately before the procedure.
* Chlorhexidine-alcohol, rather than povidone-iodine, should be used to clean the skin before incision.
* 4% chlorhexidine or povidone-iodine should be used to clean the vagina before hysterectomy, vaginal surgery, and before cesarean delivery in laboring patients or those with ruptured membranes.
* Implement perioperative glycemic control with target levels of blood glucose less than 200 mg/dL for diabetic and nondiabetic patients.
* Maintain perioperative normothermia.
* The placenta should be removed by manual traction rather than manual extraction.
* Abdominal wounds greater than 2 cm in depth should be closed with a running suture.
* Use appropriate prophylactic antibiotics.

Procedure[a]	Antibiotic	Dose[b]
Cesarean delivery	Cefazolin	1 g IV (2 g IV for weight greater than 80 kg, 3 g IV for weight greater than 120 kg)
	Clindamycin[c] plus gentamicin	900 mg IV 5 mg/kg IV
Hysterectomy, colporrhaphy, vaginal sling placement; consider for laparotomy without bowel/vaginal entry or vulvectomy	Cefazolin	2 g IV (3 g IV for weight greater than 120 kg)
	Clindamycin[c] plus gentamicin or aztreonam	900 mg IV 5 mg/kg IV 2 g IV
	Metronidazole[c] plus gentamicin or aztreonam	500 mg IV 5 mg/kg IV 2 g IV
Induced abortion/dilation and evacuation	Doxycycline	200 mg orally 1 hour before procedure
Hysterosalpingography (HSG), chromopertubation[d]	Doxycycline	100 mg orally twice daily for 5 days
Repair of obstetric anal sphincter injuries	Cefotetan or Cefoxitin or Clindamycin[c]	1 g IV 1 g IV 900 mg IV

[a] Antibiotic prophylaxis is not recommended for diagnostic or operative laparoscopy or hysteroscopy.

[b] Administration of IV antibiotics is within 1 hour of incision. Single-dose therapy is recommended. Redosing is recommended if surgery exceeds the following durations: 4 hours for cefazolin or aztreonam; 6 hours for clindamycin; metronidazole and gentamicin are not redosed. Redosing of IV antibiotics is recommended if blood loss exceeds 1500 mL.

[c] Recommended for patients with an immediate hypersensitivity to penicillin. For gentamicin dosing, in patients weighing > 20% above ideal body weight (IBW), body weight calculations are adjusted as follows: weight in kg = IBW + 0.4 (actual weight-IBW).

[d] Antibiotic prophylaxis is recommended only for patients with a history of PID or abnormal tubes noted on HSG or laparoscopy.

Diagnosis

> **BOTTOM LINE/CLINICAL PEARLS**
> - The diagnosis of SSI is based on history and physical exam findings suggestive of infection.
> - Blood tests, wound culture, and imaging can help establish the severity and extent of infection, thus guiding treatment.

Differential diagnosis

Differential diagnosis	Features
Urinary tract infection	Pain may be localized to the pelvis, but dysuria and/or frequency of urination are key features. Urinalysis will reveal leukocytes, blood, or bacteria.
Wound seroma/hematoma	Localized pain and swelling at the incision that may be accompanied by spontaneous drainage. The fluid drained will be sterile.
Retained products of conception	Persistent pain and bleeding following surgical abortion, with blood and debris seen in the endometrial cavity on ultrasound. Can be further complicated by infection of the retained products, with resulting fever, leukocytosis, and possible sepsis.
Septic pelvic thrombophlebitis	Typically, postpartum presentation of fever, leukocytosis, with or without abdominal pain, unresponsive to antibiotics. Computed tomography (CT) or magnetic resonance imaging (MRI) sometimes demonstrates thrombus. Anticoagulation is necessary for resolution.
Appendicitis, diverticulitis	Localized pain, nausea, possible change in bowel habits; diagnosis best differentiated by CT imaging.

Typical presentation
- Superficial and deep incisional SSIs will present with pain, redness, and swelling at the incision at least 2 days after surgery; there may be purulent drainage. Organ/space SSIs can present with abdominal/pelvic pain, fever, and possibly a tender pelvic mass on physical exam.

Clinical diagnosis
History
- History should focus on onset of symptoms (usually 48 hours after surgery but most often 5 days postoperatively), and any associated symptoms, such as nausea/vomiting or change in bowel or urinary habits.

Physical examination
- Classic indicators of infection should be assessed: fever (calor) defined as a temperature of 38 °C or higher on two separate occasions taken at least 6 hours apart, or an isolated temperature of 38.3 °C; swelling (tumor); and erythema (rubor) at or near the incision. Tachycardia may be present.
- Exam may reveal purulent drainage at the incision or a tender mass on pelvic exam; there may be fundal tenderness if the uterus has not been removed.

Disease severity classification
- Superficial incisional SSI: involving skin or subcutaneous tissue.
- Deep incisional SSI: involving fascial and muscle layers.

- Organ/space SSI: involving tissue deeper than the muscle/fascial layer that was opened or manipulated during surgery.

Laboratory diagnosis
List of diagnostic tests
- Complete blood count: an elevated white blood count with a left shift suggests an acute infection.
- Metabolic panel: assessment of renal function and acidemia in the setting of infection.
- Gram stain and culture of wound drainage: bacterial identification and sensitivities will guide antibiotic selection.

List of imaging techniques
- Imaging may be obtained if physical examination fails to localize the SSI.
- Pelvic ultrasound is often the first choice and can identify superficial and deep pelvic fluid collections as well as retained products of conception.
- CT imaging with contrast is particularly useful for visualizing pelvic abscesses or evaluating for perforated viscus.

Potential pitfalls/common errors made regarding diagnosis of disease
- Fever in the immediate 48 hours after surgery is less likely due to infection and most often due to atelectasis or pyogenic cytokine release.
- Beyond 48 hours after surgery, other common sources for fever such as urinary tract infection, deep venous thrombosis, and pneumonia should be considered.

Treatment
Treatment rationale
- Superficial SSI can often be managed with oral antibiotics.
- The presence and amount of purulent drainage may necessitate opening the wound for debridement.
- Deep incisional and organ/space SSI may require IV antibiotics, percutaneous pelvic drain placement, or surgical exploration.

When to hospitalize
- Patients with peritonitis, pelvic abscess, or signs of sepsis or who require IV antibiotics should be admitted.

Managing the hospitalized patient
- IV antibiotics should be administered until afebrile for 24–48 hours and then transitioned to oral antibiotics.
- For postpartum endometritis, additional treatment with oral antibiotics has not been found to be beneficial.
- For pelvic abscess, CT or ultrasound-guided percutaneous drainage should be considered for size > 8 cm diameter, or if fevers persist beyond 48 hours of treatment with IV antibiotics.
- Surgical exploration may be necessary if conservative measures fail, if there is clinical deterioration or sepsis, for ruptured abscess or perforated viscus, or for necrotizing fasciitis.
- See Algorithm 17.1.

Algorithm 17.1 Management/treatment of surgical site infections

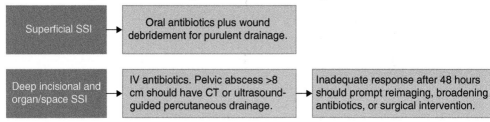

Table of treatment

Treatment	Comments
Medical	
Superficial SSI: Dicloxacillin 500 mg PO every 6 h. Trimethoprim-sulfamethoxazole 160–800 mg PO every 12 h (for suspected MRSA). Amoxicillin-clavulanate 875–125 mg PO every 12 h (for vaginal cuff cellulitis).	Duration of treatment is 7–14 days.
Deep incisional and organ/space SSI: Gentamicin 5 mg/kg every 24 h plus clindamycin 900 mg every 8 h. Ceftriaxone 2 g IV every 24 h plus metronidazole 500 mg every 12 h. Piperacillin-tazobactam 3.375 g IV every 6 h. Vancomycin 20 mg/kg IV every 12 h (can be added to the above regimens for suspected MRSA).	Duration of treatment is 14 days.[a]
Surgical	
Wound debridement Laparoscopy or exploratory laparotomy	May be necessary for purulent drainage. May be necessary if conservative measures fail, if there is clinical deterioration or sepsis, for ruptured abscess or perforated viscus, or for necrotizing fasciitis.
Radiological	
CT or ultrasound-guided percutaneous drainage	For abscess > 8 cm or abscess not responding to IV antibiotics after 48 hours treatment.

[a]Postpartum endometritis is treated with IV antibiotics until afebrile for 24–48 h. Pelvic abscess may require more than 14 days treatment depending on resolution of abscess.

Prevention/management of complications
- Necrotizing fasciitis is a rare polymicrobial complication of wound infection that can spread rapidly along the fascial planes and subcutaneous tissue.
- Clostridium and group A Streptococcus are frequently involved, producing crepitation on physical exam or gas in the subcutaneous tissue on imaging.
- Mean time to diagnosis is 10 days from surgery, with mortality as high as 50%.
- Mainstays of treatment are extensive debridement and broad-spectrum antibiotics.

> **CLINICAL PEARLS**
> - Prompt recognition and initiation of appropriate antibiotics are key to treating SSI.
> - Clinical presentation or lack of improvement should prompt wound debridement, pelvic imaging, broadened antibiotics, percutaneous drainage, or surgical intervention.

Special populations
- Patients with known MRSA colonization or at high risk for MRSA colonization (e.g. nursing home residents, hemodialysis patients) should have vancomycin (15 mg/kg) added to the preoperative antibiotic prophylaxis regimen. Universal screening for MRSA is not recommended.
- Patients receiving therapeutic antibiotics for infection before surgery should be administered an extra dose 60 minutes before surgical incision if the agents used are appropriate for surgical prophylaxis.
- Patients with bacterial vaginosis who are undergoing hysterectomy, vaginal surgery, or surgical abortion should be treated preoperatively.

Prognosis

> **BOTTOM LINE/CLINICAL PEARLS**
> - Prompt and appropriate treatment of SSI can shorten hospital stay and reduce morbidity and mortality.

Reading list
Bakkum-Gamez JN, Dowdy SC, Borah BJ, et al. Predictors and costs of surgical site infections in patients with endometrial cancer. *Gynecol Oncol* 2013 Jul;130(1):100-6.

Black JD, de Haydu C, Fan L, et al. Surgical site infections in gynecology. *Obstet Gynecol Surv* 2014 Aug;69(8): 501-10.

Darouiche RO, Wall MJ Jr, Itani KM, et al. Chlorhexidine-alcohol versus povidone-iodine for surgical-site antisepsis. *N Engl J Med* 2010 Jan 7;362(1):18-26.

Duggal N, Mercado C, Daniels K, et al. Antibiotic prophylaxis for prevention of postpartum perineal wound complications: a randomized controlled trial. *Obstet Gynecol* 2008 Jun:111(6):1268-73.

Fitzwater JL, Tita AT. Prevention and management of cesarean wound infection. *Obstet Gynecol Clin North Am* 2014 Dec;41(4):671-89.

Kao LS, Phatak UR. Glycemic control and prevention of surgical site infection. *Surg Infect (Larchmt)* 2013 Oct;14(5): 437-44.

Lachiewicz MP, Moulton LJ, Jaiyeoba O. Pelvic surgical site infections in gynecologic surgery. *Infect Dis Obstet Gynecol* 2015;2015:614950.

Lake AG, McPencow AM, Dick-Biascoechea MA, et al. Surgical site infection after hysterectomy. *Am J Obstet Gynecol* 2013 Nov;209(5):490.e1-9.

Mittendorf R, Aronson MP, Berry RE, et al. Avoiding serious infections associated with abdominal hysterectomy: a meta-analysis of antibiotic prophylaxis. *Am J Obstet Gynecol* 1993 Nov;169(5):1119-24.

Opøien HK, Valbø A, Grinde-Andersen A, et al. Post-cesarean surgical site infections according to CDC standards: rates and risk factors. A prospective cohort study. *Acta Obstet Gynecol Scand* 2007;86(9):1097-102.

Steiner HL, Strand EA. Surgical-site infection in gynecologic surgery: pathophysiology and prevention. *Am J Obstet Gynecol* 2017 Aug;217(2):121-28.

Zuarez-Easton S, Zafran N, Garmi G, et al. Postcesarean wound infection: prevalence, impact, prevention, and management challenges. *Int J Womens Health* 2017 Feb 17;9:81-88.

Suggested websites
American College of Obstetricians and Gynecologists. www.ACOG.org
American Society of Hospital Pharmacists. www.ASHP.org
Centers for Disease Control and Prevention. www.CDC.gov
The Joint Commission. www.JointCommission.org

Guidelines
National society guidelines

Title	Source	Date/URL
Prevention of infection after gynecologic procedures: ACOG practice bulletin no. 195.	ACOG	June 2018 https://www.acog.org/Clinical-Guidance-and-Publications/Practice-Bulletins/Committee-on-Practice-Bulletins-Gynecology/Prevention-of-Infection-After-Gynecologic-Procedures
Use of prophylactic antibiotics in labor and delivery: ACOG practice bulletin no. 199.	ACOG	August 2018 https://www.acog.org/Clinical-Guidance-and-Publications/Practice-Bulletins/Committee-on-Practice-Bulletins-Obstetrics/Use-of-Prophylactic-Antibiotics-in-Labor-and-Delivery
Prevention of surgical site infection	Centers for Disease Control and Prevention	2017 http://jamanetwork.com/journals/jamasurgery/fullarticle/2623725
Clinical practice guidelines for antimicrobial prophylaxis in surgery	American Society of Health-System Pharmacists (ASHP) Therapeutic Guidelines.	2013 https://academic.oup.com/ajhp/article/70/3/195/5112717?sso-checked=true

Evidence

Type of evidence	Title and comment	Date/URL
Systematic review	Cochrane Database. Active body surface warming systems for preventing complications caused by inadvertent perioperative hypothermia in adults.	2016 Apr 21 https://www.ncbi.nlm.nih.gov/pubmed/27098439
Systematic review	Cochrane Database. Preoperative bathing or showering with skin antiseptics to prevent surgical site infection.	2015 Feb 20 https://www.ncbi.nlm.nih.gov/pubmed/25927093
Systematic review	Cochrane Database. Antibiotic regimens for postpartum endometritis.	2015 Feb 2 https://www.ncbi.nlm.nih.gov/pubmed/25922861
Systematic review	Cochrane Database. Vaginal preparation with antiseptic solution before cesarean delivery for preventing postoperative infections.	2014 Dec 21 https://www.ncbi.nlm.nih.gov/pubmed/25528419
Systematic review	Cochrane Database. Preoperative hair removal to reduce surgical site infection.	2011 Nov 9 https://www.ncbi.nlm.nih.gov/pubmed/22071812

CHAPTER 18

Vaginitis, Cervicitis, and Pelvic Inflammatory Disease

Janine A. Doneza[1] and Lisa Dabney[2]

[1] Robotic and Minimally Invasive Gynecologic Surgery, MIGS/Urogynecology Fellowship Program, Fibroid Center, Bronxcare Hospital, Bronx, NY; Icahn School of Medicine at Mount Sinai, New York, NY

[2] Division of Female Pelvic Medicine and Reconstructive Surgery, Department of Obstetrics, Gynecology and Reproductive Science, Icahn School of Medicine at Mount Sinai, New York, NY

OVERALL BOTTOM LINE
- Abnormal vaginal discharge has a broad differential diagnosis and successful treatment requires an accurate diagnosis.
- The most common causes of abnormal vaginal discharge are bacterial vaginosis (BV), candidiasis (yeast), and trichomoniasis.
- Cervicitis may be acute or chronic. Acute cervicitis is often associated with a sexually transmitted chlamydia or gonorrhea infection.
- Untreated cervicitis can result in pelvic inflammatory disease (PID), an ascending pelvic infection that can involve the uterus, fallopian tubes, ovaries, and peritoneal cavity.
- The major consequences of PID are chronic pelvic pain, infertility, and ectopic pregnancy.

Background

Definition of disease
- Vaginitis is a disorder of the vagina caused by infection, inflammation, or changes in the normal vaginal flora. Most common causes are bacterial vaginosis (BV), candida, and trichomoniasis.
- Cervicitis refers to inflammation that affects the columnar epithelial cells of the endocervical glands. Acute cervicitis is usually due to infection (e.g. chlamydia, gonorrhea).
- Pelvic inflammatory disease (PID) comprises a spectrum of inflammatory disorders of the upper female genital tract including any combination of endometritis, salpingitis, and/or tubo-ovarian abscess.

Incidence/prevalence
- Chlamydia is the most commonly reported STD in the United States. Gonorrhea is the second most commonly reported STD. Chlamydia and PID occur most commonly in women aged 16 to 24.
- Pregnant, premenarchal, and postmenopausal women less commonly present with PID. PID is prevalent in women with prior STI.

Economic impact
- PID accounts for approximately 106 000 outpatient visits and 60 000 hospitalizations each year and is a frequent cause for emergency department visits.
- Candidiasis and BV are some of the most frequent causes of vaginal symptoms, resulting in healthcare visits.

Mount Sinai Expert Guides: Obstetrics and Gynecology, First Edition. Edited by Rhoda Sperling.
© 2020 John Wiley & Sons Ltd. Published 2020 by John Wiley & Sons Ltd.
Companion Website: www.wiley.com/go/sperling/mountsinai/obstetricsandgynecology

Etiology
- Yeast infections are most commonly caused by *Candida albicans*; occasionally other candida species may be involved including *C. tropicalis* and *C. glabrata*.
- Bacterial vaginosis is characterized by a shift in the vaginal flora from the dominant *Lactobacillus* to a polymicrobial flora. The microbial pathogens, singularly and in combination, that have been linked to BV continues to expand and include *Gardnerella, Atopobium, Prevotella, Peptostreptococcus, Mobiluncus, Sneathia, Leptotrichia, Mycoplasma*, and BV-associated bacterium 1 (BVAB1) to BVAB3.
- Trichomoniasis is caused by the protozoa *Trichomonas vaginalis*. It commonly occurs as coinfection with other sexually transmitted infections (STIs), especially gonorrhea.
- Gonorrhea/Chlamydia/PID: caused by *Neisseria gonorrhea* or *Chlamydia trachomatis*. PID can also be associated with anaerobic organisms, enteric gram-negative rods, streptococci, genital mycoplasmas, and BV-associated microbes.

Pathology/pathogenesis
- The healthy vaginal microbiome is dominated by *Lactobacillus sp*. This bacterium converts glucose into lactic acid, creating an acidic vaginal environment that helps to maintain the normal vaginal flora and inhibits growth of pathogenic organisms. Disruption of this process can lead to conditions favorable for development of vaginitis.
- Some of these potentially disruptive factors include phase of the menstrual cycle, sexual activity, contraceptive choice, pregnancy, foreign bodies, estrogen level, sexually transmitted diseases, and use of hygienic products or antibiotics.
- Cervical infection is clinically important because it can ascend and cause pelvic inflammatory disease.

Predictive/risk factors

Candidiasis	Gonorrhea/chlamydia/PID	Trichomoniasis	Bacterial vaginosis
Immunosuppression	Age < 25	High-risk sexual behaviors	Multiple male or
Diabetes	History of STI/PID	(prostitution)	female partners
Obesity	New/multiple partners	Incidence increases with age	Presence of other STI
Antibiotic use	Lack of barrier protection	Presence of other STI's	Douching
	Drug and alcohol use	Drug and alcohol use	Smoking

Prevention

> **BOTTOM LINE/CLINICAL PEARLS**
> - Barrier contraception and annual screening decreases incidence of sexually transmitted infections.

Screening
- Women presenting with abnormal vaginal discharge should be screened for candidiasis, trichomoniasis, and BV.
- Annual screening for chlamydia and gonorrhea is recommended for all sexually active women < 25 years of age.
- Annual screening for chlamydia and gonorrhea is recommended for women > 25 if they are at increased risk for acquiring a new infection (e.g. those who have a new sex partner, or more than one sex partner, or a sex partner with a sexually transmitted infection.

Primary prevention

- Prevention of chlamydia and gonorrhea – abstinence, safe sex practices, correct and consistent use of condoms. Safe sex practices should include alcohol and drug abuse counseling, if appropriate.

Secondary prevention

- Secondary prevention of candidiasis is possible by addressing modifiable conditions associated with recurrent infections. Women with underlying immunodeficiency, those with poorly controlled diabetes, and those receiving immunosuppressive agents are at risk for recurrent or severe infections.
- Male sex partners of women with sexually transmitted cervicovaginal infections (trichomoniasis, gonorrhea, and/or chlamydia) should be treated to decrease the risk of reinfection.
- Treatment of BV reduces the risk of acquiring chlamydia and gonorrhea.
- Prompt treatment of chlamydia and gonorrhea reduces the risk of developing PID.
- Vaginal douching, menses, cigarette smoking, and substance abuse likely influence the risk of developing PID.

Diagnosis

> **BOTTOM LINE/CLINICAL PEARLS**
> - Diagnosis relies on culture and microscopy

Differential diagnosis of vaginitis and cervicitis
Vaginal atrophy/atrophic vaginitis
Foreign body
Allergens
Chronic inflammatory process (lichen sclerosus, Behcet's syndrome)
Other STIs (syphilis, herpes, mycoplasma genitalium)

Typical presentation

- Candidiasis: itching, burning, dyspareunia, thick white "cottage cheese" discharge
- Bacterial vaginosis: abnormal vaginal discharge and a fishy odor
- Trichomoniasis: abnormal foul, thin green discharge; postcoital bleeding
- Gonorrhea/chlamydia: can be asymptomatic or present as a mucopurulent discharge or symptoms of urethritis.
- PID: bilateral, acute lower abdominal pain is the cardinal presenting symptom and can occur during coitus or after menses. A minority of patients will develop a pelvic abscess, which presents with more severe pain and fever. Perihepatitis (Fitz-Hugh–Curtis Syndrome) occurs in the setting of PID when there is inflammation of the liver capsule and presents with right upper quadrant pain and tenderness.

Clinical diagnosis

History

- Elicit information about vaginal symptoms, including characteristics of discharge, presence of malodor, itching, burning, dyspareunia (Figure 18.1).

- Questions about the location of pain, duration, the relation to the menstrual cycle, the response to prior treatment, and a sexual history can help determine etiology.

Physical examination
- Vulvar, vaginal, and speculum examination to identify lesions and presence of discharge, collect samples for microscopy and/or culture.
- Purulent endocervical discharge and a friable cervix are characteristic of endocervicitis.
- Bimanual pelvic exam to assess for acute cervical motion tenderness, uterine, and adnexal tenderness.
- Abdominal exam to determine location of pain.

Disease severity classification
- Candidiasis
  - Uncomplicated: sporadic episodes, mild symptoms suspected *Candida albicans*, nonpregnant without medical complications.
  - Complicated: four or more candida infections per year, severe symptoms, non-albicans infection, history diabetes, immunosuppression, pregnancy.

Laboratory diagnosis
- Candidiasis: visualization of pseudohyphae on microscopy or a positive culture. Culture usually done in cases of recurrent/persistent yeast infection or possible non-albicans infection (Figure 18.2).
- BV: Amsel's criteria – abnormal gray discharge, vaginal pH greater than 4.5, a positive amine whiff test, and more than 20% of the epithelial cells being clue cells. Nugent score assigns a value to different bacterial morphotypes seen on gram stain of vaginal secretions; considered the criterion standard for diagnosing BV (Figure 18.1).
- Trichomoniasis: visualization of motile flagellated trichomonads on saline microscopy. Culture can be considered in patients with persistent symptoms after therapy (Figure 18.3).
- Gonorrhea/chlamydia: cultures or nucleic acid amplification testing (NAAT) for *N. gonorrhoeae* and *C. trachomatis*. Gram stain for gram-negative diplococci seen from cervical discharge can also be a useful diagnostic tool but is often not available. Specimen can be collected from swab of cervix or vagina or from urine sample.
- PID: temperature > 101 °F, abnormal mucopurulent discharge, presence of abundant numbers of white blood cells on saline microscopy of vaginal secretions, documentation of cervical infection with *N. gonorrhoeae* or *C. trachomatis*.

Imaging techniques
- Pelvic sonogram: may see thickened, fluid-filled fallopian tubes or complex thick-walled, multilocular cystic adnexal collection.

Potential pitfalls
- Self-diagnosis of vulvovaginal candidiasis is often inaccurate and can lead to a delay in diagnosis. In addition, history alone has been shown to be insufficient for diagnosis of vaginitis; patients with symptoms of vaginitis should be asked to come into the office to be evaluated.

Treatment
Treatment rationale
- Treatment of STI decreases occurrence of complications associated with infection, including development of PID, infertility, and adverse pregnancy outcomes.

- Antimicrobial resistance can limit treatment success and facilitate the transmission of sexually transmitted infections. Combination therapy for gonorrhea and chlamydia is thus recommended to prevent antimicrobial resistance.
- Treatment of partner for gonorrhea, chlamydia, and trichomonas decreases risk of reinfection and decreases spread of infection. Treatment of BV and candidiasis does not routinely require treatment of partners.

When to hospitalize
- Hospitalization indicated for pregnancy, lack of response, non-adherence or intolerance to oral medications; severe clinical illness (high fever, nausea, vomiting, severe abdominal pain), pelvic abscess (including tubo-ovarian abscess).

Management of hospitalized patients
- Parenteral antibiotics are given until the patient exhibits 24 hours of clinical improvement.

Table of treatment

Candida	Bacterial vaginosis	Trichomoniasis	Gonorrhea, chlamydia, PID
Uncomplicated: fluconazole 150 mg x1 dose; intravaginal treatment options include clotrimazole, miconazole, nystatin, terconazole **Complicated**: fluconazole 150 mg q72 hours for 2 or 3 doses **Recurrent**- fluconazole 150 mg weekly for 6 months **Non-albicans**: intravaginal boric acid for *C. glabrata*	Clindamycin 2% cream 5 g intravaginally at bedtime for 7 days **OR** Metronidazole 500 mg oral twice daily for 7 days **OR** Metronidazole gel 0.75% 5 g intravaginally once daily for 5 days	Metronidazole **OR** tinidazole as a single oral dose of 2 grams	**Outpatient**: Gonorrhea can be treated with ceftriaxone (250 mg intramuscularly in a single dose) **plus** azithromycin 1 g orally once Chlamydia can be treated with azithromycin 1 g orally once or doxycycline 100 mg orally BID x7 days **PID inpatient**: Cefoxitin (2 g intravenously every 6 hours) or cefotetan (2 g IV every 12 hours) plus doxycycline (100 mg orally every 12 hours). Transition from parenteral to oral therapy after 24 hours of sustained clinical improvement. Patients should complete a 14-day course of treatment with doxycycline (100 mg twice daily)

Prevention/management of complications
- Treatment for BV before abortion or hysterectomy significantly decreases the risk of postoperative infectious complications. Treatment in pregnancy decreases risk of low birth weight, premature rupture of membranes, and prematurity.
- PID can cause adhesions and damage to the fallopian tube, which can result in chronic pelvic pain, infertility, and ectopic pregnancy. Prompt diagnosis and treatment of PID are important to reduce the risk of long-term complications.

Management/treatment algorithm
Treatment of gonorrhea/chlamydia/PID should result in symptomatic improvement within 3 days of initiating therapy. In those who do not improve, the patient should be reevaluated to assess for reinfection or treatment failure. Patients with PID may need hospitalization, and those with tubo-ovarian abscess (TOA) may need surgical intervention. See Algorithm 18.1.

Algorithm 18.1 Management of vaginal discharge

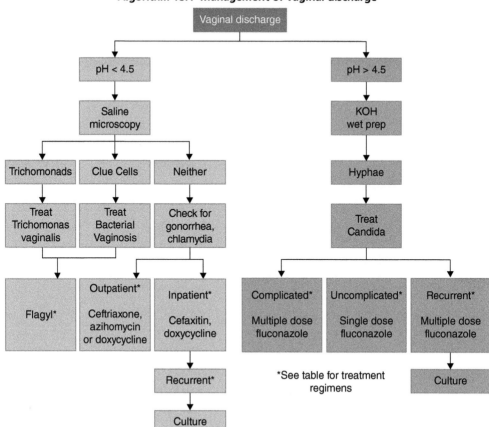

> **CLINICAL PEARLS**
> - Most women with cervicitis should receive empiric antibiotic therapy at the time of initial evaluation, without waiting for results of laboratory tests.
> - Expedited partner therapy: delivery of prescription by persons infected with an STD to their sexual partners without clinical assessment of the partners. Sex partners of women with chlamydia, gonorrhea, or trichomoniasis should be treated for the infection for which the woman received treatment.
> - Test of cure for chlamydia and gonorrhea is not required unless symptoms persist or the woman is pregnant.

Special populations
Pregnant women
- Candida species colonization may occur more commonly in pregnant women. Low-dose short-term fluconazole use is not associated with known birth defects.
- BV in pregnancy is associated with adverse pregnancy outcomes and treatment is recommended.
- Pregnancy is an indication for hospitalization and parenteral antibiotics for PID. A second-generation cephalosporin (intravenous cefoxitin) and azithromycin 1 g orally is given instead of doxycycline.

Children and adolescents
- Vulvovaginitis is one of the most common gynecologic problems in prepubertal girls but etiologies differ from the adult population.
- Most cases are thought to be noninfectious in origin organisms such as group A streptococci and *Hemophilus influenzae.*
- Bacterial culture should be obtained by introducing a swab blindly through the hymen; urine testing can be performed for gonorrhea and chlamydia.

HIV patients
- Antibiotic regimens for HIV-infected women with acute PID are similar to those for HIV-uninfected women.

Prognosis

> **BOTTOM LINE/CLINICAL PEARLS**
> - The major consequences of PID are chronic pelvic pain, infertility, and ectopic pregnancy. Treatment of PID may not prevent long-term sequelae.

Natural history of untreated disease
- Untreated trichomoniasis and BV increase risk of postoperative and pregnancy complications and may increase women's susceptibility to HIV infection.

Prognosis for treated patients
- Recurrences/reinfection are common with vaginitis and cervicitis.
- Risk of developing complications of PID occur even in treated patients; this risk increases with the number of episodes and severity of PID.

Follow-up
- Nonpregnant women who are asymptomatic do not require routine reevaluation. Women with persistent/recurrent symptoms should be reevaluated with culture and NAAT.

Reading list
ACOG committee opinion no. 645: Dual therapy for gonococcal infections. *Obstet Gynecol.* 2016 May;127(5):e95–9.
ACOG practice bulletin no. 215: Vaginitis in Nonpregnant Patients. *Obstet Gynecol.* 2020 Jan;135(1):e1–e17.
Hoffman BL, Schorge JO, Bradshaw KD, Halvorson LM. Chapter 3: gynecologic infection. In: *Williams gynecology.* 4th ed. New York: McGraw-Hill Education; 2020.
Soper DE. Pelvic inflammatory disease. *Obstet Gynecol* 2010;116:419.
Workowski KA, Bolan GA, Centers for Disease Control and Prevention. Sexually transmitted diseases treatment guidelines, 2015. *MMWR Recomm Rep* 2015;64:1.

Suggested website
Centers for Disease Control and Prevention. https://www.cdc.gov/std/tg2015/default.htm

Guidelines

Title	Source	Date/URL
STD treatment guidelines	Centers for Disease Control and Prevention	2015 https://www.cdc.gov/std/tg2015/tg-2015-print.pdf
Final recommendation statement on gonorrhea and chlamydia screening	U.S. Preventive Services Task Force	2014 http://www.uspreventiveservicestaskforce.org/Page/Document/RecommendationStatementFinal/chlamydia-and-gonorrhea-screening

Evidence

Type of evidence	Title and comment	Date/full reference
Meta-analysis	Screening for genital chlamydia infection Comment: Cochrane review showing that there is moderate quality evidence that detection and treatment of chlamydia infection can reduce the risk of PID in women.	Low N, Redmond S, Uusküla A et al. *Cochrane Database Syst Rev* 2016;Sep 13;9.
Review	Control of *Neisseria gonorrhoeae* in the era of evolving antimicrobial resistance Comment: *Neisseria gonorrhoeae* has developed resistance to first-line antimicrobial therapy; treatment now consists of dual antibiotic therapy.	Barbee LA, Dombrowski JC. *Infect Dis Clin North Am* 2013;Dec;27(4):723-37.
Review	Recurrent vulvovaginal candidiasis Comment: Recurrent Candida infection can be controlled with fluconazole maintenance therapy but cure is still elusive.	Sobel JD. *Am J Obstet Gynecol* 2016;Jan;214(1):15-21.

Images

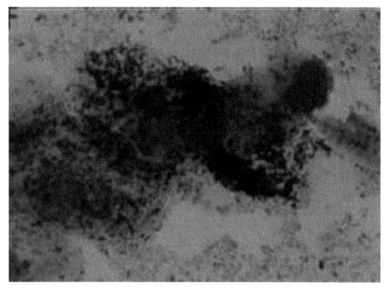

Figure 18.1 Bacterial vaginosis – presence of gram negative rods and absence of lactobacilli on gram stain. From https://www.std.uw.edu/go/syndrome-based/vaginal-discharge/core-concept/all. See color version on website.

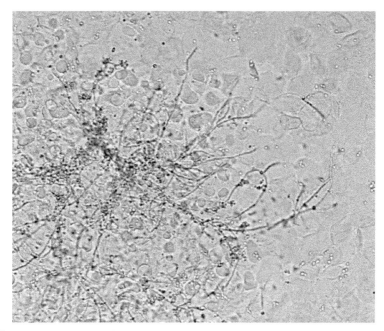

Figure 18.2 Vulvovaginal candidiasis (yeast and hyphae) on a 10% hydrogen peroxide wet mount preparation (10% magnification). From https://www.std.uw.edu/go/syndrome-based/vaginal-discharge/core-concept/all

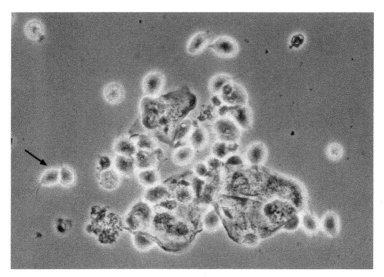

Figure 18.3 Trichomonas vaginalis on wet mount. From https://www.std.uw.edu/go/syndrome-based/vaginal-discharge/core-concept/all

---

Additional material for this chapter can be found online at:
www.wiley.com/go/sperling/mountsinai/obstetricsandgynecology

This includes multiple choice questions, advice for patients, and ICD codes. The following image is available in color: Figure 18.1.

CHAPTER 19

Abnormal Uterine Bleeding

Karina Hoan[1] and Charles Ascher-Walsh[2]
[1] FMIGS Faculty, Division of Minimally Invasive Gynecology, The Portland Clinic, Portland, OR
[2] Division of Female Pelvic Medicine and Reconstructive Surgery, Department of Obstetrics, Gynecology and Reproductive Science, Icahn School of Medicine at Mount Sinai, New York, NY

OVERALL BOTTOM LINE
- Abnormal uterine bleeding (AUB) is a term that refers to menstrual bleeding of abnormal quantity, duration, or schedule.
- Most common etiologies of nonpregnant females are structural uterine pathology, anovulation, blood-clotting disorders, neoplasia, or medications.
- Endometrial biopsy is performed in women with AUB and have an age greater than 45 or have risk factors for endometrial cancer.
- Pelvic imaging is useful if a structural lesion is suspected. Pelvic ultrasound is the first-line study.

Background
Definition of disease
- Abnormal uterine bleeding is a term that refers to menstrual bleeding of abnormal quantity (>80 mL), duration (>8 days), or schedule (<24 days/>38 days).

Disease classification
- The classification system in non-gravid reproductive-age women is referred to by the acronym PALM-COEIN (polyp, adenomyosis, leiomyoma, malignancy and hyperplasia, coagulopathy, ovulatory dysfunction, endometrial, iatrogenic, and not yet classified). See Algorithm 19.1 from the ACOG Committee opinion 557.

Incidence/prevalence
- A population-based survey of American women ages 18 to 50 years reported an annual prevalence rate of 53 per 1000 women.

Etiology
- Structural abnormalities such as uterine leiomyomas (see Figure 19.1), endometrial polyps, adenomyosis
- Ovulatory dysfunction such as anovulation or oligo-ovulation
- Bleeding disorders: most common being von Willebrand deficiency
- Endocrine disorders such as thyroid dysfunction or hyperprolactinemia
- Iatrogenic can be caused by anticoagulation or hormonal contraception (especially progestin only)
- Neoplasia-hyperplasia, endometrial intraepithelial neoplasia or carcinoma, or uterine sarcoma
- Endometritis
- Not otherwise specified

Mount Sinai Expert Guides: Obstetrics and Gynecology, First Edition. Edited by Rhoda Sperling.
© 2020 John Wiley & Sons Ltd. Published 2020 by John Wiley & Sons Ltd.
Companion Website: www.wiley.com/go/sperling/mountsinai/obstetricsandgynecology

Algorithm 19.1 PALM and COEIN classification for causes of abnormal uterine bleeding

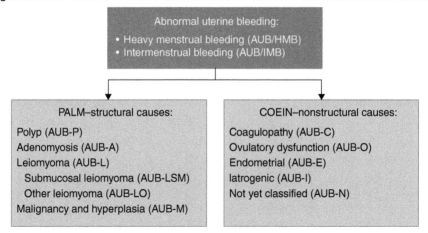

http://www.acog.org/Resources-And-Publications/Committee-Opinions/Committee-on-Gynecologic-Practice/Management-of-Acute-Abnormal-Uterine-Bleeding-in-Nonpregnant-Reproductive-Aged-Women

Pathology/pathogenesis

- Heavy menstrual bleeding (HMB) is defined as regular cyclic bleeding that is heavy or prolonged can be caused by any structural abnormality, bleeding disorder, or hyperplasia or malignancy.
- Intermenstrual bleeding can be caused by endometrial polyps, hormonal contraceptives, endometrial hyperplasia or malignancy, or endometritis. Conditions of the cervix are ruled out prior to endometrial investigations.
- Irregular bleeding is commonly associated with ovulatory dysfunction secondary to extremes of reproductive age, polycystic ovarian syndrome, and other endocrine disorders.

Predictive/risk factors

- Most common causes of abnormal uterine bleeding are intrauterine fibroid, polyp, and early pregnancy.

Prevention

- No interventions have been demonstrated to prevent the development of abnormal uterine bleeding.

Screening

- No screening methods have been shown to be effective in preventing abnormal uterine bleeding.

Diagnosis

- A patient's gynecological and obstetrical history is taken. The location, amount, color, and bleeding pattern are identified. Sexual history, contraceptive history, and history of a bleeding disorder are elicited.
- Physical exam is performed and potential sites of bleeding from the vulva, vagina, cervix, uterus, urethra, anus, or perineum are evaluated.
- Labs are ordered to rule out pregnancy, bleeding disorder, and severe anemia.
- Endometrial and cervical sampling are performed in indicated patients.

Differential diagnosis

Differential diagnosis	Features
Cervical pathology	Friable cervix
Urethral	Hematuria. Blood visualized only after urination
GI tract bleeding	Bleeding during defecation
Pregnancy of unknown location	Positive human chorionic gonadotropin (hCG) serum or urine sample

Typical presentation
- Women with AUB tend to present with strong concerns over changes in menstrual blood loss. The most common presentation is heavy menstrual bleeding, which refers to heavy cyclic menses. Women may also complain of bleeding between their menses. Ovulatory dysfunction causes irregular bleeding; women can have phases of no bleeding, spotting, and heavy bleeding.

Clinical diagnosis
History
- Obstetrical, gynecological, and medical history is elicited. Medications are reviewed. Last menstrual period, number of days of heavy vaginal bleeding, presence of intermenstrual bleeding, number of tampons/pads used per day are determined. It is established whether the patient is premenarchal, perimenopausal, or having postmenopausal bleeding. Pregnancy is excluded.

Physical examination
- The physical examination includes an abdominal and pelvic examination as well as vital signs. The exact site of vaginal bleeding is determined (uterine, genitourinary, rectal). A bimanual exam is performed and the size and contour of the uterus are evaluated. If there is active uterine bleeding, the volume and color are noted. The adnexa are palpated to rule out adnexal mass. A speculum examination should be performed to rule out a prolapsed submucosal fibroid or cervical pathology.

Useful clinical decision rules and calculators
- A patient who has acute heavy vaginal bleeding is assessed for hemodynamic stability. Patients who are hemodynamically unstable or who have copious, ongoing blood flow from the uterus should be managed in an emergency care facility.

Laboratory diagnosis
List of diagnostic tests
- β-human chorionic gonadotropin level to exclude pregnancy.
- Complete blood count to assess anemia.
- Thyroid function tests and prolactin level are considered in women with anovulatory cycles.
- Coagulation studies such as prothrombin time (PT), partial thromboplastin time (PTT), and von Willebrand factor are considered.
- Pap smear is performed.
- Endometrial biopsy is performed in nonpregnant women age greater than 45 with change in menstrual cycle. Any age with risk factors are evaluated for endometrial carcinoma (obesity, anovulation, unopposed estrogen).

List of imaging techniques

- Pelvic ultrasound is the first-line imaging study in women with AUB. Ultrasound is effective at characterizing anatomic as well as vascular uterine pathology and adnexal lesions (see Figure 19.1).
- Saline infused sonohystogram is used to evaluate intracavitary lesions.
- Hysteroscopy is both diagnostic and therapeutic. It is used to evaluate intracavitary lesions and allows targeted biopsy or excision of lesions identified during the procedure.
- Magnetic resonance imaging is considered as a follow-up imaging test and only when structures or characteristics of a mass cannot be visualized on ultrasound.
- Computed tomography is used to evaluation the pelvis for metastatic disease.

Potential pitfalls/common errors made regarding diagnosis of disease

- Endometrial biopsy is performed in nonpregnant women aged greater than 45 with change in menstrual cycle or at any age with risk factors such as obesity, anovulation, or exposure to unopposed estrogen.
- A Pap smear is obtained in women with new onset abnormal bleeding.
- Rapid growth of the uterus without clear evidence of uterine fibroids warrants a consultation by a gynecological oncologist.

Treatment

Treatment rationale

- Treatment should not be initiated until the etiology of AUB has been determined. The goal of treatment is to control bleeding, treat anemia, and restore quality of life. First-line management for women with AUB are combined oral contraceptive (OC) pills. They typically make bleeding more regular, lighter, and reduce dysmenorrhea, as well as provide contraception. OCs may be prescribed in a cyclic (with a monthly withdrawal bleed), extended (for instance, with a withdrawal bleeding every 3 months), or continuous (no withdrawal bleed) regimen. Levonorgestrel intrauterine device may be used for treatment of AUB in women who do not desire pregnancy in immediate future. Depot-medroxyprogesterone acetate and high-dose oral progestins are used to treat AUB in women who have a contraindication or prefer to avoid estrogen. Tranexamic acid is an option for women who do not desire or should not use hormonal treatment.
- Secondary approaches are used for women who fail or cannot tolerate medical therapy. For women who desire uterine conservation, myomectomy is the only surgical option. For women who do not desire to preserve fertility, a minimally invasive option such as endometrial ablation or uterine artery embolization may be appropriate. Hysterectomy is appropriate for women who desire definitive treatment.

When to hospitalize

- Severe anemia
- Symptomatic patient with alterations in vital signs
- Acute heavy bleeding

Managing the hospitalized patient

- Determine primary etiology of AUB.
- Assess vital signs, complete blood count (CBC), hCG, transvaginal ultrasound, +/- endometrial biopsy.
- Treat with IV estrogen or tranexamic acid.
- Consider blood transfusion in symptomatic patients.

Table of treatment

Treatment	Comment
Conservative	Asymptomatic patients
Medical: Combined OCs, oral or injectable progestin-only, levonorgestrel-releasing intrauterine device (IUD)	Estrogen is contraindicated in patients with risk factors for thromboembolism.
Surgical: Resection of endometrial polyp or submucosal myoma, endometrial ablation, hysterectomy	Resection performed in symptomatic patients with structural lesion. Endometrial ablation is used in women who have prolonged AUB and failed medical management. Hysterectomy is definitive treatment and considered in patients who fail more conservative measures.
Radiological: Uterine artery embolization	Women with uterine leiomyomas and completed childbearing
Psychological	N/A
Complementary	N/A
Other	Endometrial carcinoma should be ruled out prior to offering hormonal treatment.

Prevention/management of complications
- Combined oral contraceptive pills are contraindicated in women with breast cancer, liver cirrhosis, increased risk of deep vein thrombosis, uncontrolled diabetes, and history of migraines with aura. Common side effects such as breakthrough bleeding, headache, or breast tenderness can be controlled by changing type and/or dose of hormonal ingredients.
- Levonorgestrel-releasing intrauterine system (IUS) increases risk of pelvic infections. Women are tested for gonorrhea and chlamydia prior to placement of IUS and if culture is positive, the infection is treated with IUS in situ.
- Progestin-only therapy causes breakthrough bleeding and amenorrhea. Small dose of estrogen therapy is given to minimize these side effects.

> **BOTTOM LINE/CLINICAL PEARLS**
> - Determine primary etiology for AUB prior to initiating treatment.
> - First-line treatment for AUB is estrogen-progestin contraceptives. Progestin containing IUD is also reasonable option.
> - Estrogen-progestin OCs can be prescribed as cyclic with a monthly withdrawal bleed, extended with a withdrawal bleed every 3 months, or continuous regimen.
> - High-dose oral or injectable progestin-only medications are reasonable options but often cause breakthrough bleeding.
> - Hysterectomy is the only definitive treatment for uterine fibroids.

Special populations
Pregnancy
- Patient with AUB and positive serum pregnancy test should be evaluated for a threatened abortion/nonviable pregnancy.

Children
- Adolescents with AUB evaluated for pregnancy, bleeding disorders, and ovulatory dysfunction. Complete history and physical are obtained followed by hCG, CBC, thyroid stimulating hormone, PT/PTT, von Willebrand assays, and pelvic ultrasound.

Elderly

- Elderly patients with AUB or postmenopausal bleeding are evaluated for endometrial malignancy.

Prognosis

> **BOTTOM LINE/CLINICAL PEARLS**
> - Identifying the underlying cause of AUB is the most important aspect of determining prognosis.
> - Patients with structural lesions that are resected have resolution of AUB.
> - Multiple effective medical therapies are available to ameliorate abnormal uterine bleeding symptoms. On the cessation of medical therapy, regrowth of fibroids to pretreatment size occurs fairly quickly. In perimenopausal patients, medical therapy can bridge the gap to naturally occurring menopause.

Natural history of untreated disease

- Asymptomatic endometrial polyps contain underlying malignancy in approximately 1% of pre-menopausal patients and 3% of postmenopausal patients. Without surgical resection, endometrial polyps less than 1 cm resolve in approximately 50% of patients.
- Uterine fibroids are most prevalent during a woman's reproductive years. The majority of fibroids shrink with the onset of menopause.
- Untreated blood clotting disorders can cause life-threatening anemia.
- Anovulation increases risk of endometrial hyperplasia and malignancy.
- Undiagnosed and untreated endometrial carcinoma can cause systemic spread and death.

Prognosis for treated patients

- Patient who are willing to try various medical and surgical approaches to treat abnormal uterine bleeding have a good prognosis. Medical management gives the majority of women relief from their primary complaints.
- Prognosis for women who undergo treatment for endometrial carcinoma is dependent on the histology, stage, and grade of tumor at time of diagnosis.

Follow-up tests and monitoring

- Women who have resolution of symptoms after medical or surgical treatment, do not need additional follow-up testing.
- Patients who are diagnosed with uterine polyp or fibroid and do not undergo treatment are scheduled for a follow-up pelvic ultrasound in 12 months.
- Women who are treated for endometrial malignancy are followed postoperatively by gynecological oncologist.

Reading list

2016 update on abnormal uterine bleeding. *OBG Manage* 2016 March;28(3).

ACOG practice bulletin no. 110: Noncontraceptive uses of hormonal contraceptives. *Obstet Gynecol* 2010 Jan;115(1) 206-18.

ACOG committee opinion no. 557: Management of acute abnormal uterine bleeding in nonpregnant reproductive-aged women. *Obstet Gynecol* 2013 Apr;121(4) 891-6.

Annan JJ, Aquilina J, Ball E. The management of endometrial polyps in the 21st century. *Obstet Gynaecol* 2012;14:33-38.

Suggested websites

AAGL Practice Report: Practice Guidelines for the Diagnosis and Management of Endometrial Polyps. https://www.aagl.org/wp-content/uploads/2013/03/aagl-Practice-Guidelines-for-the-Diagnosis-and-Management-of-Endometrial-Polyps.pdf

Abnormal Uterine Bleeding. A Management Algorithm: http://www.jabfm.org/content/19/6/590.full

Guidelines
National society guidelines

Title	Source	Date/URL
Management of acute abnormal uterine bleeding in nonpregnant reproductive-aged women: ACOG committee opinion no. 557	American College of Obstetricians and Gynecologists	April 2013 https://www.acog.org/Clinical-Guidance-and-Publications/Committee-Opinions/Committee-on-Gynecologic-Practice/Management-of-Acute-Abnormal-Uterine-Bleeding-in-Nonpregnant-Reproductive-Aged-Women?IsMobileSet=false
Practice guidelines for the diagnosis and management of endometrial polyps: AAGL practice report	American Association of Gynecologic Laparoscopists	August 2011 https://www.aagl.org/wp-content/uploads/2013/03/aagl-Practice-Guidelines-for-the-Diagnosis-and-Management-of-Endometrial-Polyps.pdf

Evidence

Type of evidence	Title and comment	Date/URL
Expert opinion	Management of acute abnormal uterine bleeding in nonpregnant reproductive-aged women	2013 http://www.acog.org/Resources-And-Publications/Committee-Opinions/Committee-on-Gynecologic-Practice/Management-of-Acute-Abnormal-Uterine-Bleeding-in-Nonpregnant-Reproductive-Aged-Women

Images

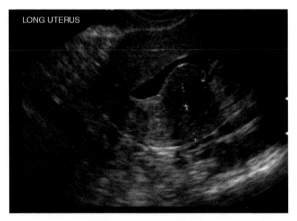

Figure 19.1 Abnormal uterine bleeding - Submucosal leiomyoma. Courtesy of UpToDate. https://www.uptodate.com/contents/image?imageKey=OBGYN%2F50777&topicKey=OBGYN%2F3263&source=outline_link&search=abnormal%20uterine%20bleeding&selectedTitle=1~150

Additional material for this chapter can be found online at:
www.wiley.com/go/sperling/mountsinai/obstetricsandgynecology

This includes a case study, multiple choice questions, advice for patients, and ICD codes.

CHAPTER 20

Fibroids

Karina Hoan[1] and Charles Ascher-Walsh[2]

[1] FMIGS Faculty, Division of Minimally Invasive Gynecology, The Portland Clinic, Portland, OR
[2] Division of Female Pelvic Medicine and Reconstructive Surgery, Department of Obstetrics, Gynecology and Reproductive Science, Icahn School of Medicine at Mount Sinai, New York, NY

> **OVERALL BOTTOM LINE**
> * Uterine fibroids are the most common pelvic tumor in women.
> * Uterine fibroids are benign growths of smooth muscle arising from the myometrium.
> * Most common presenting symptoms are abnormal uterine bleeding, infertility, pelvic pain, and pelvic pressure.
> * Asymptomatic fibroids can be followed without intervention.

Background
Definition of disease
* Uterine fibroids (leiomyomas or myomas) are abnormal growths of smooth muscle that arise from the myometrial layer of the uterus. They are classified based on their location within the myometrium.

Disease classification
* Intramural fibroids are located within the uterine wall. Submucosal myomas protrude into the endometrial cavity. Subserosal myomas are attached to the outer layer of the uterus. Cervical myomas are located in the cervix.

Incidence/prevalence
* Uterine leiomyomas are the most common pelvic tumor in females.
* Incidence is unknown because only symptomatic women are screened.
* Prevalence varies with age and ethnicity.
* Fibroids are present in approximately 26–59% of reproductive aged black women and 7–43% of reproductive aged white women.

Etiology
* Uterine fibroid growth is thought to arise from a single mutated uterine smooth muscle cell. They are monoclonal tumors.
* Initiation and promotion of abnormal growth of this single myometrial cell are not well understood.
* Estrogen and progesterone promote monoclonal myometrial cell proliferation and growth of uterine fibroids.

Pathology/pathogenesis
* Uterine fibroids arise from the myometrial layer of the uterus.
* Fibroids may remain within the muscular layer (intramural) or protrude outward to become subserosal or inward to become submucous fibroids.

Mount Sinai Expert Guides: Obstetrics and Gynecology, First Edition. Edited by Rhoda Sperling.
© 2020 John Wiley & Sons Ltd. Published 2020 by John Wiley & Sons Ltd.
Companion Website: www.wiley.com/go/sperling/mountsinai/obstetricsandgynecology

- Submucosal fibroids cause abnormal uterine bleeding (AUB) as a result of distortion of the endometrial lining.

Predictive/risk factors

Risk factor	Odds ratio
White race (age 40–44)	6.3
White race parous	0.2
African American race (age 40–44)	27.4

https://academic.oup.com/aje/article/153/1/20/107782/
Risk-Factors-for-Uterine-Fibroids-among-Women

Prevention
- No interventions have been demonstrated to prevent the development of the disease.
- Vitamin D supplementation and progesterone modulators are under investigation and show promising results in the prevention of uterine fibroids.

Screening
- Bimanual pelvic examination and pelvic ultrasound are primary screening modalities.
- Findings of an enlarged, mobile uterus with irregular contour are suggestive of uterine fibroids.

Diagnosis
- A clinical diagnosis of uterine fibroids is made based upon a pelvic examination and pelvic ultrasound findings.
- The most common presenting symptoms are AUB pelvic pain or pressure and infertility but many women are asymptomatic.
- Bimanual pelvic examination demonstrates an enlarged, mobile uterus with irregular contour.
- Pelvic ultrasound shows uterine fibroids as hypoechoic, well-circumscribed, round masses.
- Saline-infused-sonohysterogram may be used when intracavitary lesion are suspected.
- Magnetic resonance imaging may be used if ultrasound findings are not sufficient for surgical planning or if the diagnosis is uncertain.
- A definitive diagnosis is made by histological review of the myomatous tissue.

Differential diagnosis

Differential diagnosis	Features
Pregnancy	Positive β-human chorionic gonadotropin
Adnexal mass	Abnormal adnexal finding on ultrasound
Adenomyosis	Globular bulky uterus
Carcinoma	Rapidly growing fibroids, postmenopausal bleeding
Hematometria	Amenorrhea, cyclic pain
Endometriosis	Fixed uterus, menorrhagia

Typical presentation
- Patients with uterine fibroids typically seek medical attention due to symptoms such as heavy menstrual bleeding, pelvic pressure and pain, reproductive dysfunction, or because of an incidental finding on pelvic imaging. Although many uterine fibroids are asymptomatic, the number, size, and location of the myomas can influence the severity of patients' symptoms.

Clinical diagnosis
History
- Obstetrical, gynecological, and medical history is elicited. Medications are reviewed. The duration, color, volume, and pattern of vaginal bleeding are determined. Intermenstrual bleeding and postmenopausal bleeding should prompt investigation to exclude endometrial pathology. Large fibroids cause pelvic pain and pressure. Uterine fibroids that impinge or distort the endometrial cavity may cause infertility or recurrent pregnancy loss.

Physical examination
- The physical examination includes an abdominal and pelvic examination as well as vital signs. Women with prolonged heavy menstrual bleeding can become severely anemic, which may be noted in a change in heart rate and/or blood pressure. Large fibroid uteri can be palpated abdominally. The size of the uterus is described in terms of fundal height, as in a gravid uterus. For example, a uterus that reaches the level of the umbilicus is considered a 20-week size uterus. A thorough bimanual pelvic exam is performed. The size, contour, and mobility should be noted.

Laboratory diagnosis
List of diagnostic tests
- β-human chorionic gonadotropin level to exclude pregnancy
- Complete blood count to assess anemia
- Endometrial biopsy is performed in nonpregnant women age greater than 45 with menstrual cycle changes or at any age in a woman with risk factors for endometrial carcinoma (obesity, anovulation, unopposed estrogen).

List of imaging techniques
- Transvaginal ultrasound is performed in all patients with unknown cause of abnormal uterine bleeding, pelvic pain, or increased uterine size.
- Saline infused sonohysterogram is performed when there is suspicion for intracavitary leiomyoma. Helpful when planning on hysteroscopic resection.
- Hysteroscopy is both diagnostic and therapeutic. It is used to evaluate intracavitary lesions and allows targeted biopsy or excision of lesions identified during the procedure.
- Magnetic resonance imaging is considered as a follow-up imaging test and only when structures or characteristics of a mass cannot be visualized on ultrasound.
- Computed tomography is used to evaluate the pelvis for metastatic disease.

Potential pitfalls/common errors made regarding diagnosis of disease
- There is no normal rate of growth for fibroids. They may remain unchanged for years or they may grow rapidly with yearly doubling. The rate of growth has not been found to correlate with the risk of sarcoma; however, there should be more concern in patients with a change from a normal exam one year to significant uterine mass the next.

Treatment

Treatment rationale

- Expectant management is a reasonable option for asymptomatic uterine leiomyomas. The only nonhormonal therapies that have been shown in vivo and in vitro to suppress fibroid growth are vitamin D and green tea extract. Hormonal therapies, such as combined oral contraceptive pills (OCP), may be associated with decreased menstrual bleeding and are used as first-line treatment. Levonorgestrel-releasing intrauterine system (IUS) reduces uterine bleeding and increases hematocrit. Progestin implants, injections, and pills can provide relief of mild menstrual bleeding-related symptoms.
- Gonadotropin-releasing hormone (GnRH) agonists are the most effective medical therapy for uterine fibroids but have the most significant side effects. The majority of women using GnRH agonists develop amenorrhea, improved anemia, and decrease in uterine size within three months of initiating therapy. GnRH agonists may be used to decrease uterine size prior to a scheduled surgery. This is recommended if the uterine size is prohibiting a minimally invasive approach. They have been associated with less surgical blood loss but an increased risk of more rapid recurrence of fibroids after myomectomy.
- Surgical management is reserved for women whose quality of life is severely affected by symptoms of uterine fibroids. Surgical treatment is indicated in women with AUB not corrected by medical therapy, infertility, or recurrent pregnancy loss. Hysterectomy provides definitive treatment; myomectomy, uterine artery/fibroid embolization, radiofrequency ablation, and magnetic resonance-guided focused-ultrasound surgery are alternative procedures (See Figures 20.1 and 20.2).
- Ulipristal acetate, a progesterone receptor antagonist is used in many counties to treat fibroids. It has similar results as GnRH agonists with fewer side effects. It has not been approved for treatment in the US do to reports of potential liver damage. Currently, clinical trial evaluating the use of GnRH antagonists are underway and show promise for the treatment of fibroids.

Table of treatment

Treatment	Comment
Conservative	Asymptomatic patients
Medical: Combined OCP, levonorgestrel-releasing IUS, GnRH agonist	Estrogen should be avoided in patients with increased risk of developing thromboembolism. Levonorgestrel-IUS can cause AUB for first 3–6 months. Prolonged use of GnRH leads to decreased bone mass.
Surgical: Hysteroscopic resection, endometrial ablation, myomectomy, hysterectomy	Resection performed in symptomatic patients with structural lesion in endometrium. Endometrial ablation is used in women who have prolonged AUB and failed medical management. Hysterectomy is definitive treatment and considered in patients who fail more conservative measures (See Figures 20.1 and 20.2).
Radiological: Uterine artery ablation, magnetic resonance-guided focused ultrasound, radiofrequency ablation	Suitable for women who have completed childbearing and are poor surgical candidates.

Prevention/management of complications

- Combined oral contraceptive pills are contraindicated in women with breast cancer, liver cirrhosis, increased risk of deep vein thrombosis, uncontrolled diabetes, and history of migraines with aura. Common side effects such as breakthrough bleeding, headache, breast tenderness can be controlled by changing type, and/or dose of hormonal ingredients. Rare but more serious complications are increased risk of thromboembolism and breast cancer.

- Levonorgestrel-releasing IUS increases risk of pelvic infections. Women are tested for gonorrhea and chlamydia prior to placement of IUS and if culture is positive, the infection is treated with IUS in-situ.
- Progestin-only therapy causes breakthrough bleeding and amenorrhea. Small dose of estrogen therapy is given to minimize these side effects.
- GnRH agonists cause menopausal symptoms such as hot flashes, sleep disturbances, vaginal dryness, and bone loss. These symptoms can be managed by giving low dose add-back progesterone therapy.
- Surgical procedures have risk of bleeding, infection, damage to bowel or bladder or other surrounding organs. An experienced surgeon should perform the procedure to mitigate complications.

Management/treatment algorithm

- See Algorithm 20.1.

Algorithm 20.1 Diagnostic algorithm for fibroids

| Bleeding pattern | Other associated clinical features | Differential diagnosis | | Evaluation |
		Common etiologies	Less common etiologies	
Regular menses that is heavy or prolonged	Enlarged uterus on examination, discrete masses may be noted	Uterine leiomyoma		– Pelvic ultrasound – Saline infusion sonography or hysteroscopy (if intracavitary pathology is suspected)
	– Dysmenorrhea – Enlarged, boggy uterus on examination	Adenomyosis		Pelvic ultrasound
	– Family history of bleeding disorder – Symptoms of bleeding diathesis – Anticoagulant therapy	Bleeding disorder		Testing for bleeding disorder
	Risk factors for uterine malignancy		Endometrial carcinoma or uterine sarcoma	Endometrial sampling
Regular menses with intermenstrual bleeding		Endometrial polyp		– Pelvic ultrasound – Saline infusion sonography or hysteroscopy (if available)
	Risk factors for uterine malignancy		Endometrial carcinoma or uterine sarcoma	Endometrial sampling
	Recent history of uterine or cervical procedure or childbirth, particularly if infection was present		Chronic endometritis	Endometrial sampling

(Continued)

(Continued)

Bleeding pattern	Other associated clinical features	Differential diagnosis		Evaluation
		Common etiologies	Less common etiologies	
Irregular bleeding, may be more or less frequent than normal menses and volume and duration may vary		Ovulatory dysfunction:		
	Hirsutism, acne, and/or obesity	Polycystic ovary syndrome (PCOS)		Total testosterone and/or other androgens (may not be increased in all women with PCOS)
	Galactorrhea	Hyperprolactinemia		Prolactin
	− Recent weight gain or loss − Heat or cold intolerance − Family history of thyroid dysfunction	Thyroid disease		Thyroid function tests
	Risk factors for uterine malignancy		Endometrial carcinoma or uterine sarcoma	Endometrial sampling
Secondary amenorrhea	History of irregular bleeding	Ovulatory dysfunction		Refer to ovulatory dysfunction above
	Poor nutrition or intense exercise	Hypothalamic amenorrhea		− Follicle-stimulating hormone − Luteinizing hormone − Estradiol
	Hot flushes	Premature ovarian insufficiency		Follicle-stimulating hormone
	Recent history of uterine or cervical procedure or childbirth, particularly if infection was present (menses may present, but abnormally light or brief)		Cervical stenosis	On pelvic examination, instrument cannot be passed through internal cervical os
			Intrauterine adhesions (Asherman syndrome)	Hysteroscopy
Irregular or heavy bleeding in a patient using hormonal contraceptives or with an intrauterine device		Iatrogenic AUB		

> **BOTTOM LINE/CLINICAL PEARLS**
> - Hormonal therapies are the least invasive treatments and should be the first line for women without contraindications.
> - GnRH agonists can be used for 3 to 6 months to prior to surgery if the reduction in uterine/myoma volume will significantly facilitate the procedure or if there is significant anemia that has not responded to medical therapy.
> - Myomectomy is the only well-studied surgical treatment for women with symptomatic uterine fibroids and desire future fertility.
> - Hysterectomy is the only definitive treatment for uterine fibroids.
> - Poor surgical candidates can be treated with uterine artery embolization or magnetic resonance-guided focused ultrasound.

Special populations
Pregnancy
- Submucosal fibroids increase the risk of infertility as well as increase the risk of first trimester spontaneous abortion.
- Women with fibroids have an increased risk of preterm delivery and abruption at the time of delivery and have an increased risk of needing a cesarean delivery.
- Uterine myomas can cause pain and discomfort during pregnancy. Discomfort is due to fibroids outgrowing their blood supply or degenerate during the gestational period. Elective surgery is not recommended during pregnancy.

Elderly/postmenopausal
- Uterine fibroids typically shrink after menopause. In asymptomatic patients, medical or surgical intervention is not indicated. With newly diagnosed uterine fibroids or an enlarging pelvic mass, evaluation to exclude uterine malignancy takes place.

Prognosis

> **BOTTOM LINE/CLINICAL PEARLS**
> - Multiple effective medical therapies are available to ameliorate fibroid-related symptoms. On the cessation of medical therapy, regrowth of fibroids to pretreatment size occurs fairly quickly. In perimenopausal patients, medical therapy can bridge the gap to naturally occurring menopause.
> - Uterine sparing surgeries such as myomectomy and uterine artery embolization are effective in treating pelvic pressure and abnormal uterine bleeding. However, these procedures are not permanent and patients may require future treatment.
> - Pregnancy is associated with increased complications after uterine artery embolization and is not recommended. The data are unclear on how long to wait to conceive after myomectomy. Depending on the location of fibroids and type of myomectomy, there may be increased risk of preterm birth and uterine rupture.
> - Hysterectomy is the definitive approach for relief of symptoms and prevention of recurrent leiomyoma-related problems and is recommended for women who do not desire future fertility.

Natural history of untreated disease
- In premenopausal women, fibroids have an average growth rate of 1.2 cm over 2–3 years. They may grow more rapidly during pregnacy. In postpartum patients, fibroids tend to regress. In postmenopausal women, most fibroids shrink in size.

Prognosis for treated patients
- Patient who are willing to try various medical and surgical approaches to treat fibroids have a good prognosis. Medical management gives the majority of women relief from their primary complaints. The vast majority of women who undergo uterine artery embolization are satisfied with the outcome. Hysterectomy is a definitive treatment and will ameliorate symptoms related to uterine fibroids.

Follow-up tests and monitoring
- For premenopausal patients who are asymptomatic, no follow-up testing or monitoring is required. In patients with persistent or worsening symptoms, repeat pelvic ultrasound is performed and endometrial biopsy is considered.
- For postmenopausal patients with increasing size or symptoms related to a uterine mass, appropriate imaging and sampling is performed to rule out malignancy.
- Women with a uterus greater than 20 cm long who are asymptomatic and conservatively managing their fibroids should evaluate for evidence of ureteral occlusion at least annually as this can occur without symptoms.

Reading list
AAGL Practice Report: Practice guidelines for the diagnosis and management of submucous leiomyomas. *J Minim Invasive Gynecol* 2012 Mar-Apr;19(2):152-71.

ACOG practice bulletin no. 96: Alternatives to hysterectomy in the management of leiomyomas. *Obstet Gynecol* 2008 Aug;112(2 Pt 1):387-400.

ACOG practice bulletin no. 110: Noncontraceptive uses of hormonal contraceptives. *Obstet Gynecol* 2010 Jan;115(1):206-18.

Suggested website
American Family Physician. Uterine fibroid tumors: diagnosis and treatment. http://www.aafp.org/afp/2007/0515/p1503.html

Guidelines
National society guidelines

Title	Source	Date/URL
Practice guidelines for the diagnosis and management of submucous leiomyomas: AAGL practice report	American Association of Gynecologic Laparoscopists	2011 http://www.aagl.org/wp-content/uploads/2013/03/aagl-Practice-Guidelines-for-the-Diagnosis-and-Management-of-Submucous-Leiomyomas.pdf

Evidence

Type of evidence	Title and comment	Date/full reference
Clinical management guideline level A evidence	Alternatives to hysterectomy in the management of leiomyomas	August 2008 ACOG practice bulletin no. 96. *Obstet Gynecol* 2008 Aug;112(2 Pt 1):387-400.
Clinical management guideline level A evidence	Noncontraceptive uses of hormonal contraceptives	January 2010 ACOG practice bulletin no. 110. *Obstet Gynecol* 2010 Jan;115(1):206-18.

Images

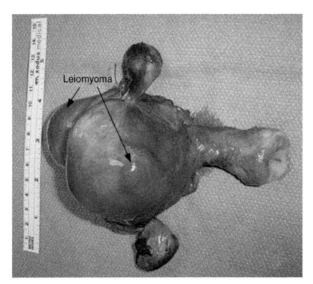

Figure 20.1 Leiomyomas - Hysterectomy specimens. Reproduced with permission from Aron Schuftan, MD. Copyright © Aron Schuftan, MD. See color version on website.

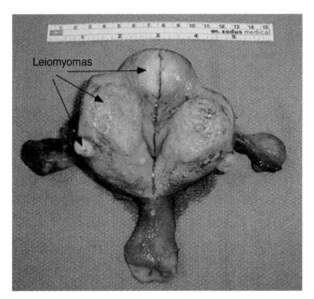

Figure 20.2 Leiomyomas - Hysterectomy specimens. Reproduced with permission from Aron Schuftan, MD. Copyright © Aron Schuftan, MD. See color version on website.

Additional material for this chapter can be found online at:
www.wiley.com/go/sperling/mountsinai/obstetricsandgynecology

This includes a case study, multiple choice questions, advice for patients, and ICD codes. The following images are available in color: Figure 20.1 and Figure 20.2.

CHAPTER 21

Pelvic Organ Prolapse

Woojin Chong[1,2] and John A. Fantl[2]
[1] Urogynecologist, Inspira Health, Vineland, New Jersey, NJ
[2] Division of Female Pelvic Medicine and Reconstructive Surgery, Department of Obstetrics, Gynecology and Reproductive Science, Icahn School of Medicine at Mount Sinai, New York, NY

OVERALL BOTTOM LINE
- Pelvic organ prolapse (POP) is the herniation of the genital tract through the vagina.
- Risk factors for POP include increasing parity, advancing age, obesity, and hysterectomy, chronic constipation, heavy lifting jobs, as well as genetic background.
- Common symptoms of POP are sensation of pelvic pressure/heaviness/protrusion of tissue from the vagina, described as "feeling a bulge" or "something is falling out of the vagina."
- Conservative treatments include vaginal pessaries and pelvic floor muscle exercises.
- Surgical managements are offered to women with symptomatic POP, who have failed or declined conservative management.

Background
Definition of disease
- Descent of one or more pelvic structures: the uterine cervix or vaginal apex, anterior vaginal wall (usually with bladder, cystocele), posterior vaginal wall (usually with rectum, rectocele), or peritoneum of the cul-de-sac (usually with small intestine, enterocele).

Incidence/prevalence
- The exact incidence and prevalence is difficult to ascertain due to (a) different criteria and classification systems, (b) various rates for symptomatic and asymptomatic women, and (c) uncertainty of the number of women with POP not reaching the health system.
- Prevalence of symptomatic POP is estimated to range from 2.9 to 8%.
- Prevalence of asymptomatic POP is probably even higher.
- In the United States, it is estimated the annual number of women undergoing surgeries for POP will reach > 190 000 by 2020.

Economic Impact
- Treatment of POP requires significant healthcare resources. The annual cost of ambulatory care of POP in the US from 2005 to 2006 was estimated at $300 million.
- The direct cost of POP surgery in 1997 was estimated to be greater than $100 million based on national average Medicare reimbursement.
- The healthcare impact of POP is likely to expand due to the growing population of elderly women.

Mount Sinai Expert Guides: Obstetrics and Gynecology, First Edition. Edited by Rhoda Sperling.
© 2020 John Wiley & Sons Ltd. Published 2020 by John Wiley & Sons Ltd.
Companion Website: www.wiley.com/go/sperling/mountsinai/obstetricsandgynecology

Etiology

- The etiology of POP is likely multifactorial. It includes advanced age, parity, familial and genetic linkage, childbirth, chronic constipation, history of prior hysterectomy, obesity, heavy lifting, chronic cough, etc.

Pathology/pathogenesis

- The full pathogenesis of POP is unknown.
- It is believed that POP is a heterogeneous condition in which disruption of the pelvic floor musculature and connective tissue result in progressive descent of pelvic organs through the vaginal canal.

Prevention

> **BOTTOM LINE/CLINICAL PEARLS**
> - No prevention strategies have been extensively studied for POP.

Screening

- Symptoms of POP may be included in annual well women's health visit. Symptoms of POP include sensation of vaginal bulge, pressure and discomfort, dyspareunia, decreased libido and orgasm, and increased embarrassment with altered anatomy affecting body image, as well as associated symptoms relating to voiding, defecatory, and sexual function.

Primary prevention

- No primary prevention strategies have been extensively studied for POP.

Secondary prevention

- It is unclear that cesarean delivery will prevent the occurrence of POP.
- Prevention of progression of POP has not been well studied either: however, some data suggest that women who use a vaginal pessary have a lower stage of POP on subsequent exam. Weight loss, treatment of chronic constipation, and avoidance of heavy lifting may reduce development in progression of POP.
- A Cochrane review shows that use of oral raloxifene in women who were 60 years or older resulted a significant reduction in the proportion of women who subsequently underwent surgery (0.8 vs 1.5%; odds ratio [OR] 0.5, 95% confidence interval [CI] 0.3–0.8).

Diagnosis

> **BOTTOM LINE/CLINICAL PEARLS**
> - POP is diagnosed during pelvic examination.
> - Taking through medical history is important to elicit POP associated symptoms.
> - The Pelvic Organ Prolapse Quantitation (POPQ) system, introduced in 1996, has become the standard classification system.

Typical presentation

- Patients with POP may present with symptoms related to the prolapsed structures, such as a bulge or vaginal pressure or with associated symptoms including urinary, defecatory, or sexual dysfunction.
- Severity of symptoms does not correlate well with the stage of prolapse.
- Symptoms are often related to position: for example, POP is less noticeable in the morning or while supine and worsen as the day progresses or women are active in an upright position.
- Many women with POP are asymptomatic: treatment is generally not indicated in such cases.

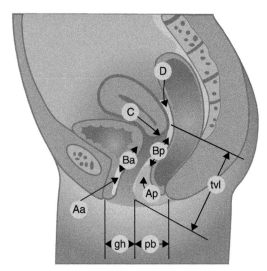

Figure 21.1 The POPQ system. Courtesy of AUGS (American Urogynecologic Society), https://www.augs.org/patient-services/pop-q-tool/. See color version on website.

Clinical diagnosis

- Physical exam should include (a) visual inspection, (b) speculum exam, (c) bimanual pelvic exam, (d) rectovaginal exam, and (e) neuromuscular exam.
- A Sims retractor or one blade of the bivalve speculum is used to assess the degree of POP.
- Patients are examined initially in the dorsolithotomy position at a 45 degree then standing position for maximum extent of POP.
- During the exam, the maximum extent of POP is determined for each point, using the POPQ system (see Figure 21.1 and Table 21.1).

Table 21.1 Description of POPQ components.

Point	Description	Range of values
Aa	Anterior vaginal wall 3 cm proximal to the external urethral meatus	−3 cm to +3 cm
Ba	Most distal (i.e. most dependent) position of any part of the anterior vaginal wall between point Aa and the vaginal cuff or anterior vaginal fornix	−3 cm to +TVL
C	Most distal (i.e. most dependent) edge of the cervix or the leading edge of the vaginal cuff (posthysterectomy)	
Ap	Posterior vaginal wall, 3 cm proximal to the posterior hymen	−3 cm to +3 cm
Bp	Most distal (i.e. most dependent) position of any part of the upper posterior vaginal wall between point Ap and the vaginal cuff or posterior vaginal fornix	−3 cm to +TVL
D	Deepest point of the posterior fornix, corresponding approximately to where the uterosacral ligaments attach to the posterior cervix (N/A if posthysterectomy)	
GH	Measured anterior-posteriorly from the middle of the external urethral meatus to the posterior midline hymen	
PB	Measured from the posterior margin of the genital hiatus to the midanal opening	
TVL	Depth of vagina when C or D point is reduced in normal position	

Proximal to hymen: measurements recorded as negative numbers ("inside the vagina"), distal to hymen: measurements recorded as positive numbers ("outside the vagina")

Table 21.2 POPQ staging.

Stage 0	Aa, Ap, Ba, Bp = −3 cm and C or D ≤ (TVL-2) cm
Stage 1	Stage 0 criteria not met and leading edge −1 cm
Stage 2	Leading edge ≥−1 cm but ≤+1 cm
Stage 3	Leading edge >−1 cm but < +(TVL-2) cm
Stage 4	Leading edge ≥ (TLV-2)cm

- For the purpose of simple clinical communication or grouping patients for research purposes, a staging system using POPQ was developed (see Table 21.2).
- The POPQ system is the POP classification system of choice of the International Continence Society (ICS), the American Urogynecologic Society (AUGS), and the Society of Gynecologic Surgeons (SGS).
- There are six points measured at the vagina with respect to the hymen and three additional measurements: total vaginal length (TVL), genital hiatus (gh), and perineal body (pb) (see Table 21.2).
- Maximal POP is defined by (a) the vaginal wall becomes tight during straining, (b) traction on the prolapse causes no further descent, and (c) patient confirms that protrusion is maximal.

Treatment
Treatment rationale
- Treatment is generally not indicated for asymptomatic POP.
- Treatment is indicated for women with symptoms of POP or associated conditions like bowel, urinary, or sexual dysfunction.
- Obstructed urination or defecation or hydronephrosis from chronic ureteral kinking are indications for treatment, regardless of degree of POP.
- Treatment is individualized according to the patient's symptoms and their impact on her quality of life.
- Establish realistic patient expectations.

Table of treatment

Expectant	**For women who can tolerate their symptoms and prefer to avoid treatment**
Conservative	Vaginal pessaries: • The mainstay of nonsurgical treatment for POP • Silicone devices in a variety of shapes and sizes, supporting the pelvic organs • Must be removed and cleaned on a regular basis • Regular vaginal exam needed to monitor for vaginal erosion • Perforation into adjacent organs is rare but may occur in neglected cases Pelvic floor muscle exercises: • Improve POP stage and POP-associated symptoms Estrogen therapy: • No data exist to support estrogen therapy (both systemic or topical) as a primary treatment of POP.
Surgical	For women with symptomatic POP who have failed or declined conservative management of POP and/or who finished with childbearing. • Various surgical approaches available for POP including vaginal, abdominal approaches with and without graft materials • The choice of a primary procedure for POP depends on a variety of factors such as reconstructive or obliterative approaches; concomitant hysterectomy; surgical route for repair of multiple sites or prolapse; concomitant anti-incontinence surgery; use of surgical mesh.

Possible complications

- Pessary use: serious complications are rare but fistula formation is possible in women with neglected pessaries.
- Apical prolapse surgical repair:
  - Sacrocolpopexy: presacral hemorrhage, mesh erosion (3.4% for all types, 0.5% for polypropylene mesh), small-bowel obstruction (0.1–5%)
  - Sacrospinous ligament suspension: ureteral kinking (2.9%), gluteal pain (2%), hemorrhage (1.9%), nerve damage (1.8%)
  - Intraperitoneal uterosacral ligament suspension: ureteral obstruction (1.8%), ureteral kinking (11% on intraop cystoscopy), sensory neuropathy and pain (3.8%)
  - Iliococcygeus suspension: similar complications as sacrospinous ligament suspension
- Anterior prolapse surgical repair: bladder, urethral and ureteral injury, hemorrhage, hematoma, dyspareunia, urinary tract infection, de novo or worsening detrusor overactivity, urinary retention, urogenital fistula
- Posterior prolapse surgical repair: dyspareunia, constipation, hematoma, inclusion cyst formation, fecal impaction. Injury to rectum, rectovaginal or rectoperineal fistula, bowel and defecatory dysfunction
- Concomitant Burch colposuspension:
  - Voiding dysfunction and urgency incontinence (2–3%)
  - Urinary tract infection (32–50%)
  - Apical prolapse (17%)
  - Incidental cystotomy (3%)

CLINICAL PEARLS
- Women with symptomatic prolapse can be managed expectantly or treated with conservative or surgical therapy.
- Treatment is generally not indicated for women with asymptomatic prolapse.
- Conservative treatment options for POP include vaginal pessaries and pelvic floor muscle exercises.
- Numerous surgical options are available for POP including vaginal and abdominal approaches (open, laparoscopic, or robotic) and with or without graft materials.

Special populations

Pregnancy
- Women may present with new symptoms or an exacerbation of POP during pregnancy.
- Pregnant women are managed conservatively with pessary or pelvic floor exercises.

Elderly
- In contrast with younger women, elderly women are at lower risk of recurrence and higher risk of surgical complications.
- The most common perioperative complications include blood transfusion or significant blood loss, pulmonary edema, postoperative congestive heart failure. The independent risk factors include length of surgery, coronary artery disease, and peripheral vascular disease.
- However, the overall perioperative morbidity rate in elderly women who undergo urogynecologic surgery is low.

Obese women
- Obesity is risk factor for new onset and recurrent POP but no difference in outcome of surgical correction of apical POP compared to nonobese women.
- Open abdominal approach in obese women increases wound complications.

Prognosis

> **BOTTOM LINE/CLINICAL PEARLS**
> • POP is a progressive condition.

Natural history of untreated disease
- Mild POP may lead to more advanced disease until menopause then the degree of POP may follow a course of alternating progression and regression.
- POP increased by at least 2 cm in 11% of women and regressed by the same amount in 3% of women in a prospective cohort study of 249 women.

Prognosis for treated patients
- Most patients have resolution of symptoms after treatment; however, recurrence after surgical management and intolerance to pessary management may occur.

Reading list

American College of Obstetricians and Gynecologists. *Urogynecology: an illustrated guide for women*. Washington, DC: ACOG; 2004.

American College of Obstetricians and Gynecologists. *Urogynecology: a case management approach [CD-ROM]*. Washington, DC: ACOG; 2005.

American College of Obstetricians and Gynecologists. Pelvic organ prolapse. ACOG practice bulletin no. 85. *Obstet Gynecol* 2007;110:717-29.

American College of Obstetricians and Gynecologists. *Pelvic support problems*. Patient education pamphlet AP012. Washington, DC: ACOG; 2010.

American College of Obstetricians and Gynecologists. Vaginal placement of synthetic mesh for pelvic organ prolapse. Committee opinion no. 513. *Obstet Gynecol* 2011;118:1459-64.

Barber MD, Maher C. Epidemiology and outcome assessment of pelvic organ prolapse. *Int Urogynecol J* 2013 Nov;24(11):1783-90.

Bradley CS, Zimmerman MB, Qi Y, et al. Natural history of pelvic organ prolapse in postmenopausal women. *Obstet Gynecol* 2007;109(4):848.

Bump RC, Mattiasson A, Bo K, et al. The standardization of terminology of female pelvic organ prolapse and pelvic floor dysfunction. *Am J Obstet Gynecol* 1996;175:10-7.

Hagen S, Stark D. Conservative prevention and management of pelvic organ prolapse in women. *Cochrane Database Syst Rev* 2011;(12). Art. No.: CD003882. DOI: 10.1002/14651858.CD003882.pub4.

Ismail SI, Bain C, Hagen S. Oestrogens for treatment or prevention of pelvic organ prolapse in postmenopausal women. *Cochrane Database Syst Rev* 2010 Sep 8;(9):CD007063.

Maher C, Feiner B, Baessler K, et al. Surgical management of pelvic organ prolapse in women. *Cochrane Database Syst Rev* 2013;(4). Art. No.: CD004014. DOI: 10.1002/14651858.CD004014.pub5.

Nygaard I, Barber MD, Burgio KL et al. Prevalence of symptomatic pelvic floor disorders in US women. Pelvic Floor Disorders Network. *JAMA* 2008;300:1311-6.

Sung VW, Hampton BS. Epidemiology and psychosocial impact of female pelvic floor disorders. Chapter 7. In: M. Walters, M. Karram eds. *Urogynecology and reconstructive pelvic surgery*. 4th ed. New York: Elsevier; 2015:96-104.

Sung VW, Washington B, Raker CA. Costs of ambulatory care related to female pelvic organ floor disorders in the United States. *Am J Obstet Gynecol* 2010;202(5):483 e1.

Walters MD. Evaluation of urinary incontinence and pelvic organ prolapse: history, physical examination and office tests. Chapter 9. In: M. Walters, M. Karram eds. *Urogynecology and reconstructive pelvic surgery*. 4th ed. New York: Elsevier; 2015:117-29.

Wu JM, Kawasaki A, Hudley AF, et al. Predicting the number of women who will undergo incontinence and prolapse surgery 2010 to 2050. *Am J Obstet Gynecol* 2011;205:230.e1-5.

Suggested websites

American Urogynecologic Society. www.augs.org

Society of Urodynamics, Female Pelvic Medicine & Urogenital Reconstruction. www.sufuorg.com

Additional material for this chapter can be found online at:
www.wiley.com/go/sperling/mountsinai/obstetricsandgynecology

The following image is available in color: Figure 21.1.

CHAPTER 22

Stress Incontinence

Nina S. Jacobson[1] and Charles Ascher-Walsh[2]

[1] Division of Female Pelvic Medicine and Reconstructive Surgery, Department of Obstetrics and Gynecology, Jersey Shore University Medical Center, Neptune City, NJ

[2] Division of Female Pelvic Medicine and Reconstructive Surgery, Department of Obstetrics, Gynecology and Reproductive Science, Icahn School of Medicine at Mount Sinai, New York, NY

OVERALL BOTTOM LINE
- Stress urinary incontinence is the involuntary leakage of urine that occurs with increases in intra-abdominal pressure.
- Stress incontinence is very common among women of reproductive age and can vary in severity.
- It is important to rule out other causes of urinary incontinence.
- There are both conservative and surgical treatment options that are very effective.

Background

Definition of disease

- The etiology of urinary incontinence includes genitourinary (filling/storage disorders, fistulas, congenital abnormalities) and nongenitourinary (functional, environmental, pharmacologic, metabolic).
- Stress urinary incontinence (SUI) is the complaint of involuntary loss of urine with effort or physical exertion or when laughing, sneezing, or coughing.
- Urodynamic stress incontinence is a diagnosis by symptoms, signs, and urodynamic testing and involves the finding of involuntary leakage with increases in intra-abdominal pressure during filling cystometry in the absence of detrusor contractions.

Disease classification

- The International Continence Society (ICS) established a committee for the standardization of terminology of lower urinary tract function and the most recent revision was in 2010.
- The lower urinary tract is composed of the bladder and urethra, which work together as a functional unit to promote storage and emptying of urine.
- The most common urine storage disorder in women is urodynamic stress incontinence and this is attributed to outlet dysfunction.

Incidence/prevalence

- It is estimated that the combined prevalence of urinary incontinence is 15–17%.
- The prevalence of stress incontinence and detrusor overactivity increases with age and affects up to 43.1% of women over 40 years old (See Figure 22.1).
- Among ambulatory incontinent women, the most common condition is urodynamic stress incontinence, which represents 50 to 70% of cases.
- Among elderly, noninstitutionalized incontinent women evaluated in referral centers, urodynamic stress incontinence is found less often (30 to 46%), and detrusor abnormalities and mixed disorders are more common.

Mount Sinai Expert Guides: Obstetrics and Gynecology, First Edition. Edited by Rhoda Sperling.

© 2020 John Wiley & Sons Ltd. Published 2020 by John Wiley & Sons Ltd.

Companion Website: www.wiley.com/go/sperling/mountsinai/obstetricsandgynecology

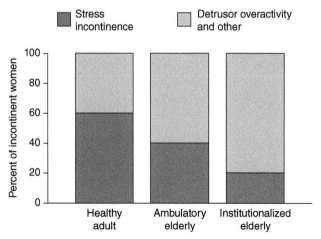

Figure 22.1 Likelihood of stress incontinence or detrusor overactivity being the predominant cause of urinary incontinence by age category Source: Karram and Walters 2014.

- Institutionalized elderly women who are incontinent have detrusor overactivity in 38 to 60% of cases and urodynamic stress incontinence in only 16 to 21% of cases.

Economic impact
- In the year 2000 the estimated total cost of urinary incontinence in the United States was $16.3 billion; $12.4 billion spent on care for women alone.
- Women with severe urinary incontinence pay approximately $900 annually for personal routine care.
- Approximately 6% of nursing home admissions of older women can be attributed to urinary incontinence, with an estimated cost of $3 billion per year.

Social impact
- Urinary incontinence can contribute to social isolation, depression, and reduction in quality of life.
- It can affect relationships and is also associated with sexual dysfunction.

Etiology
- There is a storage phase and voiding phase of urination.
- During normal storage phase the detrusor muscle in the bladder relaxes and the urethral sphincter contracts.
- During normal voiding phase the detrusor muscle contracts and the urethral sphincter relaxes.
- Stress urinary incontinence is caused by outlet dysfunction during the storage phase or reduced urethral resistance.
- This outlet dysfunction can be attributed to anatomic support defects, intrinsic sphincter deficiency, or a combination of the two.

Pathology/pathogenesis
- Integral Theory (Petros and Ulmsten 1990): Stress and urge symptoms both arise from the same anatomic defect, a lax vagina. This theory hypothesizes a complex interplay of anatomic structures that is unconventional.
- Hammock Theory (DeLancey 1994): The urethra and bladder rest on the anterior vagina, which is suspended by the levator ani muscles at the arcus tendineus fasciae pelvis. Loss of this hammock-like support leads to failed urethral compression during periods of increased abdominal pressure.

- Although slightly different, both theories explain why urethral support translates into improved closure and stress continence.

Predictive/risk factors

Risk factor	Odds ratio
Age	Women 50–54 y/o as compared to < 40 y/o: Odds ratio (OR) 2
Obesity	Body mass index > 30 kg/m2: OR 3.1
Smoking	Current smokers: OR 1.34
Vaginal Delivery	≥1 birth: OR 1.5–1.7
High Impact Exercise	Variable depending on exercise type: OR > 1
Race	Hispanic and Caucasian at higher risk than African American and Asian American (OR 0.5)

Prevention

> **BOTTOM LINE/CLINICAL PEARLS**
> - It is important to screen all women of reproductive age.
> - Weight control, pelvic floor exercises, and avoiding constipation can all help to prevent stress incontinence.
> - Systemic estrogen therapy, with or without progesterone, does not appear to be effective in the prevention of urinary incontinence.
> - Data regarding vaginal estrogen are inconclusive, although there is evidence to support it may be helpful in strengthening the urethra.

Screening
- Women of reproductive age can be screened by history alone.

Primary prevention
- Maintain a healthy weight, avoid smoking cigarettes
- High fiber diet to maintain healthy bowel habits and avoid severe constipation
- Practice pelvic floor muscle exercises, especially during pregnancy and postpartum

Diagnosis

> **BOTTOM LINE/CLINICAL PEARLS**
> - History is significant for involuntary leakage of urine with increased intra-abdominal pressure, such as with cough, laugh, or sneeze.
> - Must consider urinary tract infection in the differential.
> - A simple cough stress test is useful in the initial evaluation.
> - Post-void residual urine volume should be obtained to rule out urinary retention and overflow incontinence.
> - Specialized urodynamic studies may be necessary if complex conditions are present or the etiology of incontinence is unclear.

Differential diagnosis

Differential diagnosis	Features
Urinary tract infection	Urine leakage associated with dysuria, frequency, and urgency
Detrusor overactivity	Urinary urgency, typically accompanied by frequency and nocturia (nighttime urination), with and without urge urinary incontinence
Mixed urinary incontinence	Involuntary loss of urine associated with urgency and with physical exertion, sneezing, coughing, or laughing
Chronic urinary retention	Involuntary loss of urine when the bladder does not completely empty, associated with high residual volumes
Functional urinary incontinence	Involuntary loss of urine due to cognitive, functional, or mobility impairments in the presence of intact lower urinary tract system
Drug side effects	Alpha-adrenergic blockers can cause stress incontinence
Extraurethral urinary incontinence	Urine leakage through channels other than the urethral meatus, such as vesicovaginal, urethrovaginal, or ureterovaginal fistulas or ectopic ureter

Typical presentation

- A patient will usually present complaining of involuntary leakage of urine. This typically occurs with exertion or exercise, or with cough, laugh or sneeze. If the problem is severe the patient may also have incontinence with ambulating or heavy lifting. Symptoms associated with chronic pulmonary disease or chronic severe constipation can worsen stress incontinence. Therefore, a detailed medical history is imperative. On pelvic exam one might find a positive cough stress test. Findings of a thorough history and physical exam are often enough to establish the diagnosis with reasonable accuracy.

Diagnosis

See Algorithm 22.1 for an overview of the diagnostic process.

History

- Description of chief complaint, including duration and frequency
- "Do you leak urine when you cough, laugh, or sneeze?"
- Obtain a clear understanding of the severity of the problem and its effect on the patient's quality of life
- Thorough medical, surgical, gynecologic, neurologic, and obstetric histories should be obtained to rule out other causes of urinary incontinence.
- List of medications as there are drugs that can affect lower urinary tract function

Physical examination

- General, gynecologic, and lower neurologic examinations should be performed on every woman with urinary incontinence.
- Pelvic exam should be conducted with the patient in dorsal lithotomy position.
- After the resting vaginal examination, the patient is asked to valsalva or cough and the examiner looks for evidence of vaginal relaxation or urine leakage.
- Cough stress test: considered positive if the patient leaks with cough. This can be done with a full bladder or empty bladder ("empty cough stress test"). It can also be done while the patient is supine or while standing.
- Traditionally, urethral hypermobility was measured with the Q-tip test. However, this test is no longer considered useful in the diagnosis and treatment of incontinence. The Q-tip test involves placement of

Algorithm 22.1 Algorithm for diagnosis of stress urinary incontinence

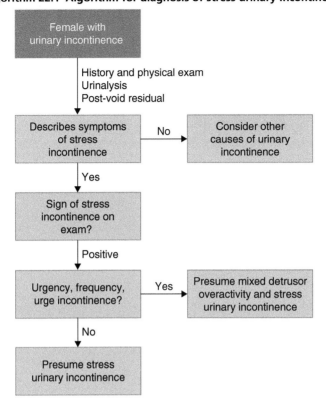

a cotton swab into the urethra to the level of the bladder neck and measurement of the axis change during valsalva. Maximum straining angle measurements > 30° are considered abnormal. Often women with "urethral hypermobility" do not have stress incontinence. Similarly, there are many women with stress incontinence who do not have urethral hypermobility.

List of diagnostic tests
- A clean midstream or catheterized urine sample should be obtained for dipstick urinalysis.
- Urine culture and sensitivity should be obtained when the dipstick test indicates possible infection.
- Post-void residual volume is a measurement of the remaining urine in the bladder after the patient voids. This can be measured using a bladder ultrasound or by catheterization, the latter of which is most accurate. Volumes less than 50 mL indicate adequate bladder emptying and volumes greater than 200 mL can be considered inadequate emptying.
- If after history and physical exam more information is needed to help determine the type of urinary incontinence, a bladder diary is a useful adjunct. This requires the patient to record volume and frequency of fluid intake and of episodes of voluntary and involuntary (i.e. leakage) voiding. Episodes of urinary incontinence and associated events or symptoms such as coughing, urgency, and pad use are noted. A 24-hour recording period is usually sufficient.
- Multichannel urodynamic testing should be reserved for complex cases. Urodynamic studies are performed in the office setting. Small catheters are placed in the bladder and either the vagina or rectum in order to obtain abdominal, intravesical, and detrusor pressures. This study provides useful information regarding the function of the bladder and urethra.

List of imaging techniques

- There are imaging techniques that can be used to evaluate the bladder and urethra but they are not clinically useful for diagnosing stress urinary incontinence.
- Cystourethrography can be used to assess the anatomy and function of the bladder base and urethra. This procedure uses an X-ray to take pictures during urination after retrograde filling of the bladder with contrast material through a urine catheter.
- Transvaginal ultrasound can be used to evaluate urethrovesical anatomy but information not clinically useful.

Potential pitfalls/common errors made regarding diagnosis of disease

- Failure to perform a urinalysis and/or urine culture to rule out infection
- Failure to obtain a post-void residual to rule out urinary retention
- Failure to consider rare etiologies, such as genitourinary fistula or ectopic ureter

Treatment

See Algorithm 22.2.

Treatment rationale

- Treatment should always begin with lifestyle modifications, including limiting fluid intake and caffeine, avoiding cigarettes, and controlling weight.
- Conservative management with pelvic floor muscle exercises is very effective. This can be performed regularly by the patient at home after instruction in the office either by a gynecologist or a pelvic floor therapist.
- Medical management is not recommended.
- Urethral bulking agents can be a great option in older patients with many comorbidities who want to avoid surgery or in patients who have failed surgery.
- The most common type of surgical management is the midurethral sling, which is a minimally invasive and relatively short procedure (<30 minutes) with minimal risk.

Algorithm 22.2 Algorithm for management of stress urinary incontinence

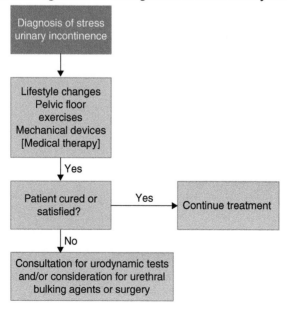

When to hospitalize
- Hospitalization is rarely necessary and would be indicated only if there was a severe surgical complication for which the patient needed to be evaluated and treated.

Managing the hospitalized patient
- If a patient is admitted for a rare complication, management should be individualized.

Table of treatment

Treatment	Comments
Conservative • Lifestyle changes • Pelvic floor muscle exercises (PFME) • Continence support pessaries or other support device • Pharmacotherapy • Urethral bulking agents (Coaptite®, Durasphere®, Macroplastique®)	• Decrease fluid intake, limit caffeine, stop smoking, lose weight • PFME can be performed with or without a physical therapist and can be combined with electrical stimulation • Examples: ring with knob, incontinence dish, Poise Impressa® disposable bladder supports • See table below regarding pharmacologic therapy. None are approved by the Food and Drug Administration (FDA) for this primary indication and in most cases potential side effects outweigh the benefits. • Synthetic materials are injected transurethrally or periurethrally around the bladder neck to increase urethral resistance

Surgical
• Burch procedure
 	
• Bladder neck slings
 	
• Midurethral slings (MUS)
	• Paravaginal tissue is attached to Cooper's ligament to keep the bladder neck in place and help support the urethra, done abdominally
	• Autologous graft (most studied), allograft, xenograft or synthetic mesh can be used
	• Most common type of surgery used today, done transvaginally
	  ○ Retropubic approach (tension-free vaginal tape)
	  ○ Transobturator approach (TOT)

Pharmacologic Therapy (none are FDA-approved for stress incontinence)

Drug type	Drug name	Dosage
Serotonin/norepinephrine reuptake inhibitor	Duloxetine	40 mg bid
α-adrenergic agonist	Midodrine Pseudoephedrine hypochloride	2.5 mg tid 15 mg bid or 30 mg bid
β-agonist/antagonist	Clenbuterol Propranolol	0.02 mg bid 10 mg bid to 40 mg bid
Tricyclic antidepressant	Imipramine hydrochloride	10 mg qhs (older patients), 25 mg tid

Prevention/management of complications
- Available pharmacologic therapy for SUI can cause significant side effects, as many of these medications were not intended to treat urinary incontinence. In general, it is better to avoid these medications if possible.
- Pessaries: An increase in bacterial vaginosis is seen with pessary use. Pessaries can also lead to irritation and erosions in the vagina. Rare complications include vesicovaginal or rectovaginal fistulas, small-bowel entrapment, bilateral hydronephrosis, and urosepsis.
- Surgery: Complications include urinary tract infection, voiding dysfunction, and injury to the bladder, bowel, blood vessels, or nerves. When comparing the different types of midurethral sling, bleeding complications are more common with retropubic slings than transobturator, and groin pain is more

common with transobturator slings. The overall rate of mesh exposure or erosion after a midurethral sling is 2%.

CLINICAL PEARLS
- Pelvic floor muscle exercises (kegels) can be effective as a first-line treatment for stress urinary incontinence.
- Incontinence pessaries may improve symptoms of SUI but objective evidence is lacking. These may be a good option for patients who prefer to avoid surgery and are unlikely to adhere to a physical therapy regimen.
- Pharmacologic therapies for SUI are not very effective and generally not recommended.
- The most common type of surgical management is a midurethral sling.
- Although PFME is considered first line it is still reasonable to offer a midurethral sling initially as an alternative primary treatment option in appropriately counseled women.

Special populations
Pregnancy
- During pregnancy and postpartum pelvic floor muscle exercises should be encouraged. Other treatment options are not advised. Stress incontinence may improve or completely resolve 6–8 weeks postpartum.

Elderly
- Urethral bulking injections may be appropriate in older women with comorbidities who cannot tolerate anesthesia or invasive surgery.

Prognosis

BOTTOM LINE/CLINICAL PEARLS
- Stress urinary incontinence is not dangerous and can go untreated without consequence.
- SUI can significantly affect one's quality of life.
- Conservative management should always be first line.

Natural history of untreated disease
- Stress urinary incontinence may worsen if untreated.
- Severe stress incontinence can lead to social isolation, depression, and reduction in quality of life.

Prognosis for treated patients
- Approximately 50% of women with stress incontinence are satisfied after 1 year of PFME.
- One study comparing pelvic floor therapy with MUS reported that 49% of women in the PFME group switched over to the surgery group. Subjective 1-year cure rates were 85% in the surgery group and 53% in the PFME group.
- Urethral bulking agents work temporarily so there is a need for repeat injections. Improvement rates range from 63 to 80% at 1 year. A Cochrane review concluded that this option is less effective than surgery, with a 1.7-fold to 4.8-fold increased likelihood of cure with surgical treatment.
- Subjective cure rates up to 1 year after midurethral sling were similar and ranged from 62 to 98% (TOT) and 71 to 97% (TVT). Short-term objective and long-term subjective and objective cure rates were also similar.

Reading list

Alling ML, Lose G, Jorgensen T. Risk factors for lower urinary tract symptoms in women 40 to 60 years of age. *Obstet Gynecol* 2000;96:446-51.

American College of Obstetrics & Gynecology/American Urogynecologic Society. ACOG practice bulletin no. 155: Urinary incontinence in women. *Obstet Gynecol* 2015 Nov;126(5):e66-81.

Anger JT, Saigal CS, Madison R, et al. Urologic Diseases of America Project. Increasing costs of urinary incontinence among female Medicare beneficiaries. *J Urol* 2006;176:247-51.

Brown JS, Seelet DG, Fong J, et al. Study of Osteoporotic Fractures Research Group. Urinary incontinence in older women: who is at risk? *Obstet Gynecol* 1996;87:715-21.

DeLancey JO. Structural support of the urethra as it relates to stress urinary incontinence: the hammock hypothesis. *Am J Obstet Gynecol* 1994 Jun;170(6):1713-20; discussion 1720-3.

Dieter AA, Wilkins MF, Wu JM, et al. Epidemiological trends and future care needs for pelvic floor disorders. *Curr Opin Obstet Gynecol* 2015 October;27(5):380-84.

Fozzatti C, Riccetto C, Hermann V, et al. Prevalence study of stress urinary incontinence in women who perform high impact exercises. *Int Urogynecol J* 2012 Dec; 23(12):1687-91. Epub 2012 May 23.

Karram MM, Walters MD. *Urogynecology and reconstructive pelvic surgery*. 4th ed. Philadelphia, PA: Saunders; 2014.

Morrison A, Levy R. Fraction of nursing home admissions attributable to urinary incontinence. *Value Health* 2006;272-4.

Petros PE, Ulmsten UI. An integral theory of female urinary incontinence. Experimental and clinical considerations. *Acta Obstet Gynecol Scand Suppl* 1990;153:7-31.

Suggested websites

Surgery for Stress Urinary Incontinence. http://www.acog.org/Patients/FAQs/Surgery-for-Stress-Urinary-Incontinence

Stress Urinary Incontinence. https://www.yourpelvicfloor.org/conditions/stress-urinary-incontinence

Guidelines
National society guidelines

Title	Source	Date/full reference or URL
Clinical management guidelines for obstetrician-gynecologists	American College of Obstetricians and Gynecologists and the American Urogynecologic Society	ACOG practice bulletin no. 155: Urinary incontinence in women. *Obstet Gynecol* 2015 Nov;126(5):e66-81.
Surgical treatment of female stress urinary incontinence (SUI): AUA/SUFU Guideline	American Urological Association	2017 https://www.auanet.org/guidelines/stress-urinary-incontinence-(sui)-guideline

CHAPTER 23

Adnexal Mass

Janine A. Doneza[1] and Tamara Kolev[2]

[1] Robotic and Minimally Invasive Gynecologic Surgery, MIGS/Urogynecology Fellowship Program, Fibroid Center, Bronxcare Hospital, Bronx, NY; Icahn School of Medicine at Mount Sinai, New York, NY

[2] Department of Obstetrics, Gynecology and Reproductive Science, Icahn School of Medicine at Mount Sinai, New York, NY

OVERALL BOTTOM LINE

The goal of the evaluation of a patient with an adnexal mass is to determine the most likely etiology of the mass. Different types of adnexal masses are more likely depending upon the age and reproductive status of the patient. It is important to exclude urgent conditions or malignancy.

Background

Definition of disease

- Mass of the ovary, fallopian tube, or surrounding connective tissues

Incidence/prevalence

- Found in women of all ages
- Age is the most important independent risk factor for ovarian cancer in the general population; incidence increases after menopause.
- Risk of ovarian cancer in the general population is 1.6%. Risk of ovarian cancer in a patient with one affected family member is 5%. Risk in patient with *BRCA1* is 41–46%. Risk with *BRCA2* is 10–27%. Risk with Lynch syndrome is 5–10%.

Economic impact

- Ovarian cysts often require excision because of symptoms or the possibility of cancer. Nearly 10% of women will undergo surgical evaluation for an adnexal mass, resulting in an estimated 60 000 surgical excisions in the US per year.

Etiology

- Children: Adnexal masses occur less frequently in this age group but when a mass is found, there should be a high suspicion for adnexal torsion or an ovarian malignancy. Germ cell tumors are the most common type of ovarian cancer in children and adolescents.
- Premenopausal women: Adnexal masses stimulated by reproductive hormones are predominantly found in this age group. These include physiologic cysts, endometriomas, and leiomyomas.
- Postmenopausal women: Ovarian or fallopian tube cancer is more likely in postmenopausal women. Urgent conditions (e.g. adnexal torsion, tubo-ovarian abscess) may also occur in postmenopausal women but are less common and are more likely to be associated with malignancy.

Pathology/pathogenesis

- Adnexal mass can result from the process of ovulation, stimulation by reproductive hormones, or unchecked cell growth.

Mount Sinai Expert Guides: Obstetrics and Gynecology, First Edition. Edited by Rhoda Sperling.

© 2020 John Wiley & Sons Ltd. Published 2020 by John Wiley & Sons Ltd.

Companion Website: www.wiley.com/go/sperling/mountsinai/obstetricsandgynecology

- In normal ovulation, a follicle develops to maturity and then ruptures to release an ovum; this is followed by formation and subsequent involution of the corpus luteum.
- Follicular cysts arise when rupture does not occur and the follicle continues to grow. Corpus luteal cysts occur when the corpus luteum fails to involute and continues to enlarge after ovulation.
- Simple cysts develop when high levels of gonadotropins or androgens cause small epithelial lined structures in the ovary to secrete fluid into their inner cavity and enlarge to become cysts.
- Endometrioma arises from the ectopic growth of endometrial tissue.
- Uterine leiomyoma arise from smooth muscle cells of the myometrium. These benign tumors are estrogen and progesterone-sensitive and thus growth occurs mostly during the reproductive years.
- Ovarian carcinogenesis is not completely understood. One hypothesis is that it originates from the ovarian surface epithelium, which undergoes malignant transformation and eventually spreads from the ovary to distant sites. Mutations in *KRAS*, *PTEN*, *TP53*, and *VEGF* genes are thought to be involved.

Predictive/risk factors

Risk factors
Age
Family history
Genetic syndromes
Nulliparity
Early menarche
Late menopause
White race
Infertility

Prevention

> **BOTTOM LINE/CLINICAL PEARLS**
> - There are no routine screening tests for ovarian cancer in patients who are at average risk for ovarian cancer. Specificity and PPV of CA 125 are consistently higher in postmenopausal women compared with premenopausal women, in whom elevations can be seen with benign processes.

Screening
- In women at average risk of ovarian cancer, adnexal masses may be detected by annual pelvic exam or during a workup for women presenting with symptoms.
- CA 125 and transvaginal ultrasound (TVUS) can be used for ovarian cancer surveillance only in patients who have a history of BRCA mutation.

Primary prevention
- There is a reduction in ovarian cancer risk associated with the use of oral contraceptive pills.
- Oral contraceptive pill use can be used to suppress the ovarian-hypothalamic axis so new cysts will not form.

Secondary prevention
- Women with *BRCA1* or *BRCA2* mutations should be offered risk-reducing salpingo-oophorectomy by age 40 years or when childbearing is complete.

Diagnosis

> **BOTTOM LINE/CLINICAL PEARLS**
> • Transvaginal ultrasonography is the most commonly used technique for evaluation of adnexal masses and is superior to other imaging modalities when used for the evaluation of adnexal masses.

Differential diagnosis

Premenopausal

physiologic cyst
endometrioma
mature teratoma
ectopic pregnancy
hydrosalpinx
tubo-ovarian abscess
GI-related disease – appendiceal abscess

Postmenopausal

fibroid
simple cysts
cystadenoma
diverticulitis/abdominal abscess
ovarian carcinoma, sex-cord stromal tumor
leiomyosarcoma
metastatic disease from uterine, gastric, or breast cancer

Pregnant women

ectopic pregnancy
luteoma
corpus luteum cyst
theca lutein cysts

See Figures 23.1–23.4.

Typical presentation
• Pelvic pain or pressure is the most common symptom associated with an adnexal mass. Women with endometriosis may have cyclic pain with menses. Severe pain may be indicative of torsion, cyst rupture, or tubo-ovarian abscess (TOA). Some women present with abnormal uterine bleeding.
• Ovarian cancer may be associated with abnormal bleeding and increased abdominal girth. For sex-cord stromal tumors, women present with symptoms related to virilization due to excess androgen production by the tumor.

Clinical diagnosis
History
• Patients should be asked about fever or vaginal discharge, pain in relation to menses, abnormal uterine bleeding, and symptoms related to androgen excess. Family history of cancer and hereditary disorders are important to elicit.

Physical examination
• Pelvic examination and imaging to confirm whether a mass is present. Rectovaginal examination is performed to allow palpation of the ovary posteriorly.

Laboratory diagnosis
List of diagnostic tests
• Pregnancy test, complete blood count (CBC), gonorrhea/chlamydia, urinalysis (UA), serum markers

- Tumor markers: alpha-fetoprotein (AFP), human chorionic gonadotropin (hCG), lactate dehydrogenase (LDH), CA 19-9, CA 125, carcinoembryonic antigen (CEA). Note: CA 125 is associated with epithelial ovarian cancer, endometriosis, pregnancy, and pelvic inflammatory disease (PID). Most useful in postmenopausal women; the combination of elevated CA 125 level and a pelvic mass in a postmenopausal woman is highly suspicious for malignancy.
- Serum biomarker panels: OVA1 and ROMA are serum-based tests used as an adjunct to clinical decision-making for women who are planning surgery for an adnexal mass. These tests are used to determine the likelihood that the pelvic mass is benign or malignant.

List of imaging techniques
- Transvaginal ultrasound is the recommended imaging modality.
- Findings that raise concern for malignancy include size > 10 cm, papillary or solid components, irregularity, presence of ascites, and high color Doppler flow.
- Computed tomography (CT) and magnetic resonance imaging (MRI) are not used in the initial evaluation of adnexal mass.

Potential pitfalls
- Failure to recognize benign conditions that can be observed from conditions that need more immediate intervention may lead to significant morbidity, and possibly mortality, for the patient. One example is the misinterpretation of findings on sonogram in evaluation of pain in early pregnancy: a simple cyst may represent corpus luteum or an ectopic pregnancy.
- Most adnexal masses are benign. For example, the incidence of simple cysts in postmenopausal women has been reported to be up to 20%. Intervention for small simple cysts in this age group may lead to unnecessary testing and surgery.
- The diagnosis of ovarian torsion can be challenging; the absence of an adnexal mass or the presence of flow on Doppler do not exclude torsion. Thus, the decision to proceed with surgery must often be made in the absence of some of these clinical features.

Treatment
Treatment rationale
- An adnexal mass may represent a condition that requires urgent intervention such as ectopic pregnancy, adnexal torsion, or an ovarian cancer.

When to hospitalize
- Patients diagnosed with PID may need to be hospitalized for parenteral antibiotics if they are pregnant, intolerant to oral medications due to nausea/vomiting, nonadherent to therapy, or have high fever or pelvic abscess/TOA.

Table of treatment

Treatment	Comment
Low-risk adnexal mass: asymptomatic, simple cyst <1% risk of malignancy	No surgical intervention; interval follow-up ultrasound at 3–6 months to assess for resolution or stability
Intermediate-risk: cyst with thin septation or low-level echoes, but lacks features of malignancy >1% risk of malignancy	Consider surgical intervention due to possibility of cancer or to prevent complications such as torsion. Surveillance may be an option as well.
High-risk adnexal mass: cyst with solid, nodular, thick septations with elevated CA 125	Surgical intervention, referral to gyn-oncologist

Algorithm 23.1 Management algorithm for adnexal masses

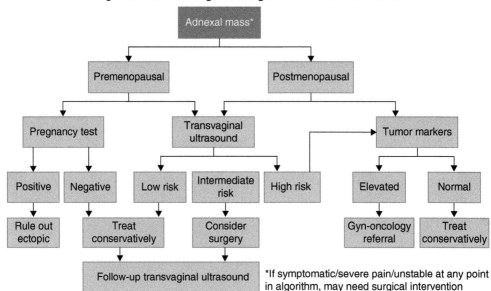

- Observation is recommended when the morphology of the adnexal mass on ultrasonography suggests benign disease. Functional cysts spontaneously resolve in 2–8 weeks.
- Repeat ultrasound imaging is recommended whenever diagnosis is uncertain or when cancer remains within the differential diagnosis. The ideal interval for ultrasound follow-up has yet to be defined.
- Women who present with acute pain and an ovarian mass should be evaluated without delay and may require urgent intervention as these cases may represent ovarian torsion and ectopic pregnancy.
- A definitive size cutoff to delineate the need for surgical intervention has not been established. Cysts of 10 cm or larger are often considered to be an indication for surgery.
- Referral to a gyn-oncologist for postmenopausal women with any elevation in CA 125 and ultrasound findings of a suspicious pelvic mass or a premenopausal woman with a very elevated CA 125 level and a suspicious pelvic mass.

Prevention/management of complications
- An ovarian cyst may rupture and bleed. Surgical management is required in cases where the patient is unstable and/or bleeding is ongoing.
- Ovarian torsion can result in ischemia and is most common if the ovary is 5 cm or larger. Adnexal torsion is managed by reduction of the torsion and ovarian cystectomy. Ovarian fixation is controversial but may be considered in recurrent cases of torsion.
- Endometriosis can be associated with infertility. Surgical excision of endometriomas may improve fertility outcomes.

Benign conditions can be followed up with repeat sonogram. If a malignancy is present, the surgeon may proceed with staging and cytoreduction. See Algorithm 23.1.

CLINICAL PEARLS
- Fertility preservation should be a priority when managing masses in adolescents and premenopausal women. Even in women who present with large ovarian cysts of 10 cm or greater, it is possible to save normal portions of the ovary.

> • Given advancements in minimally invasive surgery, laparoscopic management of presumed benign adnexal masses is generally appropriate and associated with decreased postoperative morbidity.

Special populations
Adolescents
- Management of adnexal masses in adolescents should prioritize ovarian conservation to preserve fertility.
- Transabdominal ultrasonography is recommended for virginal or prepubertal adolescents.
- Surgical indications include malignancy. Unilateral oophorectomy has not been shown to impair menstrual regularity or spontaneous pregnancy rates.

Pregnancy
- Most adnexal masses in pregnancy have a low risk of malignancy and may be managed expectantly. One of the most commonly reported pathologic diagnoses are mature teratomas.
- MRI is the modality of choice if additional imaging is needed.
- CA 125 levels are elevated in pregnancy; they peak in the first trimester and are not associated with malignancy.
- If intervention is warranted based on symptoms, laparoscopic management is safe in the second trimester.

Prognosis

> **BOTTOM LINE/CLINICAL PEARLS**
> • The goal for evaluation of pelvic mass is to exclude malignancy. However, epithelial ovarian cancer is most commonly detected in an advanced stage, when the overall 5-year survival rate is 20–30%.

Natural history of untreated benign disease
- Physiologic ovarian cysts resolve spontaneously.
- Endometriosis lesions increase throughout adolescence, persist during the reproductive years, and become less common in postmenopause.
- Tubal damage caused by PID increases the risk of tubal pregnancy, as well as infertility.

Prognosis for treated patients
- Ovarian cancer represents one of the cancers with the worst prognosis in adult women, with 40% 5-year survival in stage III disease and 18% for stage IV.
- Endometriosis has been associated with development of clear cell adenocarcinoma.

Follow-up
- Simple cysts up to 10 cm in diameter are likely benign and may be safely monitored using repeat imaging even in postmenopausal patients.
- Monitoring for women who have completed treatment for epithelial ovarian cancer include history and pelvic examinations every 3–6 months up to 5 years posttreatment, then annually. Serial measurement of CA 125 is a component of follow-up and is checked at every visit.

Reading list

ACOG practice bulletin No. 174: Evaluation and management of adnexal masses. *Obstet Gynecol* 2016 Nov;128(5):e210-e226.

ACOG practice bulletin No. 182: Hereditary breast and ovarian cancer syndrome. *Obstet Gynecol* 2017 Sep;130(3):e110-e126.

Curtin JP. Management of the adnexal mass. *Gynecol Oncol* 1994;55(3 Pt 2):S42.

Hall TR, Randall TC. Adnexal masses in the premenopausal patient. *Clin Obstet Gynecol* 2015 Mar;58(1):47-52.

Hoffman BL, Schorge JO, Schaffer JI, Halvorson LM, Bradshaw KD, Cunningham FG, Calver LE. *Williams gynecology*, 2nd ed. Chapter 9: Pelvic mass. New York: McGraw-Hill; 2012.

Rauh-Hain JA, Melamed A, Buskwofie A, et al. Adnexal mass in the postmenopausal patient. *Clin Obstet Gynecol* 2015 Mar;58(1):53-65.

Sayasneh A, Ekechi C, Ferrara L, et al. The characteristic ultrasound features of specific types of ovarian pathology (review). *Int J Oncol* 2015 Feb;46(2):445-58.

Sisodia RM, Del Carmen MG, Boruta DM. Role of minimally invasive surgery in the management of adnexal masses. *Clin Obstet Gynecol* 2015 Mar;58(1):66-75.

Guidelines
National society guidelines

Title	Source	Date/URL
Genetic/familial high-risk assessment: breast and ovarian.	National Comprehensive Cancer Network	2019 https://www2.tri-kobe.org/nccn/guideline/gynecological/english/genetic_familial.pdf
Evaluation and management of adnexal masses. ACOG practice bulletin no. 174	American College of Obstetricians and Gynecologists	2016 https://www.acog.org/Clinical-Guidance-and-Publications/Practice-Bulletins/Committee-on-Practice-Bulletins-Gynecology/Evaluation-and-Management-of-Adnexal-Masses
The role of the obstetrician–gynecologist in the early detection of epithelial ovarian cancer. ACOG committee opinion	American College of Obstetricians and Gynecologists	2017 https://www.acog.org/Clinical-Guidance-and-Publications/Committee-Opinions/Committee-on-Gynecologic-Practice/The-Role-of-the-Obstetrician-Gynecologist-in-the-Early-Detection-of-Epithelial-Ovarian-Cancer-in

Evidence

Type of evidence	Title and comment	Date/full reference
Retrospective study	Management of unilocular or multilocular cysts more than 5 cm in postmenopausal women. Comment: In postmenopausal women, cysts that are unilocular or contain septa, have a low risk of malignancy even when they are larger than 5 cm.	Guraslan H, Dogan K. *Eur J Obstet Gynecol Reprod Biol* 2016 Aug;203:40-3.
Prospective cohort	Preoperative evaluation of serum CA 125 levels in premenopausal and postmenopausal patients with pelvic masses. Discrimination of benign from malignant disease. Comment: Greater sensitivity and specificity were observed in the postmenopausal subgroup than in the premenopausal subgroup.	Malkasian GD Jr, Knapp RC, Lavin PT, et al. *Am J Obstet Gynecol* 1988 Aug; 159(2):341-6.
Prospective cohort	Frequency and disposition of ovarian abnormalities followed with serial transvaginal ultrasonography. Comment: Serial ultrasonography has shown that many ovarian abnormalities resolve. Thus, sonogram findings should not be used as the only indication for surgery	Pavlik EJ, Ueland FR, Miller RW, et al. *Obstet Gynecol* 2013 Aug;122(2 Pt 1):210-7.

Images

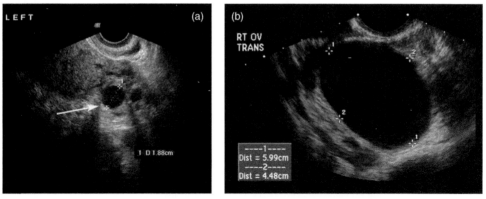

Figure 23.1 a. Normal follicle – anechoic (Courtesy of Dr. Thomas Shipp); b. Simple ovarian cyst (Courtesy of UpToDate).

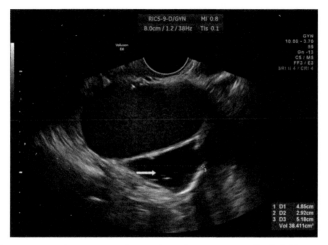

Figure 23.2 Benign mature ovarian teratoma – hyperechogenic areas representing hair (Courtesy of UpToDate). See color version on website.

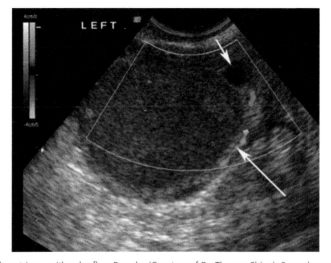

Figure 23.3 Endometrioma with color flow Doppler (Courtesy of Dr. Thomas Shipp). See color version on website.

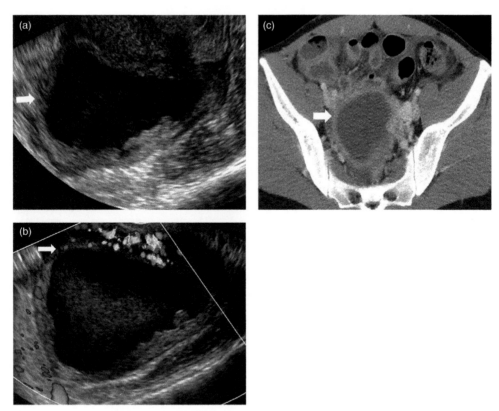

Figure 23.4 a. Ultrasound image of the pelvis of a 24-year-old woman with intermittent pelvic pain for 2 weeks shows a tubo-ovarian abscess (arrow) seen as a lesion with thick, echogenic, irregular walls and internal echoes, misinterpreted as a hemorrhagic cyst. Please note larger size and more shaggy wall of the adnexal cystic lesion. b. Corresponding color Doppler image shows a peripheral vascularity in the wall of the cystic lesion (arrow), similar to corpus luteum cyst. c. Corresponding axial contrast-enhanced CT image of the pelvis that was done because of worsening pelvic pain, fever, and elevated white count confirms a tubo-ovarian abscess (arrow) seen as a large rim-enhancing lesion in the adnexa. Source: Bonde AA, Korngold EK, Foster BR. Radiological appearances of corpus luteum cysts and their imaging mimics. *Abdom Radiol (NY)* 2016 Nov;41(11):2280. See color version on website.

Additional material for this chapter can be found online at:
www.wiley.com/go/sperling/mountsinai/obstetricsandgynecology

This includes multiple choice questions, advice for patients, and ICD codes. The following images are available in color: Figure 23.2, Figure 23.3 and Figure 23.4.

CHAPTER 24

Endometriosis

Suzanne S. Fenske
Department of Obstetrics, Gynecology and Reproductive Science, Icahn School of Medicine at Mount Sinai, New York, NY

OVERALL BOTTOM LINE
- Endometriosis is a disease characterized by presence of endometrial tissue in locations other than the uterus.
- Endometriosis is a disease of estrogen and inflammation.
- The exact pathogenesis of endometriosis is unknown; however, theories include retrograde menstruation, hematogenous or lymphatic transport, stem cells from bone marrow, and coelomic metaplasia.
- Patients can have pelvic pain, dysmenorrhea, dyspareunia, infertility, or be asymptomatic.
- Symptoms of endometriosis can be successfully managed with medical and surgical therapy.
- There is no cure for endometriosis and it can recur after medical and surgical treatment.

Background
Definition of disease
- Endometriosis is defined as the presence of endometrial-like tissue outside the uterus, which induces a chronic, inflammatory reaction. The presence of this tissue in locations other than the uterus can result in pain, infertility, and/or adhesions.

Disease classification
- The American Society for Reproductive Medicine classification is the most commonly used system. This classification system has its limitations as it is not a good predictor of pregnancy outcome and has no correlation with symptoms.

Incidence/prevalence
- Endometriosis is a gynecologic condition that occurs in 6–10% of women of reproductive age.
- It has a prevalence of 38% in infertile women.
- It has a prevalence of 71–87% in women with chronic pelvic pain.

Economic impact
- Symptoms of endometriosis contribute substantially to the burden of disease and add substantial cost to society through reduced economic and personal productivity.

Etiology
- The pathogenesis of endometriosis is complex but still thought to mainly be associated with attachment and implantation of endometrial glands and stroma on peritoneum from retrograde menstruation.
- Retrograde menstruation is unable to explain endometriosis located in distant sites and, therefore, hematogenous or lymphatic transport, stem cells from bone marrow, and coelomic metaplasia are alternative theories.

Mount Sinai Expert Guides: Obstetrics and Gynecology, First Edition. Edited by Rhoda Sperling.
© 2020 John Wiley & Sons Ltd. Published 2020 by John Wiley & Sons Ltd.
Companion Website: www.wiley.com/go/sperling/mountsinai/obstetricsandgynecology

- The endometriosis lesions are responsible for overproduction of prostaglandins by cyclooxygenase-2 activity and overproduction of estrogen by increased aromatase activity.
- This chronic inflammatory disorder with increased macrophages and cytokines may cause pain and infertility.
- Endometriosis-caused infertility is thought to occur due to oxidative stress and increase in cytokines that can affect sperm and oocyte function.

Pathology/pathogenesis

- The manifestation of endometriosis is variable.
- In some women, there are no symptoms.
- In others, there may be dysmenorrhea, dyspareunia, ovarian masses, infertility, bowel or bladder symptoms, cyclical hemothorax or epistaxis, or chronic pelvic pain.
- Familial association of endometriosis has been suggested and proposed inheritance is characteristic of a polygenic-multifactorial mechanism.

Prevention

> **BOTTOM LINE/CLINICAL PEARLS**
> - No interventions have been demonstrated to prevent the development of endometriosis; however, treatments such as surgery and medical suppression can slow the recurrence.

Screening

- There is no routine screening for endometriosis. The diagnosis of endometriosis, suspected based on history, symptoms, and signs, is corroborated by physical examination and imaging techniques and is finally proven by histological examination of specimens collected at the time of surgery.

Primary prevention

- There are no known interventions or treatments that prevent the first occurrence of endometriosis.

Secondary prevention

- No interventions prevent the reoccurrence of symptoms of endometriosis. That being said, there are treatment options that can delay the reoccurrence and/or slow the progression of disease.
- A randomized, double-blind controlled trial of laser laparoscopy in treatment of pelvic pain due to endometriosis demonstrated that at 6 months, patients who underwent surgical treatment, 62.5% of patients reported significant symptom improvement.
- In another study, patients with all stages of endometriosis had surgical excision and at 7-year follow-up 55% required additional surgery.
- Gonadotropin-releasing hormone (GnRH) agonists have been demonstrated to extend pain relief after surgical intervention for endometriosis.
- Hormonal treatment options (hormonal contraceptives, progestins, antiprogestins, or GnRH agonists) have been found to reduce endometriosis-associated pain.

Diagnosis

> **BOTTOM LINE/CLINICAL PEARLS**
> - Diagnosis of endometriosis is suspected when a patient has a history of dysmenorrhea, dyspareunia, and infertility.

- Suspicion of endometriosis is further supported when physical examination reveals ovarian cysts and/or palpable nodularity on bimanual pelvic examination.
- Although there are no confirmatory laboratory test, suspicion of endometriosis could be further supported if pelvic ultrasound or magnetic resonance imaging (MRI) demonstrates ovarian cysts that have characteristic appearance of endometriomas.
- Definitive diagnosis is made with surgical exploration and biopsies.

Differential diagnosis

Differential diagnosis	Features
Dysmenorrhea	• Painful menses without pathologic abnormality
Hemorrhagic cysts	• Cyclical physiological ovarian cyst that spontaneously resolves and does not have presence of endometrial tissue
Vulvodynia	• Painful intercourse on insertion rather than deep penetration
Infertility due to other causes	• No presence of endometriosis at the time of laparoscopy • Infertility workup may demonstrate poor ovarian reserve or abnormal semen analysis.
Pelvic pain due to gastrointestinal causes	• Review of systems demonstrates positive findings
Pelvic pain due to urologic causes	• Review of systems demonstrates positive findings
Pelvic pain due to musculoskeletal causes	• Review of systems demonstrates positive findings

Typical presentation
- Endometriosis is variable in presentation. For many, endometriosis presents as chronic dysmenorrhea or pain with ovulation. These patients report pelvic pain that is present at ovulation and, again, just before menses and during menses that resolves with conclusion of menses. Other patients report pain with intercourse on deep penetration. Still others report inability to conceive as their predominant symptom.

Clinical diagnosis
History
- A detailed history of pelvic pain and relation to menstrual cycle should be obtained.
- A careful review of symptoms should be obtained to rule out other causes such as gastrointestinal, urologic, and musculoskeletal.
- Prior treatments should be reviewed.
- Family history and, specifically, presence of a diagnosis of endometriosis.

Physical examination
- Begin by observing the patient walking and standing to assess for musculoskeletal etiology.
- Examine the patient for presence of reproducible pain on palpation of back and abdomen.
- For patients with complaints of dyspareunia, examine the introitus and vestibule with a Q-tip to assess for pain that would indicate vulvodynia.
- Perform a single digit examination of the vagina and examine the pelvic floor muscles of reproducible pain.
- Perform a bimanual examination to assess for ovarian masses, decreased mobility of the uterus, uterosacral nodularity, and palpable evidence of endometriosis nodules.
- Perform rectovaginal examination to assess for nodularity or thickening of the rectovaginal septum.

Laboratory diagnosis

List of diagnostic tests

- If pelvic pain is the presenting complaint, then an initial evaluation for sexually transmitted infections should be performed.
- If pelvic pain is the presenting complaint, then gold standard for imaging is a pelvic ultrasound to assess for anatomic abnormalities.
- If infertility is the presenting complaint, then perform semen analysis, documentation of normal ovulatory function, and a test to rule out tubal occlusion and assess uterine cavity and test for ovarian reserve.

Potential pitfalls/common errors made regarding diagnosis of disease

- The symptoms that lead to a diagnosis of endometriosis can often be multifactorial. Many providers will miss additional diagnoses such as irritable bowel syndrome, painful bladder syndrome, vulvodynia, pelvic floor muscle pain, and other causes of infertility.
- At the time of surgery, a diagnosis of endometriosis could be missed when it does not present with classic appearance. Our ability to visually detect endometriosis can often come up short and it is recommended to perform biopsies.

Treatment

Treatment rationale

- Well-tolerated, low-cost, easily accessible options such as nonsteroidal anti-inflammatory drugs (NSAIDs), other analgesics, combined oral contraceptive pills (OCP), and progestins should be considered for use as first-line empirical medical treatment.
- Second-line medical treatment such as GnRH agonist with add-back hormonal treatment or GnRH antagonist or levonorgestrel intrauterine device can be considered in patients not optimally treated with first-line treatment prior to surgical diagnosis and treatment while awaiting laparoscopic surgery.
- For patients who do not respond to medical treatment and/or want a definitive diagnosis, laparoscopic surgery is the gold standard.
- Laparoscopic excision for ovarian endometriomas is preferred when possible to minimize symptoms recurrence and endometrioma recurrence.
- Laparoscopic surgical removal of endometriosis improves fertility in stage I and II endometriosis.
- Aromatase inhibitors might be reasonable as a second-line medical treatment.
- There is some weak evidence for use of acupuncture and transcutaneous electrical nerve stimulation (TENS) for pain management associated with endometriosis.

When to hospitalize

- Hospitalization should be considered if a patient is in acute pain that is unable to be managed with outpatient therapy or if a surgical emergency presents such as ovarian torsion.

Table of treatment

Treatment	Comment
Medical - NSAIDs - OCP - Progestins - GnRH agonists - Progestin intrauterine device - Aromatase inhibitors - GnRH antagonists	NSAIDs can be considered if pain is not too severe and only present with menses. For hormonal management in patients without a contraindication to estrogen, consider OCP. As an alternative option in patients who do not want OCP or have contraindication to estrogen, consider progestin therapy either in pill, depot, or as intrauterine device. GnRH agonists should be given with add-back therapy to avoid menopausal side effects and to protect against bone loss. Add-back therapy can be combined hormonal therapy or just progestin. Aromatase inhibitors are given in combination with OCP, progestins, or GnRH agonists. GnRH antagonists have been proven to be effective, but require additional research.

(Continued)

Treatment	Comment
Surgical • Laparoscopic excision • Laparoscopic ablation	Laparoscopic surgical removal of endometriosis is an effective first-line approach for treating pain related to endometriosis. Randomized controlled trials have failed to demonstrate benefit of excision over ablation. Laparoscopic approach is always recommended over laparotomy.
Complementary • Acupuncture • TENS • Vitamin B1 and B6 • Magnesium	There is some evidence that acupuncture is effective; however, it requires repeated treatments and effects are not long-lasting. TENS has been demonstrated to effective in short term for dysmenorrhea. Vitamin B1 and B6 have been demonstrated to relieve dysmenorrhea, but safety concerns exist. Magnesium has been proven to reduce pain.

Prevention/management of complications
- Patients on GnRH agonists/antagonists without add-back therapy will have menopausal side effects including, but not limited to, hot flashes, insomnia, vaginal dryness, and loss of bone mineral density.
- Surgery for endometriosis faces risks of damage to surrounding organs including bowel, bladder, ureters, vessels, etc. If these complications occur during surgery, timely recognition is key and should be treated with immediate repair with a specialist.

CLINICAL PEARLS
- Medical suppressive therapy improves pain symptoms; however, pain will recur with cessation of medication.
- Surgical treatment improves pain symptoms; however, over time, pain will recur and patients should be put on medical suppression after surgery.
- Excision of endometrioma is recommended over drainage of the cyst.
- GnRH agonist should be used in combination with hormonal therapy to avoid side effects and prevent against bone mineral loss.

Prognosis

BOTTOM LINE/CLINICAL PEARLS
- There is no cure for endometriosis.
- Endometriosis symptoms and its effects on patients are variable.
- Pain from endometriosis can be treated with medical management and surgical management, but recurrence of symptoms is likely.

Reading list

Committee opinion no. 663: Aromatase inhibitors in gynecologic practice. *Obstet Gynecol* 2016;127:e170.

Committee opinion no. 760. Dysmenorrhea and endometriosis in the adolescent. *Obstet Gynecol* 2018 Dec;132(6):e249-e258.

Dunselman G, Vermeulen N, Becker C, et al. ESHRE guideline: management of women with endometriosis. *Hum Reprod* 2014:29(3):400-12.

Hickey M, Ballard K, Farquhar C. Endometriosis. *BMJ* 2014;348:g1752.

Johnson N, Hummelshoj. Consensus on current management of endometriosis. *Hum Reprod* 2013:28(6):1552-68.

Lobo R, Endometriosis. In: Katz VL, Lentz GM, Lobo RA, Gershenson DM. *Comprehensive gynecology.* 5th ed. Philadelphia, PA: Mosby Elsevier; 2007.

Practice bulletin no. 114. Management of endometriosis. *Obstet Gynecol* 2010;116:223.

Practice Committee of American Society for Reproductive Medicine. Treatment of pelvic pain associated with endometriosis: a committee opinion. *Fertil Steril* 2014;101:927.

Schorge JO, Schaffer JI, Halvorson LM, et al. *Williams gynecology.* Dallas, TX: McGraw-Hill; 2008.

Guidelines
National society guidelines

Title	Source	Date/full reference
Treatment of pelvic pain associated with endometriosis: a committee opinion	American Society for Reproductive Medicine Comment: Endometriosis should be viewed as a lifelong disease with a goal of maximizing the use of medical treatment over surgery. Definitive treatment is a hysterectomy with removal of ovaries.	2014 *Fertil Steril* 2014 Apr;101(4):927-35.
Dysmenorrhea and endometriosis in the adolescent: a committee opinion	American College of Obstetricians and Gynecologists Comment: First-line therapy is NSAIDs and hormonal suppression. Pelvic imaging should be considered for secondary dysmenorrhea. Recommendation is for conservative surgical management for diagnosis with medical suppression. If recalcitrant, consider GnRH agonist with add-back therapy for at least 6 months	2018 *Obstet Gynecol* 2018 Dec;132(6):e249-e258.
Management of endometriosis: practice bulletin	American College of Obstetricians and Gynecologists Comment: Transvaginal ultrasound is the imaging of choice for evaluation. Medical treatment improves symptoms but recurrence occurs with cessation. Surgical treatment improves pregnancy rates, but magnitude is unclear.	2010 (reaffirmed 2018) *Obstet Gynecol* 2010 Jul;116(1):223-36.

CHAPTER 25

Anogenital HPV

Eric M. Ganz[1], Shannon Tomita[2], and Rhoda Sperling[3]

[1] Department of Obstetrics, Gynecology and Reproductive Science, Icahn School of Medicine at Mount Sinai, New York, NY

[2] Division of Gynecologic Oncology – Department of Obstetrics, Gynecology and Reproductive Science, Icahn School of Medicine at Mount Sinai, New York, NY

[3] Department of Obstetrics, Gynecology and Reproductive Science – Department of Medicine, Division of Infectious Diseases, Icahn School of Medicine at Mount Sinai, New York, NY

OVERALL BOTTOM LINE

- Anogenital human papillomavirus (HPV) types are divided into low-risk and high-risk types based on their ability to cause cancer.
- Infection with low-risk HPV types can cause genital warts as well as low-grade cell changes of cervical, vaginal, vulvar, or anal tissue.
- Persistent infection with high-risk HPV types can cause high-grade (precancerous) lesions and cancer.
- Prevention of HPV infection and HPV-associated precancer and cancer is possible with vaccination.
- Treatment of warts and precancerous lesions typically involves destruction or excision of lesions.

Background
Definition of disease
- Anogenital HPV is a viral sexually transmitted infection.

Incidence/prevalence
- 80% of sexually active women will contract HPV over their lifetime.
- Incidence: ~14 million new cases of HPV annually in the United States.
- Prevalence: ~79 million women ages 14–59 in the United States with the highest prevalence among those ages 20–24 years of age.

Economic impact
- In the United States, direct annual medical costs associated with genital HPV infection, including treatment of genital warts, precancers, and cancers and screening for cervical cancer, are estimated to be $1.7 billion.

Etiology
- There are over 40 HPV types that can infect the anogenital skin and mucus membranes.
- Low-risk HPV types can cause genital warts as well as low-grade (benign) changes of cervical, vaginal, vulvar, or anal tissue.
- Persistent infection with high-risk HPV can cause high-grade (also known as precancerous or high-grade dysplastic) lesions and cancer.

Mount Sinai Expert Guides: Obstetrics and Gynecology, First Edition. Edited by Rhoda Sperling.
© 2020 John Wiley & Sons Ltd. Published 2020 by John Wiley & Sons Ltd.
Companion Website: www.wiley.com/go/sperling/mountsinai/obstetricsandgynecology

- HPV 6, 11 cause ~ 90% of genital warts.
- HPV 16, 18 cause ~ 70% of the cervical dysplasias/cervical cancers.

Pathology/pathogenesis

- HPV is transmitted during sexual activity, including oral sex.
- HPV uses the host cellular machinery to replicate and this process is guided by viral regulatory genes. The proteins encoded by the HPV viral regulatory genes E6 and E7 mediate much of the virus's oncogenic potential. The production of E6 and E7 related onco-proteins represent a key difference between high-risk and low-risk types.
- Most infections (both high risk and low risk) are asymptomatic and will clear spontaneously.
- For symptomatic infections, the incubation period (the time from initial infection to clinically recognized disease) is variable.
- The incubation period for genital warts (also known as condyloma or condyloma acuminata) typically ranges from 3 weeks to several months.
- The incubation period for the development of dysplastic lesions (abnormal cell changes) typically ranges from several months to years. If cancer develops, it typically occurs decades after the initial infection.
- Dysplastic lesions can spontaneously regress; estimates are 20–40% of dysplastic lesions will regress without treatment.
- Persistent infection with high-risk HPV types is essential in the process of oncogenesis.
- Persistent infection with high-risk HPV types is the most important risk factor for progression of dysplasia to cancer. Additional factors associated with disease progression include older age, HPV types 16 and 18, and immunodeficiency.

Clinical disease	HPV types
Anogenital warts	6,11,42,44
Anal dysplasia	6,16,18,31,53,58
Cervical, vaginal, and vulvar high-grade dysplasia and cancer	Highest risk types – 16,18,31,45 Other high-risk types – 33,35,39,51,52,56,58,59

Predictive/risk factors

Risk factor	Odds ratio
Multiple sex partners	1.4
Age under 30	2.3
Immunosuppression/HIV	4.1
Cigarette smoking	5.0

Prevention

> **BOTTOM LINE/CLINICAL PEARLS**
> - Primary prevention with routine HPV vaccination is a highly successful strategy to prevent type-specific HPV infections and their sequelae.
> - Correct and consistent condom can reduce the risk of both transmitting and acquiring HPV.

Screening
- Anogenital warts are diagnosed by visual inspection and confirmed by biopsy (Workowski et al. 2015).
- Vulvar and vaginal dysplasia are diagnosed by visual inspection and confirmed by biopsy.
- Pap smear cytology and HPV testing are accepted screening techniques for cervical dysplasia and cervical cancer. Screening recommendations differ by age. Current recommendations: (a) no screening before age 21; (b) ages 21–29 cytology screening every 3 years; (c) ages 30–65 cytology every 3 years or with HPV co-testing every 5 years; and (d) after age 65, no routine screening (Massad et al. 2013).
- Anal dysplasia can be detected by anal Pap and/or digital rectal examination. Anal cytology is recommended for HIV-infected women and may be useful for other high risk populations such as women with persistent condyloma or women with other HPV-related cancers (Leeds and Fang 2016).
- Screening guidelines continue to evolve. Primary HPV screening is being evaluated as an alternative strategy to traditional Pap smear cytology screening (Huh et al. 2015).

Primary prevention
- HPV vaccines have been shown to be highly effective in preventing type-specific HPV infection and disease.
- There are three prophylactic HPV vaccines that have been licensed in the United States: a bivalent HPV 16/18 vaccine, a quadrivalent HPV 6/11/16/18 vaccine, and the newest 9-valent vaccine.
- Currently the only HPV vaccine available in the US is the 9-valent HPV vaccine (9vHPV, Gardasil9), which offers protection against seven oncogenic HPV types (16, 18, 31, 33, 45, 52, and 58) that account for approximately 80% of cervical cancers, and 2 HPV types (6 and 11) that cause approximately 90% of genital warts.
- Condoms, if used consistently and correctly, can lower the chances of acquiring and transmitting HPV and developing HPV-related diseases.
- Limiting the number of sexual partners can reduce the risk for HPV. However, even persons with only one lifetime sexual partner can get HPV.

Secondary prevention
- Treatment of anogenital warts and anogenital (vulvar, vaginal, and cervical) dysplasia involves the destruction or excision of infected tissue and will reduce the risk of recurrence.

Diagnosis

BOTTOM LINE/CLINICAL PEARLS
- History should include a discussion of sexual activity, STD history, smoking history, and HIV history.
- Anogenital warts can be flat, papular, or verrucous/pedunculated growths on the genital mucosa.
- Diagnosis of anogenital warts is made by visual inspection and confirmed by biopsy.
- Vulvar and vagina dysplasia is often clinically indistinguishable from benign genital warts.
- Cervical warts and dysplastic lesions may be apparent as raised, irregular lesions on speculum examination of the cervix but more often are subclinical.
- Cervical dysplasia is identified by screening with Pap cytology/HPV testing and confirmed by colposcopy and biopsy.
- Anal dysplasia is identified by digital rectal examination or by screening with Pap cytology/HPV testing and confirmed by high-resolution anoscopy and biopsy.

Differential diagnosis

Differential diagnosis	Features
Condyloma lata	• Moist, wart-like papules associated with secondary syphilis • Lesions are highly contagious and diagnosis can be made by dark-field microscopy or positive syphilis serology
Folliculitis (vestibular papillae)	• Pink, fine, frond-like projections of the vestibular epithelium or labia minora • Not infectious. • Most often asymptomatic but can present with itching, stinging, or burning • Definitive diagnosis is made by biopsy
Molluscum contagiousum	• Cluster of discrete small, raised, pearly papules with central dimpling • Viral infection, DNA poxvirus • Most often asymptomatic but may present with itching • Diagnosis based on clinical appearance
Endocervicitis	• Typically asymptomatic but may present with intermenstrual bleeding, postcoital spotting, and/or pelvic pain • Inflammation and friability of the ectocervix seen on speculum exam • Often accompanied by a mucopurlent discharge • Associated with sexually transmitted gonorrhea and/or chlamydia • Diagnosis based on polymerase chain reaction (PCR) testing and Pap/HPV results
Endocervical polyp	• Typically asymptomatic but may present with intermenstrual bleeding, postcoital spotting • Smooth, polypoid tissue seen protruding through the endocervical canal on speculum examination • Removal of polyp and histopathological confirmation rules out HPV-related dysplasia/malignancy

Typical presentation
- Vulvovaginal infections (both warts and dysplastic lesions) are typically asymptomatic but may be painful or pruritic depending on the size and distribution of lesions.
- Cervical HPV infections (both warts and dysplastic lesions) are typically asymptomatic and incidentally found on screening examination. Occasionally patients present with irregular bleeding including postcoital bleeding.
- Anal HPV infections (both warts and dysplastic lesions) are usually asymptomatic but may present with pruritis, bleeding, or tenesmus.

Clinical diagnosis
History
- A comprehensive sexual and medical history should be obtained.
- The sexual history should include information about age at first coitus, the number and gender of the patient's sexual partners, condom use, type of sexual contacts (oral, vaginal, anal, etc.), and history of sexually transmitted infections.
- The medical history should include tobacco use and any comorbid medical conditions or therapies associated with immunosuppression (for example, HIV infection, transplant recipient, or use of biologics).
- The gynecology history should elicit any concerning symptoms including abnormal vaginal or anal bleeding or discharge, vulvovaginal or anal pruritis/irritation, or any new concerning bumps or lesions in the anogenital area.

Physical examination
- A careful visual examination of the external genitalia (labia, vulva, mons, and perianal area) should be performed to identify lesions suspicious of HPV disease.
- A speculum examination should be performed to visualize the vaginal mucosa (including the vaginal fornices) as well as the cervix/ectocervix for lesions suspicious of HPV disease and also areas with erosive/friable tissue.
- A digital rectal examination should be performed to assess for nodularity or friable masses.

Useful clinical decision rules and calculators
- Management of cervical cellular abnormalities is complex and requires synthesis of patient age, Pap test results, biopsy pathology, and high-risk HPV DNA testing. The American Society for Colposcopy and Cervical Pathology (ASCCP) has developed a comprehensive, user-friendly app for the Updated Consensus Guidelines for Managing Abnormal Cervical Cancer Screening Tests and Cancer Precursors. https://www.asccp.org/store-detail2/asccp-mobile-app
- New algorithms are being developed by ASCCP to provide a more individualized approach to cervical cancer screening, surveillance, and treatment. The algorithms will incorporate patient-specific information about HPV vaccination history, past history of high-grade cervical dysplasia, previous type-specific HPV test results, and comorbid medical conditions that could alter immune responses. This shift in paradigm is needed because a failure to adequately assess individualized risk factors has contributed to overtesting and overtreatment in low-risk women and undertesting and undertreatment in high-risk women.

Laboratory diagnosis
List of diagnostic tests
- Cervical Pap smear cytology. The Pap smear is obtained by gently scraping cells from the cervix using a small brush or spatula.
  - Starting at age 21
  - Continuing every 3 years until age 30
- Cervical Pap smear cytology with HPV co-testing
  - Starting at age 30
  - Continuing every 5 years until age 65
- Anal Pap smear cytology. The anal Pap is obtained by introducing a polyester or dacron swab 2–3 inches into the anus and gently rotating.
  - Routine screening is not recommended
  - For patients at high risk for anal dysplasia
- Colposcopy – Used as a follow-up test to evaluate patients with an abnormal Pap smear and/or HPV test results. Colposcopy is performed using a special microscope, called a colposcope, that gives a magnified view of the tissue and identifies lesions requiring biopsy.
- High-resolution anoscopy (HRA) – Performed on all patients with an abnormal anal Pap smear for the identification of lesions requiring biopsy or ablative treatment.
- Cervical biopsy – Obtained when a patient has a visible grossly abnormal lesion or an abnormal lesion(s) detected on colposcopic evaluation.
- Anal biopsy – Obtained when a patient has a visible abnormal lesion or an abnormal lesion(s) detected on HRA.
- Vulva or vaginal biopsy – Obtained when patient has a visible lesion(s) suspicious for genital warts, dysplasia, or malignancy.

Potential pitfalls/common errors made regarding diagnosis of disease
- Diagnostic errors can occur with histopathologic evaluation of biopsy specimens with inconsistencies attributable to differences in reviewer skills.
- Colposcopy and high-resolution anoscopy are highly specialized skills that have inherent human error involved in their use.

Treatment
Treatment rationale
- Treatment of anogenital warts should be guided by wart size, number, anatomic site, patient preference, cost of treatment, convenience, side effects, and provider experience. There is no evidence that any one treatment is superior to another. Repeated treatments are often necessary.
- Low-grade dysplasia of the cervix (cervical intraepithelial neoplasia grade 1 or CIN1) does not need to be treated as most of these lesions will regress.
- High-grade dysplasia of the cervix (CIN 2/CIN3) is a precancer and should be treated. Treatment can be either ablative (cryosurgery) or excisional – either a loop electrosurgical excision procedure (LEEP) or cold knife cone biopsy. Excisional treatment is preferred as there is a surgical specimen available for pathologic review.
- Vulvar dysplasia (vulvar intraepithelial neoplasia or VIN) is also divided into low-grade and high-grade lesions. For high-grade lesions, wide local excision is the most effective treatment. Low-grade lesions can be treated with excision, laser ablation, or topical imiquimod.
- Vaginal dysplasia (vaginal intraepithelial neoplasia or VaIN) is also divided into low- grade and high-grade lesions. First-line treatment for high-grade lesions (VaIN II-III lesions) is ablative surgical treatment.
- Anal dysplasia (anal intraepithelial neoplasia or AIN) is also divided into low-grade and high-grade lesions. Treatment choice depends on size, number, and location of lesions and/or symptoms. Small, isolated high-grade lesions can be treated with trichloroacetic acid (TCA). For lesions too large/extensive for TCA, anoscopy-directed lesion ablation with electrocautery can be used in a series of multiple treatments.

Table of treatment

Treatment of anogenital warts

Treatment	Comments
Conservative	If left untreated, anogenital warts can resolve spontaneously, remain unchanged, or increase in size and number.
Medical	Local treatment is recommended for patients with limited disease. Moderate pain and local irritation is common for all the local medical treatments.
Imiquimod 3.75% or 5% cream	Topically active immune enhancer. Patient applied; 3 times a week up to 16 weeks.
Podofilox 0.5% solution or gel	Topically active antimitotic drug. Patient applied; twice a day for 3 days followed by no therapy. May be repeated. Healthcare provider often provides initial treatment.
Sinecatechins 15% ointment	Green tea extract. Patient applied 3 times daily until lesions resolve; can be used for up to 16 weeks.
Trichloroacetic acid (TCA)	Caustic agent. Provider applied.

(Continued)

Treatment	Comments
Surgical	For patients with extensive disease or refractory to local therapy.
Surgery	Either scalpel or CO_2 laser. Has the advantage of eliminating most warts in a single visit. Requires local or general anesthesia.
Cryotherapy	Posttreatment tissue necrosis and blistering common.
Electrocautery	Care must be taken to control the depth of electrocautery to prevent scarring.

CLINICAL PEARLS
- Anogenital warts can be treated by topical medicines, cryosurgery, laser, or surgical excision.
- High-grade cervical dysplasia is precancerous and is typically treated by LEEP or cone biopsy.
- High-grade vulvar, vaginal, and anal dysplasia are precancerous lesions that also require treatment.

Special populations
Pregnancy
- HPV can proliferate more rapidly and become more friable during pregnancy. During pregnancy, TCA, cryotherapy, and surgical removal may be used. Cytotoxic agents should not be used.
- Mother-to-child HPV transmission can occur but is infrequent, and cesarean delivery should not be performed solely to prevent transmission to the neonate. A rare condition, juvenile-onset recurrent respiratory papillomatosis (RRP) is associated with vertical HPV transmission.
- Cesarean delivery may be indicated if lesions are extensive and judged to be at risk for avulsion and hemorrhage with a vaginal delivery.

Others
- Persons living with HIV infection, particularly those individuals with advanced immunosuppression, often have larger or more numerous anogenital warts that do not respond as well to therapy and recurrences occur more frequently after treatment.
- Women with HIV infection have an increased risk of cervical precancers and cancers and require more frequent Pap screening.

Prognosis

BOTTOM LINE/CLINICAL PEARLS
- After initial treatment, anogenital warts often recur.
- Cervical cytology/HPV screening utilized in combination with treatment of cervical dysplasia is a successful strategy to prevent cervical cancer.
- After initial treatment of vaginal, vulvar, and anal high-grade dysplasia, recurrence is common.

Prognosis for treated patients
- Anogenital warts – commonly recur within 3 months of treatment.
- High-grade cervical dysplasia – 10% risk of recurrence after treatment.
- High-grade vulvar dysplasia – 9–50% risk of recurrence after treatment.
- High-grade vaginal dysplasia – 0–50% risk of recurrence after surgical treatment in an 18-year follow-up study.
- High-grade anal dysplasia – after ablation, 30–40% residual disease in mean follow-up of ~ 14 months.

Reading list

Drolet M, Benard E, Perez N, et al., on behalf of the HPV Vaccination Impact Study Group. Population-level impact and herd effects following the introduction of human papillomavirus vaccination programs: updated systematic review and meta-analysis. *Lancet* 2019 Aug 10;394(10197):497-509. Published online 2019 Jun 26 http://dx.doi.org/10.1016/S0140-6736(19)30298-3

Dunne EF, Unger ER, Sternberg M, et al. Prevalence of HPV infection among females in the United States. *JAMA* 2007;297:813–9.

Huh WK, Ault KA, Chelmow D, et al. Use of primary high-risk human papillomavirus testing for cervical cancer screening: interim clinical guidance. *Obstet Gynecol* 2015;125:330–7.

Leeds IL, Fang SH. Anal cancer and intraepithelial neoplasia screening: A review. *World J Gastrointest Surg* 2016;8(1):41-51.

Lehtinen M, Paavonen J, Wheeler CM, et al. Overall efficacy of HPV-16/18 AS04-adjuvanted vaccine against grade 3 or greater cervical intraepithelial neoplasia: 4-year end-of-study analysis of the randomised, double-blind PATRICIA trial. HPV PATRICIA Study Group. *Lancet Oncol* 2012;13:89-99.

Massad LS, Einstein MH, Huh WK, et al. 2012 updated consensus guidelines for the management of abnormal cervical cancer screening tests and cancer precursors. *Obstet Gynecol* 2013; 121:829-46.

Park IU, Introcaso C, Dunne EF. Human papillomavirus and genital warts: a review of the evidence for the 2015 Centers for Disease Control and Prevention sexually transmitted diseases treatment guidelines. *Clin Infect Dis* 2015 Dec 15;61(Suppl 8):S849-55.

Quadrivalent vaccine against human papillomavirus to prevent high-grade cervical lesions. FUTURE II Study Group. *N Engl J Med* 2007;356:1915-27.

Schiffman M, Kjaer SK. Chapter 2: Natural history of anogenital human papillomavirus infection and neoplasia. *J Natl Cancer Inst Monogr* 2003;(31):14-9.

Workowski KA, Bolan GA; Centers for Disease Control and Prevention. Sexually transmitted diseases treatment guidelines, 2015. Human papillomavirus (HPV) infection. *MMWR Recomm Rep* 2015;64(No. RR-3):1-137.

Suggested websites

American Society for Colposcopy and Cervical Pathology (ASCCP). www.asccp.org

Centers for Disease Control and Prevention (CDC). www.cdc.gov

University of Wisconsin National STD Curriculum. www.std.uw.edu

American College of Obstetricians, and Gynecologists (ACOG). www.acog.org

American Cancer Society (ACS). www.cancer.gov

Guidelines
National society guidelines

Title	Source	Date/full reference
Cervical cancer screening and prevention	American College of Obstetricians, and Gynecologists	Cervical cancer screening and prevention. Practice bulletin no 168. ACOG. *Obstet Gynecol* 2016:128;e111-30.
American Cancer Society, American Society for Colposcopy and Cervical Pathology, and American Society for Clinical Pathology screening guidelines for the prevention and early detection of cervical cancer.	ACS-ASCCP-ASCP Comment: This document includes current recommendations for cervical cancer screening	Saslow D, Solomon D, Lawson HW, et al. American Cancer Society, American Society for Colposcopy and Cervical Pathology, and American Society for Clinical Pathology screening guidelines for the prevention and early detection of cervical cancer. *Am J Clin Pathol* 2012;137:516-42.
Use of 9-valent human papillomavirus (HPV) vaccine	Advisory Committee on Immunization Practices, CDC	Petrosky E, Bocchini JA Jr, Hariri S, et al. Use of 9-valent human papillomavirus (HPV) vaccine: updated HPV vaccination recommendations of the advisory committee on immunization practices. Centers for Disease Control and Prevention (CDC). *MMWR Morb Mortal Wkly Rep* 2015;64:300-4.

(*Continued*)

Title	Source	Date/full reference
Human papillomavirus vaccination	ACOG – Committee of Adolescent Healthcare ACOG – Immunization Expert Work Group	Human papillomavirus vaccination. Committee opinion no. 704. American College of Obstetricians and Gynecologists. *Obstet Gynecol* 2017;129:e173-8.
Sexually transmitted diseases treatment guidelines, 2015	CDC Comment: This document includes guidance and scientific rationale for the treatment of anogenital condyloma	http://www.cdc.gov/std/tg2015
Management of vulvar intraepithelial neoplasia	ACOG & ASCCP Comment: This document includes guidance and rationale for the management of VIN	ACOG committee opinion no. 675 summary: management of vulvar intraepithelial neoplasia. *Obstet Gynecol* 2016;128(4):937-8.

Evidence

Type of evidence	Title and comment	Date/full reference
Cross-sectional survey	Prevalence of human papillomavirus among females after vaccine introduction—National Health and Nutrition Examination Survey, United States, 2003–2014 Comment: Within 8 years of vaccine introduction, 4vHPV-type prevalence decreased 71% among 14- to 19-year-olds and 61% among 20- to 24-year-olds.	Oliver, SE, Unger ER, Lewis R, et al. *J Infect Dis* 2017 Sep 1; 216(5):594-603.

Images

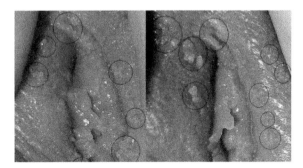

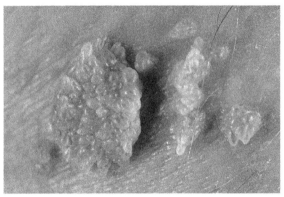

Figure 25.1 Visual inspection – Condyloma acuminata. See color version on website.

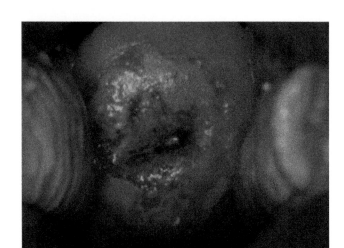

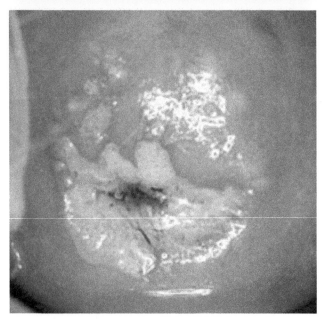

Figure 25.2 Colposcopy – Cervical dysplasia. See color version on website.

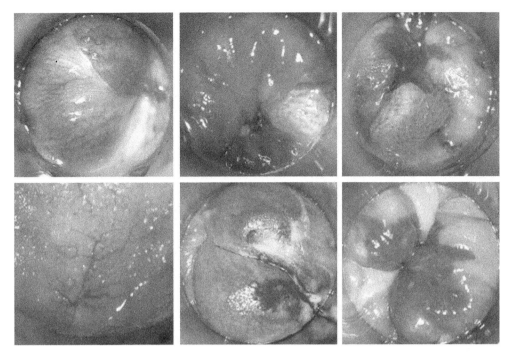

Figure 25.3 High-resolution anoscopy – Anal dysplasia. See color version on website.

Additional material for this chapter can be found online at:
www.wiley.com/go/sperling/mountsinai/obstetricsandgynecology

The following images are available in color: Figure 25.1, Figure 25.2, and
Figure 25.3.

CHAPTER 26

Genitourinary Syndrome of Menopause

Karen F. Brodman
Department of Obstetrics, Gynecology and Reproductive Science, Icahn School of Medicine at Mount Sinai, New York, NY

OVERALL BOTTOM LINE
- Genitourinary syndrome of menopause (GSM) is a common condition caused by decreased or absent estrogen, typically occurring during menopause.
- Symptoms include vaginal dryness, pain with sex, vulvar and vaginal irritation, and urinary symptoms such as urinary tract infections (UTIs), urgency, and incontinence.
- Treatment includes hormonal and nonhormonal therapies, plus newly introduced laser technology.

Background
Definition of disease
- GSM results from decreased sex steroids, primarily estrogen, in the vagina, vulva, and adjacent urogenital tract.
- This decline induces vulvar, vaginal, and urinary changes that foster irritation, infection, dyspareunia, cystitis, urgency, and incontinence.

Disease classification
- In 2014, the North American Menopause Society (NAMS) and the International Society for the Study of Women's Sexual Health (ISSWSH) introduced the terminology genitourinary syndrome of menopause as a less stigmatizing and more inclusive description of vulvovaginal atrophy, atrophic vaginitis, and urogenital atrophy.
- In the literature, the older terminology vulvovaginal atrophy (VVA) is frequently used.

Incidence/prevalence
- GSM affects more than 50% of all menopausal women, 75% of sexually active menopausal women, and 15% of premenopausal women.
- It has been underdiagnosed and undertreated due to patient embarrassment and physician unawareness; this is changing with new attention to the disorder.

Economic impact
- With over 50% of menopausal women experiencing GSM, the economic impact of recurrent vaginal and urinary infections and decreased quality of life is substantial.

Etiology
- Estrogen decline is responsible for GSM.
- Typically, low estrogen occurs during perimenopause and menopause.
- Other causes of hypoestrogenism include:
  - Surgical menopause
  - Pelvic radiation therapy

Mount Sinai Expert Guides: Obstetrics and Gynecology, First Edition. Edited by Rhoda Sperling.
© 2020 John Wiley & Sons Ltd. Published 2020 by John Wiley & Sons Ltd.
Companion Website: www.wiley.com/go/sperling/mountsinai/obstetricsandgynecology

- Chemotherapy
- Medications: aromatase inhibitors, gonadotropin-releasing hormone (GnRH) analogs
- Prolonged lactation
- Endocrine disorders: hypothalamic amenorrhea, hyperprolactinemia

Pathology/pathogenesis
- Vaginal squamous epithelium contains three layers: immature parabasal cells, intermediate cells, and mature superficial cells. The lower genital tract is rich in hormone receptors.
- Estrogen:
  - Maintains mature superficial cells that form a protective layer, which enhances vaginal integrity
  - Promotes blood flow to vaginal tissue, which increases collagen production and elasticity in underlying connective tissue
  - Supports a lactobacilli rich vaginal microbiome that converts glycogen to lactic acid, thus maintaining a pH <4.5
- Testosterone:
  - Vagina and vulva respond to this hormone; vestibule is rich in testosterone receptors.
- Lack of hormones:
  - Causes loss of lactobacilli dominant flora, raising pH > 5
  - Decreases blood flow causing vaginal and labial atrophy
  - Reduces collagen, which diminishes elasticity
  - Results in thin fragile walls that are subject to trauma and inflammation
  - Produces similar changes in adjacent urethra and bladder

Predictive/risk factors
- Risk factors include
  - premature menopause
  - infrequent sexual intercourse
  - nulliparity or delivery exclusively by cesarean delivery
  - cigarette smoking

Prevention
- Frequent sexual intercourse maintains vaginal patency and enhances blood flow.
- Addressing symptoms promptly offers best outcome, limiting potentially irreversible structural changes.

Screening
- All perimenopausal and menopausal women should be proactively questioned about new-onset GSM symptoms at yearly checkups.
- Symptoms may occur in any hypoestrogenic state; these women should be screened for vaginal atrophy.

Primary prevention
- Maintain vaginal health by avoiding excessive douching or vaginal products containing chemical additives.
- Continue active sexual activity, either with a partner or by masturbation.
- Discontinue smoking, which decreases blood flow to vaginal tissue.

Secondary prevention
- Therapeutic interventions reduce severity of GSM and often prevent progression.

Diagnosis

- Diagnosis is clinical, based on typical symptoms and physical findings in the context of amenorrhea or oligomenorrhea.
- Lab tests are used if diagnosis is unclear.

Differential diagnosis

Differential diagnosis	Features
Vulvovaginal infection	Vaginal wet prep or vaginal nucleic acid amplification test (NAAT) to diagnose vaginal infections, which frequently coexist with GSM
Vulvar lesions or skin conditions such as condyloma, lichen sclerosis, or malignancy	Focal lesions or discolorations should be biopsied if diagnosis is unclear
Vulvodynia	Absent vaginal infection, Q-tip test positive

Typical presentation

- Symptoms start during perimenopause, when estrogen decline starts. The patient complains of typical symptoms: sex is painful; her vagina feels dry; there are unprovoked vaginal burning or discomfort, new onset vaginal infections, and increased number of postcoital UTIs. Frequently, women do not complain to their doctor about dyspareunia – they are too embarrassed to discuss it or attribute it to just getting older, although they are deeply troubled by their new symptoms. Without treatment, the symptoms worsen; a vicious cycle of sex avoidance leads to marital discord and aversion to intimacy.

Clinical diagnosis

History

- Review menstrual history for missed or absent periods.
- Inquire about new-onset dyspareunia and its effect on patient.
- Ask if there is vulvovaginal discomfort, burning, or discharge.
- Genitourinary symptoms of urgency, frequency, and incontinence should be assessed.
- Determine extent of irritant exposure (chronic urine leakage, use of over-the-counter [OTC] products).
- See Algorithm 26.1.

Physical examination

- Vulvar inspection reveals thin, pale labia and contracted introitus.
- Speculum insertion elicits pain from decreased elasticity.
- Vaginal walls appear pale with absent rugae, mucosa is friable with petechiae, vaginal discharge is yellow and watery.
- If desired, obtain a vaginal pH and wet prep specimen while the speculum is in place.

Disease severity classification

- GSM is designated as either mild or moderate to severe.
- Classification is made in context with the patient's exam and severity of symptoms.

Laboratory diagnosis

List of diagnostic tests

Office tests

- Vaginal pH: Value > 5 suggests GSM and/or vaginal infection.
- Wet prep: microscopic exam of vaginal secretions; helpful in assessing parabasal cells and diagnosing infection.

Algorithm 26.1 GSM diagnostic algorithm

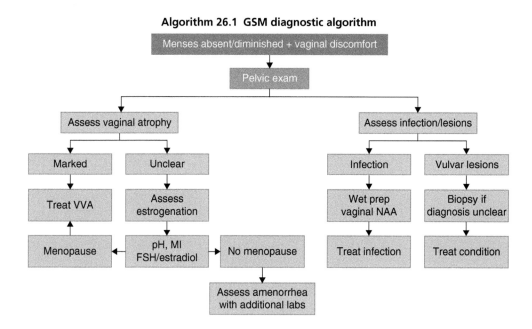

Laboratory tests
- Maturation Index (MI): quantifies percentage of superficial and parabasal cells.
- Vaginal NAAT or culture to evaluate infection.
- Blood tests: Low estradiol (E2) with elevated follicle stimulating hormone (FSH) suggests menopause or perimenopause.
- Vulvar biopsy: sample lesions with unclear diagnosis

Potential pitfalls/common errors made regarding diagnosis of disease
- Treating vaginal infection without addressing underlying VVA hinders recovery; treat both simultaneously.
- Failure to appreciate GSM in perimenopause is common.
- Menopause patients using low-dose systemic hormone therapy with refractory VVA may need additional local therapy.
- Lichen sclerosus frequently presents and worsens during menopause and if present needs to be treated along with GSM.

Treatment
Treatment rationale
- Vaginal moisturizers and lubricants are first line of treatment.
- If symptoms persist add low-dose vaginal estrogen.
- For those unable or unwilling to use estrogen consider oral selective estrogen receptor modulator (SERM) such as ospemifene or laser therapy.
- DHEA vaginal suppository is approved by the Food and Drug Administration (FDA) for GSM; stimulates estrogen and testosterone receptors.
- Use vaginal dilator therapy as needed.
- See Algorithm 26.2.

Algorithm 26.2 GSM management/treatment algorithm

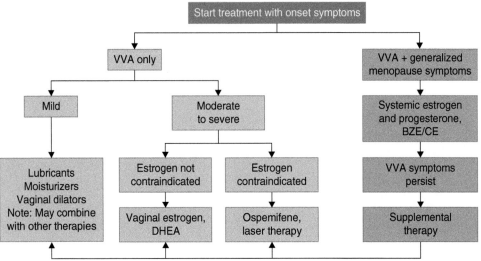

Table of treatment

Treatment	Comments
Conservative/OTC: Vaginal moisturizers and lubricants Hyaluronic acid (HA)	Nonhormonal, use alone or with other therapies Readily available, decreases coital irritation HA: moisturizes, acidifies pH, promotes lactobacilli
Medical: *Local vaginal:* Low-dose estrogen cream, tablet, or gel cap: insert vaginally twice weekly Vaginal ring (Estring): insert 1 ring every 3 months Dehydroepiandrosterone (DHEA): vaginal insert, one daily	Local therapy with minimal systemic levels, no progesterone needed, effective after 12 weeks, excellent safety profile DHEA converts intravaginally to estrogen and testosterone
Medical: *Systemic:* Estrogen: oral tablet, transdermal patch or gel, vaginal ring (Femring) Bazedoxifene/conjugated estrogen (BZE/CE): daily oral tablet Ospemifene: daily oral tablet	Higher dose estrogen treats general menopause symptoms plus GSM. If uterus present, add progesterone BZE: SERM that protects endometrium Ospemifene: SERM that treats GSM, no effect on other menopause symptoms
Other: Laser: fractionated CO_2 laser for vagina and external vulva Pelvic physical therapy, vaginal dilators	Treatment not yet FDA approved for GSM, studies are ongoing; stimulates connective tissue, restores elasticity,lowers pH; can be used on vulva as well as vagina; high cost may limit access for some Use to expand introitus, enhances medical therapy

Prevention/management of complications
- Estrogen is contraindicated in undiagnosed vaginal/uterine bleeding. Low dose vaginal estrogen use in patients with breast or uterine cancer is controversial but may be appropriate for select patients; consult with oncologist.

CLINICAL PEARLS
- Unlike other menopause symptoms, GSM is progressive and does not resolve without treatment. DHEA is a precursor hormone; converts to estrogen and testosterone intravaginally; minimal systemic exposure; stimulates both estrogen and testosterone receptors.
- Vaginal estrogen ring comes in two strengths, low dose for GSM (Estring) and high dose for systemic treatment (Femring); be sure to prescribe properly.
- Vaginal estrogen dosage is far lower than systemic estrogen; use without progesterone; excellent safety profile.

Special populations

Pregnancy
- With lactation, estrogen plummets. Treat atrophy with lubricants; low-dose vaginal estrogen is safe and effective while nursing.

Elderly
- Symptoms progress with age; low-dose vaginal therapy can be continued indefinitely.

Others
- Risk of thrombosis with low-dose vaginal estrogen in at-risk women has not been studied.
- Use lowest dose vaginal estrogen in those at high risk of endometrial cancer and monitor carefully.

Prognosis

BOTTOM LINE/CLINICAL PEARLS
- Early and effective treatment yields best long-term results.
- Proactively evaluate and treat this highly prevalent condition.
- Local hormone therapy – estrogen or DHEA – is effective; has excellent safety profile.
- Nonhormonal laser treatment is promising; further studies pending.
- Vaginal dilators and physical therapy are useful adjunct to treat a tight introitus.
- Encourage lubricants with sex, even for those using other therapies.

Natural history of untreated disease
- Systemic menopausal symptoms improve with time, whereas untreated GSM progresses.
- The vagina contracts, labia atrophy and fuse, and elasticity declines, making sexual intercourse painful.
- Vulvovaginal scarring and loss of connective tissue may eventually be irreversible.

Prognosis for treated patients
- Symptoms often recur when treatment is discontinued; ongoing therapy is typically needed.

Follow-up tests and monitoring
- Monitor patient for symptomatic improvement.
- Vaginal bleeding requires further evaluation.
- Objective findings include acid pH, improved elasticity, mucosal integrity.

Reading list

Athanasiou S, Pitsouni E, Antonopoulou S, et al. The effect of microablative fractional CO_2 laser on vaginal flora of postmenopausal women. *Climacteric* 2016 Oct;19(5):512-8.

Bhupathiraju SN, Grodstein F, Stampfer MJ, et al. Vaginal estrogen use and chronic disease risk in the Nurses' Health Study. *Menopause* 2018 Dec 17;26(6):603-10.

Calleja-Agius J, Brincat MP. The urogenital system and the menopause. *Climacteric* 2015;18(Suppl 1):18-22.

Edwards D, Panay N. Treating vulvovaginal atrophy/genitourinary syndrome of menopause: how important is vaginal lubricant and moisturizer composition? *Climacteric* 2016;19(2):151-61.

Labrie D, Archer DF, Koltun W, et al. Efficacy of intravaginal dehydroepiandrosterone (DHEA) on moderate to severe dyspareunia and vaginal dryness, symptoms of vulvovaginal atrophy, and of the genitourinary syndrome of menopause. *Menopause* 2016;23(3):243-56.

Nappi RE, Biglia N, Cagnacci A, et al. Diagnosis and management of symptoms associated with vulvovaginal atrophy: expert opinion on behalf of the Italian VVA study group. *Gynecol Endocrinol* 2016;32(8):602-6.

Portman DJ, Goldstein SR, Kagan R. Treatment of moderate to severe dyspareunia with intravaginal prasterone therapy: a review. *Climacteric* 2019 Feb;22(1):65-72.

Sokol ER, Karram MM. An assessment of the safety and efficacy of a fractional CO2 laser system for the treatment of vulvovaginal atrophy. *Menopause* 2016 Oct;23(10):1102-7.

Suggested websites

North American Menopause Society. www.menopause.org
Excellent source for menopause information plus educational videos
International Society for the Study of Vulvovaginal Disease. www.issvd.org
Offers information on a wide variety of vulvovaginal disorders
Good source for vaginal dilators. www.hopeandher.com
Popular laser product. www.monalisatouch.com

Guidelines
National society guidelines

Title	Source	Date
Management of menopausal symptoms: practice bulletin no. 141	ACOG	January 2014 (reaffirmed 2018)
Use of vaginal estrogen in women with a history of estrogen dependent breast cancer: committee opinion 659	ACOG Comment: Data show no increase in cancer recurrence when using low-dose vaginal estradiol for GSM	March 2016, (reaffirmed 2018)
Fractional laser treatment of vulvovaginal atrophy and U.S. Food and Drug Administration clearance: ACOG position statement	ACOG Comment: CO2 fractional laser is not FDA approved as treatment for GSM, studies are pending	May 2016 (reaffirmed July 2018)
Management of genitourinary syndrome of menopause in women with or at high risk for breast cancer	Consensus recommendation from NAMS and ISSWSH Comment: Individualize treatment, start nonhormonal, local hormone treatment may be option for some, include oncologist in decision to treat	March 2018

International society guidelines

Title	Source	Date/full reference
Management of symptomatic vulvovaginal atrophy	North American Menopause Society (NAMS)	*Menopause* 2013 Sep;20(9):888-902.
Vulvovaginal Atrophy Terminology Consensus Conference Panel. Genitourinary syndrome of menopause: new terminology for vulvovaginal atrophy	International Society for the Study of Women's Sexual Health (ISSWSH) and NAM	*Menopause* 2014;Oct;21(10):1063-8.

Evidence

Type of evidence	Title and comment	Date/full reference
Review	Genitourinary syndrome of menopause: an overview of clinical manifestations, pathophysiology, etiology, evaluation, and management Comment: excellent overview	*Am J Obstet Gynecol* 2016:704-11.

Additional material for this chapter can be found online at:
www.wiley.com/go/sperling/mountsinai/obstetricsandgynecology

This includes a case study, advice for patients, and ICD codes.

CHAPTER 27

Menopausal Hot Flashes

Elissa Gretz Friedman
Department of Obstetrics, Gynecology and Reproductive Science, Icahn School of Medicine at Mount Sinai, New York, NY

OVERALL BOTTOM LINE
- Menopause is a natural transition that every female experiences during midlife, at the end of her ovarian reserve.
- The hot flash is a common symptom of menopause, experienced by 75% of women.
- Hot flashes can affect quality of life (Avis et al. 2003), memory (Maki et al. 2008), and sleep (Kravitz et al. 2003), and 60–86% of women seek medical care.
- The most effective treatment for hot flashes is menopausal hormone therapy (MHT), which should be used at the lowest effective dose.

Background
Definition of disease
- The hot flash is a feeling of heat that develops and spreads over the chest, neck, and head, and may or may not be followed by sweating. It occurs as a symptom of the menopause transition.

Incidence/prevalence
- Hot flashes occur in 75% of women during the menopause transition. They vary in number, intensity, and bother.
- Hot flashes persist for an average of 7.4 years and can last for greater than a decade in some women (Avis et al. 2015).

Etiology
- The mechanism of the hot flash is unknown although it is most often characterized as a thermoregulatory heat dissipating event. In menopausal women, the thermoregulatory zone is narrowed. When the core body temperature is outside the zone, a homeostatic mechanism like shivering or sweating is triggered.
- Hot flashes occur in women during the menopause transition when the estrogen level drops, although there is no correlation of hot flashes to an absolute estrogen level. Endogenous estrogen levels do not vary between women with and without hot flashes.

Pathology/pathogenesis
- There is evidence linking hot flash activity to the autonomic nervous system, including increased norepinephrine (Freedman 2001), as well as the serotonergic, opioid, and adrenal systems.
- The kisspeptin-neurokinin B (NKB)-dynorphin (KNDy) signaling system in the hypothalmus might be a key pathway in the mechanism of the hot flash (Rance 2013).

Mount Sinai Expert Guides: Obstetrics and Gynecology, First Edition. Edited by Rhoda Sperling.
© 2020 John Wiley & Sons Ltd. Published 2020 by John Wiley & Sons Ltd.
Companion Website: www.wiley.com/go/sperling/mountsinai/obstetricsandgynecology

Predictive/risk factors

Risk factor	Odds ratio
African American (AA) women are more likely to have hot flashes than White, Hispanic, or Asian women (Freeman et al. 2001; Gold et al. 2006) and additionally have more frequent, severe, persistent and bothersome hot flashes (Thurston et al. 2008).	
Obesity: adipose tissue possibly acts as an insulator, preventing the heat dissipation action of vasomotor menopausal symptoms (VMS), and increasing their occurrence.	
Smoking:	Current smokers 60% increased likelihood of reporting VMS relative to nonsmokers
Negative mood or affect; higher level of anxiety, depressive symptoms and perceived stress were associated with increased VMS in the SWAN study (Bromberger et al. 2013).	

Diagnosis

> **BOTTOM LINE/CLINICAL PEARLS**
> - Hot flashes are diagnosed by history or a patients description of the symptom. There are no specific physical findings.
> - Hot flashes should be correlated to age and changes in menstrual bleeding pattern to distinguish from other possible causes as listed below.

Differential diagnosis

Differential diagnosis	Features
Hyperthyroidism	
Carcinoid	Flushing, no sweating
Pheochromocytoma	Flushing and profuse sweating and hypertension
Alcohol or alcohol withdrawal	
Chronic opiate use or withdrawal	
Antidepressants – selective serotonin reuptake inhibitors (SSRIs)	Sweating
Nicotic acid	Intense warmth and itching
Ca channel blockers	
Antiestrogens: anastrozole, tamoxifen, raloxifene, leuprolide	
Chronic infection	
Post gastric surgery	Dumping syndrome
Mast cell disorders	Associated with GI symptoms
Lymphoma	Specifically night sweats
Renal cell cancer	
Pancreatic islet cell cancer	
Medullary cancer of thyroid	
Anxiety disorders	

Typical presentation

- Typically a midlife woman will present complaining of frequent hot flashes disrupting her life during the day and awakening her during the night. She may be emotionally labile and may complain of difficulty concentrating. Upon questioning, her menstrual bleeding pattern may be consistent with perimenopause or menopause. Early perimenopause is defined as a change in menstrual cycle length of +/- 7 days. Late perimenopause is defined as skipping cycles by at least 60 days. Vasomotor symptoms are most likely to occur during this stage. A patient is considered menopausal when she has not had a period for 1 year.

Clinical diagnosis

History

- Complete health evaluation is indicated with history, including symptoms that may indicate a workup for an alternative diagnosis as stated in the differential section. A complete medication history is important. For example, the SSRIs can cause sweating, which can be confused with hot flashes by the patient. GYN bleeding history should be consistent with either perimenopause or menopause. At this time, also evaluate the patient for any possible contraindications to hormonal treatment of hot flashes, including history of breast or other estrogen-dependent cancer, thromboembolic disease, undiagnosed abnormal vaginal bleeding, pregnancy, smoking, and significant cardiac history.

Physical examination

- There are no physical findings pathognomonic of the hot flash.
- Complete examination, including breast and pelvic examinations, are indicated. Signs of hypoestrogenism would be expected: pale dry vaginal mucosa with loss of rugae.

Useful clinical decision rules and calculators

- The patient's information may be put into the MenoPro/NAMS app developed by the North American Menopause Society available in the Apple App store and options for therapy are listed based on the patient's data. The recommendations and information sheets can then be e-mailed directly to the patient for consideration.

Disease severity classification

- Symptom severity is related to the degree to which a patient's quality of life is affected. The decision to treat is based upon a patient's need for relief of symptoms.

Laboratory diagnosis

List of diagnostic tests

- Follicle-stimulating hormone (FSH) and anti-Müllerian hormone reflect ovarian reserve. They may be checked if menopause symptoms are atypical or occur at an early age. Ovarian function is erratic during the transition. It is not recommended to check FSH, luteinizing hormone, or estradiol as they are difficult to interpret and only indicative of that moment in time. Salivary testing of hormone levels are inaccurate and have no indication.
- Lipid panel, HgA1C. Used to calculate cardiovascular risk prior to considering MHT. Results can be used in the MenoPro app.
- Endometrial biopsy. Recommended if patient is having an abnormal bleeding pattern. These include: any postmenopausal bleeding, in perimenopause, frequent (closer than 21 days) or prolonged (greater than 7 days) of bleeding.

List of imaging techniques

- Transvaginal ultrasound should be performed if the patient is having abnormal vaginal bleeding. With postmenopausal bleeding, a normal endometrial stripe is less than 5 mm.
- Mammogram should be up to date prior to considering hormonal treatment for hot flashes.

Treatment

Treatment rationale

- When a patient desires treatment for hot flashes, recommend lifestyle changes for 3 months. If a patient can be treated adequately with lifestyle changes, medications, with possible side effects, are avoided.
- Lifestyle changes include
  - avoid common triggers such as alcohol, stress, hot foods, spicy foods, and caffeine.
  - Keep core body temperature down; Dress in layers, use a fan, keep room temperature cool, drink ice cold drinks.
  - Weight loss
  - Regular exercise, yoga, paced respirations (slow deep rhythmic abdominal breathing, 6–8 times per minute with onset of flash).
- If after 3 months the patient is still symptomatic medication can be considered.

Table of treatment

Treatment			Comments
Conservative Lifestyle Changes. Described in the treatment rationale section.			
Medical			
Oral estrogen preparations			May be used alone if patient had a hysterectomy. If patient has a uterus must be used with a progesterone. If the patient is within 1–2 years of final menses sequential estrogen/progesterone is preferred. If without menses for greater than 2 years continuous combined is recommended
Active ingredient	Product	Dosage (mg/d)	
17B estradiol *	Estrace	0.5, 1.0, 2.0	
Conjugated estrogens	Premarin	0.3, 0.45, 0.625, 0.9, 1.25	
Synthetic conjugated estrogen	Enjuvia	0.3, 0.45, 0.625, 0.9, 1.25	
Conjugated estrogens, CSD	C.E.S pms-Conjugated Est	0.3, 0.625, 0.9, 1.25	
Esterified estrogens	Menest	0.3, 0.625, 1.25, 2.5	
	Estropipate generic avail	0.625 (0.75 estropipate), 1.25 (1.5), 2.5 (3.0)	
Transdermal estrogen products			Transdermal preparation is preferred in most women to avoid the first-pass effect. Patients with moderate CVD risk 5–10%, well-controlled BP, smokers, remote history of situational thrombotic event, transdermal is recommended
Patches 17B-estradiol*	Product	Dosage (mgE2/day)	
	Alora	0.025	
	Climara	0.025, 0.0375, 0.05, 0.06 0.075, 0.1, once/week	
	Estraderm	0.05, 0.1 twice/week	
	Minivelle	0.025, 0.375, 0.05, 0.075, 0.1 twice/week	
	Vivelle-dot	0.025, 0.375, 0.05, 0.075, 0.1 twice/week	
Transdermal gels 17B-estradiol*	Divigel	0.25, 0.5, 1.0	
	Estrogel	0.75	
	Elestrin	0.52 (adjust based on clinical response	

(Continued)

(*Continued*)

Treatment			Comments
Transdermal spray 17B-estradiol*	Evamist	1.53 (1 spray/d initially, adjust dose based on clinical response)	
Systemic vaginal estrogen			
Vaginal ring Estradiol acetate*	Femring	0.05 mg/d, 0.10 mg/d for 90 days	This is a systemic dose of estrogen and a progesterone must be used if the patient has a uterus
Progestogens			
Active ingredient	Product name	Dosage (mg/d)	
Medroxyprogesterone	Provera	2.5 (administered daily), 5, 10 (administered cyclically 12/14d/mo)	
Micronized progesterone*	Prometrium	100 (administered daily), 200 (administered cyclically 12d/mo) (cannot be used in patients with peanut allergy)	Peanut oil—do not use in patient with peanut allergy
Levonorgestrel IUD	Mirena	52 mg intrauterine device	Effective for 5 years. Avoids most systemic progesterone effects
Combination estrogen-progestogen products			
Active ingredient	product name	Dosage	
Oral continuous-cyclic	Premphase	0.625 mgE+5.0mg (2 conjugated estrogens(E)+ tablets: E days 1–14, Medroxyprogesterone acetate (P)	Recommended in recently menopausal patient to decrease unscheduled bleeding
		E +P days 15–28)	
Oral continuous-combined			Recommended in patient with a uterus who is greater than 2 years since final menses
Estradiol*/Progesterone*	Bijuva	1 mg/100 mg/day	Only oral bioidentical combination medication
Conjugated estrogens(E)+			
Medroxyprogesterone acetate (P)	Prempro	0.3 or 0.45 mgE + 1.5 mgP, 0.625 mgE + 2.5 or 5.0 mgP	
Ethinyl estradiol(E) +northindrone acetate(P)	Femhrt	0.5 mg/2.5 mg 1.0 mg/5 mg	
17B-estradiol+ norethindrone acetate (P)	Activella	0.5 mg/0.1 mg 1.0 mg/0.5 mg	
17B-estradiol(E)+drospirenone (P)	Angeliq	0.25 mg/0.5 mg 0.5 mg/1.0 mg	

(Continued)

Treatment			Comments
Oral Intermittent-combined			
17B-estradiol(E)+norgestimate(P)	Prefest	1 mgE and 1 mgE+0.09P (E alone for 3d, followed by E+P for 3d, repeated continuously)	
Transdermal Continuous-combined			
17B-estradiol(E)+northindrone acetate(P)	Combipatch	0.05 mgE+ 14 mgP twice/wk	
17B-estradiol(E)+levonorgestrel(P)	Climara Pro	0.045 mgE + 0.015 mgP once/wk	
Other oral products			
conjugated estrogens+bazedoxifene	Duavee	0.45(E)+10(bazedoxifene)	Do not need progesterone in patient with uterus
*bioidentical			

Treatment			Comments
Non-Hormonal Treatments for Vasomotor Symptoms (Pinkerton 2020)			
(with positive benefits in randomized clinical trials not FDA approved except where noted) On average 20–40% less effective than hormonal treatment			
Selective serotonin reuptake inhibitors (SSRI)			Taper to discontinue
*Paroxitine SSRI	Brisdelle	7.5 mg/d	*Only FDA approved for treatment of HF
Escitalopram	Lexapro		10-20 mg/d
Citalopram	Celexa		10-20 mg/d
Fluoxitine	Prozac or Sarafem		20 mg/d
Selective norepinephrine reuptake inhibitors (SNRI)			
Venlafaxine	Effexor	37.5 to 75 mg/d	
Desvenlafaxine	Pristiq	75 mg/d to BID	
Other			
Gabapentin	Neurotin	300-900 mg	Sedative effect use at night
Pregabalin	Lyrica	75-150 mg BID	Caution interacts ace inhibitors
Clonidine patch	Catapres-TTS	0.1 mg to 0.3 mg weekly	
Psychological			
Cognitive behavioral therapy			Ayres et al. 2012
Hypnosis			Elkins et al. 2013
Complimentary			
Soy, black cohosh, acupuncture, yoga			Similar to placebo 30-50% benefit

Prevention/management of complications

- The most common complication from treatment with hormones for hot flashes is vaginal bleeding. Unscheduled bleeding can be reduced by using a sequential regimen, if hormones are prescribed within 1–2 years of the final menstrual period. Any bleeding on a continuous combined regimen is considered abnormal and should be evaluated with endovaginal ultrasound and if the endometrium is 5 mm or greater, an endometrial biopsy.
- Deep vein thrombosis/pulmonary embolus. Caution should be used when a patient is on hormone therapy and is to be immobilized for a period of time. In general, thrombosis is a rare complication of hormonal therapy. It most commonly occurs during the first 1–2 years after initiation of therapy and the risk decreases over time. Observational data show lower risk with transdermal estrogen than oral estrogen.
- Both estrogen therapy (ET) and estrogen-progestogen therapy (EPT) increase the risk of ischemic stroke in postmenopausal women. HT should be avoided for women with elevated baseline risk of stroke.
- Breast cancer risk increases with EPT use beyond 3–5 years of use although it is viewed as rare. Estrogen alone showed no increased risk in the Women's Health Initiative after 7.1 years.

Management/treatment

- Women with mild to moderate hot flashes—lifestyle changes for 3 months are recommended.
- For women with moderate to severe hot flashes in whom lifestyle changes have failed MHT can be considered.
- A patient starting hormonal therapy should be less than age 60 and less than 10 years from her final menstrual period. Age and time since menopause are critical modifiers of the effect of systemic hormone therapy on cardiovascular disease with more favorable effect in patients aged 50–59 and within 10 years of menopause (Shifren and Gass 2014).
- If a patient continues to have moderate to severe hot flashes and desires treatment with menopausal hormone therapy:

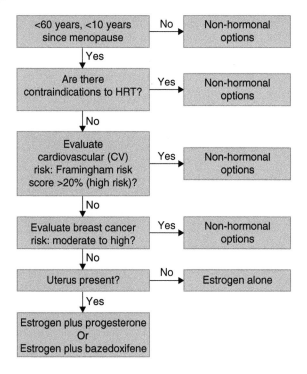

Adapted from Stuenkel et al. 2015.

- A patient's information may be put into the MenoPro/NAMS app developed by the North American Menopause Society available in the Apple App store and options for therapy are listed based on the patient's data. The recommendations and information sheets can be e-mailed directly to the patient for consideration.
- Adequate progestogen must be given in addition to estrogen if the patient has an intact uterus. Continuous progestin is preferred, if possible, as bleeding is the number one indication for discontinuation of MHT. Progestogen is not indicated with estrogen if the patient has had a hysterectomy.
- If the patient has new onset of hot flashes greater than 10 years from the final menstrual period look for other causes.

Special populations
Others
- Breast cancer: Systemic hormone therapy is not recommended in patients with a history of breast cancer.
- In a patient with increased breast cancer risk alternatives to hormonal therapy should be considered. A patient for whom risk reducing medication is indicated would not be a good candidate for hormone therapy. Breast cancer risk score: http://www.cancer.gov/bcrisktool/

Prognosis
Natural history of untreated disease
- Hot flashes last, on average, 7.4 years and will resolve without treatment.
- SWAN data showed that in women with more hot flashes there was evidence of increased subclinical CV disease, specifically aortic calcification, compared to women without flashes (Thurston et al. 2012).
- Women with more hot flashes have been found to have increased CV events. There are no data to show that this is prevented by treatment of hot flashes.

Prognosis for treated patients
- Hormonal treatment is the most effective treatment for hot flashes. Hormonal treatment is recommended at the lowest effective dose. After 3-5 years, attempts should be made to discontinue treatment.

Follow-up tests and monitoring
- Patients should undergo annual examination and mammograms while on hormone therapy.
- In a patient on thyroid medication, check level 3 months after starting hormonal therapy.
- Consideration to stopping menopausal hormone therapy should be evaluated on an annual basis. There is no difference in return of symptoms if the hormones are tapered or stopped abruptly.
- Any abnormal vaginal bleeding should be fully evaluated.

Reading list

Avis NE, Ory M, Matthews KA, et al. Health-related quality of life in a multiethnic sample of middle-aged women: Study of Women's Health Across the Nation (SWAN). *Med Care* 2003;41(11):1262-76.

Avis NE, Crawford SL, Greendale G, et al. Duration of menopausal vasomotor symptoms over the menopause transition. *JAMA Intern Med* 2015;175(4):531-9.

Ayres B, Smith M, Hellier J, et al. Effectiveness of group and self-help cognitive behavior therapy in reducing problematic menopausal hot flashes and night sweats (MENOS2): a randomized controlled trial. *Menopause* 2012;19(7):749-59.

Bromberger JT, Kravitz HM, Chang Y, et al. Does risk for anxiety increase during the menopausal transition? Study of women's health across the nation. *Menopause* 2013;20(5):488-95.

Elkins B, Fisher WI, Johnson AK, et al. Clinical hypnosis in the treatment of postmenopausal hot flashes: a randomized controlled trial. *Menopause* 2013;20(3):291-8.

Freedman RR. Physiology of hot flashes. *Am J Hum Biol* 2001;13(4):453-64.

Freeman EW, Sammel MD, Grisso JA, et al. Hot flashes in the late reproductive years: risk factors for African American and Caucasian women. *J Womens Health Gend Based Med* 2001;10(1):67-76.

Gold EB, Colvin A, Avis N, et al. Longitudinal analysis of the association between vasomotor symptoms and race/ethnicity across the menopausal transition: study of women's health across the nation. *Am J Public Health* 2006;96(7):1226-35.

Kravitz HM, Ganz PA, Bromberger J, et al. Sleep difficulty in women at midlife: a community survey of sleep and the menopausal transition. *Menopause* 2003;10(1):19-28.

Maki PM, Drogos LL, Rubin LH, et al. Objective hot flashes are negatively related to verbal memory performance in midlife women. *Menopause* 2008;15(5):848-56.

North American Menopause Society. *Menopause practice: a clinician's guide*. 6th ed. Pepper Pike, OH: NAMS; 2019.

Pinkerton JV. Hormone therapy for postmenopausal women. *N Eng J Med* 2020;382:446-55.

Rance NE, Dacks PA, Mittelman-Smith MA, et al. Modulation of body temperature and LH secretion by hypothalamic KNDy (kisspeptin, neurokinin B and dynorphin) neurons: a novel hypothesis on the mechanism of hot flushes. *Front Neuroendocrinol* 2013;34(3):211-27.

Shifren JL, Gass ML. The North American Menopause Society recommendations for clinical care of midlife women. *Menopause* 2014;21(10):1038-62.

Stuenkel CA, Davis SR, Gompel A, et al. Treatment of symptoms of the menopause: an Endocrine Society Clinical Practice Guideline. *J Clin Endocrinol Metab* 2015;100(11):3975-4011.

Thurston RC, Bromberger JT, Joffe H, et al. Beyond frequency: who is most bothered by vasomotor symptoms? *Menopause* 2008;15(5):841-7.

Thurston RC, Kuller LH, Edmundowicz D, et al. History of hot flashes and aortic calcification among postmenopausal women. *Menopause* 2010;17(2):256–61.

Suggested website

North American Menopause Society. www.menopause.org

Guidelines
National society guidelines

Title	Source	Date/full reference
Management of menopausal symptoms: ACOG practice bulletin no. 141	American College of Obstetrics and Gynecology	January 2014 *Obstet Gynecol* 2014 Jan;123(1):202-16. PMID 24463691.

International society guidelines

Title	Source	Date/full reference
The 2017 hormone therapy position statement of The North American Menopause Society	The North American Menopause Society	*Menopause* 2017;24(7):728-53.
Treatment of symptoms of the menopause: An Endocrine Society Clinical Practice Guideline	The Endocrine Society	*J Clin Endocrinol Metab* 2015;100(11):3975-4011.
The North American Menopause Society recommendations for clinical care of the midlife woman	Menopause Practice: A Clinician's Guide Key points and clinical recommendations	*Menopause* 2014;21(10).

Evidence

Type of evidence	Title and comment	Date/URL
Randomized clinical trial and observational trial	Women's Health Initiative (WHI). Comment: The clinical trials were designed to test the effects of postmenopausal hormone therapy (E + P or E alone), diet modification, and calcium and vitamin D supplements on heart disease, fractures, and breast and colorectal cancer. E + P lead to increase risk Heart attack, stroke, blood clots, breast cancer, decreased risk colon cancer. E alone, no increased risk of heart attack or breast cancer but did show increased risk of stroke and blood clots	1993–present www.whi.org

(*Continued*)

Type of evidence	Title and comment	Date/URL
Multisite longitudinal, epidemiologic study designed to examine the health of women during their middle years	The Study of Women's Health Across the Nation (SWAN). Comment: 20-year study of women in diverse ethnic and racial groups thru midlife. Over 440 scientific publications. African American women have greater number of hot flashes than white. Asian women have the fewest.	1994–present www.swanstudy.org
Multicenter, 5-year clinical trial	Kronos Early Estrogen Prevention Study (KEEPS) Trial. Comment: To evaluate the effectiveness of 0.45 mg of conjugated equine estrogens, or 50 microgram weekly transdermal estradiol (both in combination with cyclic oral, micronized progesterone, 200 mg for 12 days each month), and placebo in preventing progression of carotid intimal medial thickness and the accrual of coronary calcium in women aged 42–58 years who are within 36 months of their final menstrual period. Noninvasive imaging of atherosclerosis using carotid ultrasound studies and coronary artery calcium (CAC) by CT was performed. The carotid ultrasound studies showed similar rates of progression of arterial wall thickness in all three treatment groups. A nonstatistically significant trend toward lower rates of CAC with HT, compared to placebo, was seen.	2012 https://www.menopause.org/annual-meetings/2012-meeting/keeps-report

Additional material for this chapter can be found online at:
www.wiley.com/go/sperling/mountsinai/obstetricsandgynecology

This includes a case study and multiple choice questions.

CHAPTER 28

Urinary Tract Infection

Annacecilia Peacher and Anne Hardart
Division of Female Pelvic Medicine and Reconstructive Surgery; Department of Obstetrics, Gynecology and Reproductive Science, Icahn School of Medicine at Mount Sinai, New York, NY

> **OVERALL BOTTOM LINE**
> - Urinary tract infections (UTIs) are common and increase in incidence with age.
> - They typically arise from fecal flora that ascend into the bladder via the periurethral tissue.
> - Estrogen, low vaginal pH, and acidic urine aid in defense against UTIs.
> - Nitrofurantoin is a first line treatment for uncomplicated UTI, or cystitis, but should be avoided in pyelonephritis.
> - Asymptomatic bacteriuria should be treated in pregnancy but not in the general population.

Background
Definition of disease
- Urinary tract infection includes cystitis (infection of the lower urinary tract/bladder) and pyelonephritis (upper tract infection).
- Acute cystitis or simple UTI: sudden onset of bladder symptoms (pain, dysuria, frequency) with or without hematuria.
- Complicated UTI: signs or symptoms of upper tract infection; underlying urologic abnormalities.
- Recurrent UTI: Two or more UTIs in a 6-month period, or three or more UTIs in 12 months.

Incidence/prevalence
- Approximately 50% of women experience a urinary tract infection during their lifetime, with 5% experiencing frequent infections.
- The prevalence of UTI increases with age: it is approximately 1–2% in young children, 2–4% among 15–24 year-olds, 15% at 60 years old, 25–50% after age 80 (Frick 2014).

Economic impact
- Urinary tract infections account for 500 000 nosocomial infections per year, and 1% of these become life threatening (Frick 2014).
- There were 11 million adult outpatient visits for UTI in 2000 (ACOG 2008).

Etiology
- Most infections are caused by ascending fecal flora that initially colonize the vaginal introitus and periurethral area and ascend into the urethra and bladder.

Mount Sinai Expert Guides: Obstetrics and Gynecology, First Edition. Edited by Rhoda Sperling.
© 2020 John Wiley & Sons Ltd. Published 2020 by John Wiley & Sons Ltd.
Companion Website: www.wiley.com/go/sperling/mountsinai/obstetricsandgynecology

Pathology/pathogenesis
- The most common pathogen is *Escherichia coli*
- The virulence of the bacteria depends on factors such as fimbria type and adhesion factors that aid in ascension up the urinary tract.
- A short urethra makes women more susceptible.
- Estrogen and low vaginal pH are protective; they promote lactobacilli and other gram-positive bacteria that replicate poorly in urine.
- Postmenopausal status promotes UTI with decreased acidic vaginal environment, decrease in protective lactobacilli.

Predictive/risk factors
- Reduced urine flow (neurogenic; obstructive, such as related to pelvic organ prolapse)
- Sexual activity
- Estrogen depletion
- Catheterization
- Urinary incontinence
- Fecal incontinence
- Urinary tract abnormalities
- Diabetes mellitus

Prevention
- Antibiotic prophylaxis in patients with a history of recurrent urinary tract infections.
- Topical estrogen in postmenopausal women with a history of recurrent urinary tract infections.
- Cranberry, including juice and tablet formulations, may have some benefit.
- Other agents, including probiotics, D-mannose are of unproven benefit.

Screening
- Not recommended for asymptomatic individuals, except during pregnancy.
- In symptomatic patients, urine dipstick for nitrites and leukocyte esterase have sensitivity of 75% and specificity of 82% (Frick 2014).

Primary prevention
- Avoid indwelling catheters
- Avoid urethral instrumentation

Secondary prevention
- Antibiotic prophylaxis, including post-coital or daily, for recurrent urinary tract infections
- Topical estrogen for postmenopausal women with recurrent urinary tract infections
- Lack of definitive data on post-coital voiding, probiotics, cranberry supplements, D-mannose, and methenamine hippurate

Diagnosis
- One or more symptoms of UTI, including dysuria, with varying degrees of urinary frequency, urgency, hematuria and suprapubic pain.
- Fever, chills and flank pain suggest pyelonephritis.
- Physical exam may or may not show suprapubic or costovertebral angle tenderness.

- Urinalysis may show nitrites, leukocyte esterase or blood.
- A positive urine culture has been traditionally defined as > 100 000 CFU/mL of bacteria, but thresholds of 10^3–10^4 improve sensitivity.

Differential diagnosis

Differential diagnosis	Features
Vaginitis, including yeast, bacterial vaginosis	Vaginal discharge and/or pruritis
Vaginal atrophy	Vaginal dryness and irritation
Interstitial cystitis/painful bladder syndrome	Chronic symptoms, perhaps triggered by certain foods, sterile urine
Urethritis	Consider sexually transmitted pathogens such as chlamydia, gonorrhea, genital herpes simplex, trichomonas
Lower urinary tract neoplasm	Persistent symptoms or hematuria after treatment

Typical presentation
- Short duration of increasing urinary frequency and urgency, usually with worsening dysuria and often suprapubic pain. Patients may report a feeling of urgency with small volumes voided. Hematuria is a less common symptoms.

Clinical diagnosis
History
- A clinician should inquire about duration of symptoms, presence of a history of recurrent UTIs, current medications, including analgesics, and any recent antibiotic use, as well as any recent instrumentation of their urethra.

Physical examination
- A pelvic exam is not usually required, but may be performed to elicit suprapubic tenderness and to rule out incomplete bladder emptying, urethral diverticulum and to exclude other causes of symptoms, such as vaginitis.
- Costovertebral angles tenderness can be assessed if upper tract infection is suspected.

Disease severity classification
- Uncomplicated UTI: infection in a healthy patient with functionally and anatomically normal lower urinary tract.
- Complicated UTI: infection with factors that may increase colonization or decrease efficacy of treatment such as anatomic or functional abnormality of lower urinary tract, immunocompromised host, or multidrug resistant bacteria.
- Recurrent UTI: two or more infections in a 6-month period or three or more infections in one year.

Laboratory diagnosis
List of diagnostic tests
- An office urine dipstick should be performed when there is high clinical suspicion for infection.
- A laboratory urinalysis will more accurately indicate pyuria, hematuria, and epithelial cells for signs of contamination.
- A urine culture with sensitivities should be performed for complicated or recurrent UTI.

List of imaging techniques
- Not usually required.
- Consider CT without contrast to evaluate for suspected renal calculi or CT urogram as part of workup for persistent hematuria.
- Consider MRI if high suspicion for urethral diverticulum.

Potential pitfalls/common errors made regarding diagnosis of disease
- Overuse of antibiotics, with potential side effects and resulting resistance, if treating presumptively.
- Potential prolonged discomfort, but low risk of upper tract infection, when withholding treatment while awaiting cultures.
- Concurrent lower urinary symptoms (such as overactive bladder or painful bladder syndrome) especially in the presence of asymptomatic bacteriuria.

Treatment
Treatment rationale
- In a shared decision making approach, and depending on severity of symptoms, empiric therapy may be initiated versus analgesics and hydration while awaiting cultures.
- For uncomplicated UTIs: nitrofurantoin (100 mg twice daily for 5–7 days), trimethoprim-sulfamethoxazole (160/180 mg twice daily for 3 days), or Fosfomycin (3 g sachet in a single dose) are first line treatment options, depending on the patient's allergy profile and culture sensitivities.
- For complicated UTIs, such as pyelonephritis, using a local antibiogram may be useful to determine prevalence of antibiotic resistance and optimal antibiotic regimens. Possible regimens include: Ciprofloxacin (twice daily for 5–7 days), trimethoprim-sulfamethoxazole (twice daily for 7–14 days).
- Asymptomatic bacteriuria should be treated when patient is pregnant, in patients with renal transplant, before urologic surgery.

When to hospitalize
- Inability to tolerate oral medication
- Pyelonephritis in patients with comorbidities, signs or urosepsis or urinary tract obstruction

Managing the hospitalized patient
- Positive blood cultures in 20–40% of patients of pyelonephritis
- Options include parenteral fluoroquinolone, aminoglycoside +/- ampicillin, 3rd generation cephalosporin, or carbapenem
- Switch from parenteral to oral antibiotics 48 hours after clinically well
- Treat pyelonephritis for a total of 5–14 days, depending on response and antibiotic

Table of treatment

Medical	Comment
Uncomplicated UTI:	
nitrofurantoin (100 mg twice daily for 5 days)	Common side effects nausea/vomiting
	Long-term exposure can lead to pneumonitis and peripheral neuropathy
trimethoprim-sulfamethoxazole or TMP-SMX (160/180 mg twice daily for 3 days)	TMP-SMX should be used with caution, in some areas resistance exceeds 20%
Fosfomycin (3 g sachet in a single dose)	Low rates of multidrug resistance

(Continued)

(Continued)

Medical	Comment
Pyelonephritis:	
Ciprofloxacin (twice daily for 7 days) or other fluoroquinolone	Fluoroquinolones not recommended as first line for uncomplicated UTI Not used in pregnant women or children High rate of multidrug resistance, and potential for serious side effects including tendinitis and tendon rupture
Consider TMP-SMX (160/180 mg twice daily)	If contraindication to fluoroquinolone and can tolerate oral therapy; 10–14 days
Ceftriaxone 1 g IV daily	Transition to oral fluoroquinolone for 7–14 day course
Consider carbapenem in cases of multidrug resistance (MDR)	Transition to oral fluoroquinolone for 7–14 day course

Prevention/management of complications
- Antibiotic resistance should be kept in mind and sensitivities of urine culture should be used to tailor treatment regimen.
- Consider treating with analgesics and hydration while awaiting culture, depending on severity of symptoms.

Management/treatment algorithm
- See Algorithm 28.1.

> **CLINICAL PEARLS**
> - Uncomplicated UTIs are best treated with 5–7 days of nitrofurantoin.
> - Treat asymptomatic bacteriuria in pregnancy but not in nonpregnant individuals.
> - Use urine culture sensitivities to alter antibiotic regimen when necessary.

Special populations
Pregnancy
- Asymptomatic bacteriuria is treated.
- Fluoroquinolones should not be used in pregnancy.

Children
- Short-term treatment for acute infections. The most common pathogen for uncomplicated UTI in children is *Enterobacteriaceae*; trimethoprim is often used without the sulfonamide.

Elderly
- Diagnosis can be difficult since underlying urinary symptoms (frequency urgency and incontinence) are common. Treatment is the same. Asymptomatic bacteriuria is not an indication for treatment.

Prognosis

> **BOTTOM LINE/CLINICAL PEARLS**
> - When treated with appropriate antibiotics and for the correct duration, UTIs are usually easily treated.
> - Recurrent UTI require more care: consider patient-initiated treatment or prophylaxis (antibiotic or non-antibiotic) in cases of recurrent UTI.

Algorithm 28.1 Algorithm for diagnosis and management of acute dysuria in women

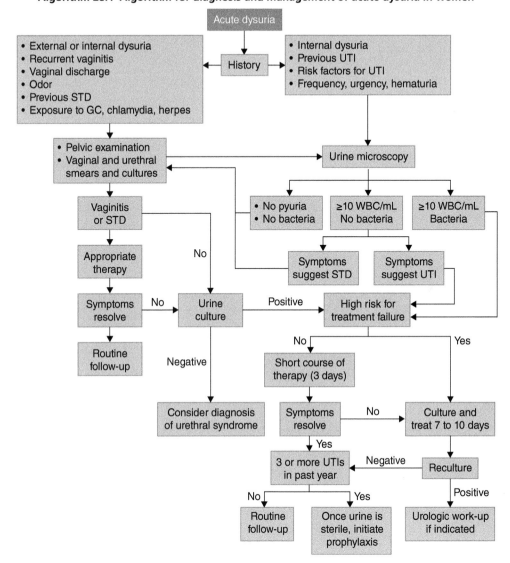

Source: Frick, AC. Chapter 39: Lower urinary tract infection. In: Walters MD, Karram MM, eds. *Urogynecology and reconstructive pelvic surgery*. 4th ed. Philadelphia: Saunders; 2014:583-90.

Natural history of untreated disease
- Contrary to popular belief, most cases of uncomplicated UTI are self-limited, and progression to systemic infection is uncommon (American Urological Association).

Follow-up tests and monitoring
- A test of cure is not indicated if symptoms resolve. Repeat cultures may be considered in pregnancy, pyelonephritis, or recurrent UTIs to guide management.
- If hematuria is present, repeat urinalysis to assure resolution of hematuria.

Reading list

ACOG practice bulletin no. 91: Treatment of urinary tract infection in the nonpregnant women. *Obstet Gynecol* 2008 Mar;111(3):785-94.

American Urological Association. Adult UTI. https://www.auanet.org/education/adult-uti.cfm.

Anger J, Lee UA, Ackerman L, et al. Recurrent uncomplicated urinary tract infections in women: AUA/CUA/SUFU guideline. *J Urol* 2019 Aug;202(2):282-9.

Frick AC. Chapter 39: Lower urinary tract infection. In: Walters MD, Karram MM, eds. *Urogynecology and reconstructive pelvic surgery*. 4th ed. Philadelphia: Saunders; 2014:583-90.

Guidelines
National society guidelines

Title	Source	Date/URL
ACOG Practice Bulletin Number 91: Treatment of Urinary Tract Infection in the Nonpregnant Women.	ACOG	American College of Obstetrics & Gynecology. (2008). ACOG practice bulletin no. 91: Treatment of Urinary Tract Infection in the Nonpregnant Women. *Obstet Gynecol* 111:785-94.
Adult UTI	American Urological Association	2016 https://www.auanet.org/education/adult-uti.cfm
Recurrent Uncomplicated Urinary Tract Infections in Women: AUA/CUA/SUFU Guideline	American Urological Association, Canadian Urological Association, Society of Urodynamics, Female Pelvic Medicine and Urogenital Reconstruction	2019 https://www.auanet.org/guidelines/recurrent-uti

CHAPTER 29

Ectopic Pregnancy

Amanda M. Silbermann[1] and Peter G. McGovern[2]

[1] Department of Obstetrics and Gynecology, New York University School of Medicine, New York, NY
[2] Division of Reproductive Endocrinology and Infertility, Department of Obstetrics, Gynecology and Reproductive Science, Icahn School of Medicine at Mount Sinai, New York, NY

> **OVERALL BOTTOM LINE**
> - Ectopic pregnancy should be suspected in any reproductive-aged woman with abdominal pain and/or vaginal bleeding; however, patients may be asymptomatic.
> - Risk factors for ectopic pregnancy include pelvic inflammatory disease, prior tubal surgery, smoking, and infertility.
> - The diagnosis is made based on clinical presentation, β-hCG (beta-human chorionic gonadotropin), and transvaginal ultrasound findings.
> - Depending on the clinical scenario, treatment can be medical or surgical.
> - Although symptoms may vary, ectopic pregnancies that rupture may lead to a life-threatening situation and should be monitored closely.

Background

Definition of disease

- An ectopic pregnancy is an extrauterine pregnancy, most often found in the fallopian tubes; however, it can be found in the uterine cornua, cervix, ovary, abdomen, or prior hysterotomy site.

Disease classification

- Whereas some ectopic pregnancies may be considered clinically stable, if an ectopic pregnancy ruptures, it can result in a life-threatening hemorrhage and become a surgical emergency.

Incidence/prevalence

- The incidence of ectopic pregnancy is estimated to be 20 in 1000 pregnancies.
- Over half of the ectopic pregnancies in the United States occur in women aged 25 to 34, with only 11% of ectopics occurring in women aged 35 to 44.

Etiology

- Pelvic inflammatory disease (PID), most often caused by previous *Chlamydia trachomatis* infection, is the major factor contributing to the risk of ectopic pregnancy.
- Other factors that can alter tubal motility include prior tubal surgery such as sterilization, or a hormonal imbalance, where elevated estrogen or progesterone levels can alter tubal contractility.
- In 40% of cases, the cause is unknown.

Mount Sinai Expert Guides: Obstetrics and Gynecology, First Edition. Edited by Rhoda Sperling.
© 2020 John Wiley & Sons Ltd. Published 2020 by John Wiley & Sons Ltd.
Companion Website: www.wiley.com/go/sperling/mountsinai/obstetricsandgynecology

Pathology/pathogenesis

- In patients with salpingitis, the inflammation of the endosalpinx causes damage to the cilia that normally propel the embryo through the fallopian tube into the uterus. This damage may be segmental or universal, transient or irreversible. Delayed or interrupted transport of the embryo can lead to implantation within the fallopian tube.

Predictive/risk factors

Risk factor	Odds ratio
Salpingitis	2
1–9 cigarettes per day	2
10–19 cigarettes per day	3
≥ 20 cigarettes per day	4
History of tubal surgery	3.5
History of intrauterine device (IUD)	1.5
Previous infertility	2.5
Prior ectopic pregnancy	5 (one prior) –10 (two or more prior)

Prevention

> **BOTTOM LINE/CLINICAL PEARLS**
> - No interventions have been demonstrated to prevent ectopic pregnancy.

Screening

- There is no screening performed for ectopic pregnancies.

Primary prevention

- Reliable contraception decreases the risk of all pregnancies, including ectopic pregnancy.

Secondary prevention

- Bilateral salpingectomy

Diagnosis

> **BOTTOM LINE/CLINICAL PEARLS**
> - The patient's history often includes irregular vaginal bleeding associated with abdominal pain and absence of menses.
> - Exam findings that support diagnosis of ectopic pregnancy include abdominal tenderness, vaginal spotting, and adnexal tenderness on bimanual pelvic exam. In the event of a ruptured ectopic, exam findings may include hypotension and tachycardia secondary to acute blood loss, with possible acute abdomen due to hemoperitoneum.
> - In order to confirm the diagnosis of ectopic pregnancy, the combination of β-hCG and transvaginal ultrasound is used.

Differential diagnosis
See Algorithm 29.1.

Algorithm 29.1 Algorithm for diagnosis and management of ectopic pregnancy in women
- In patients with β-hCG less than 1500, an appropriate rise in hCG in 48 hours is at least 49%. If the hCG is within the discriminatory zone, an appropriate rise is at least 40%. If the hCG is > 3000, an appropriate rise is at least 33% in 48 hours.

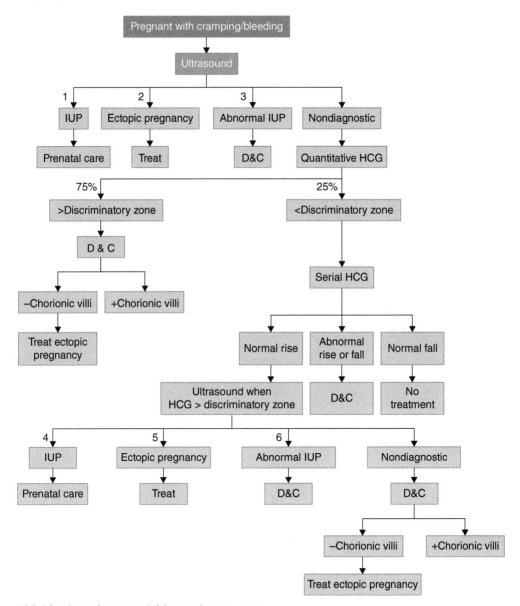

D&C, Dilatation and curettage; IUP, intrauterine pregnancy.

Source: Gracia C, Barnhart KT. Diagnosing ectopic pregnancy. *Obstet Gynecol* 2001;97:465. Reproduced with permission of Elsevier.

Legend: "Discriminatory zone" = 1500–3000 mIU/mL depending upon the center.

"Normal rise" in β-hCG is at least 50% rise every 48 hours (when initial level is ≤ 1500 mIU/mL).

Differential diagnosis	Features
Ruptured corpus luteum	Hemoperitoneum or free fluid on ultrasound. +/− intrauterine pregnancy. Appropriately rising β-hCG, or negative urine pregnancy test.
Threatened abortion	Visible intrauterine gestation on ultrasound with irregular vaginal bleeding.
Incomplete abortion	Previously documented intrauterine gestation on ultrasound, with irregular vaginal bleeding.
Ovarian torsion	Urine pregnancy test likely negative. Adnexal mass seen with absent or intermittent blood flow to adnexa on Doppler.
Endometriosis	Urine pregnancy test negative. History of chronic cyclic pain.
Salpingitis	Vaginal discharge, cervical motion tenderness, +/− fever and leukocytosis.

Typical presentation

- Typically, an ectopic pregnancy will present with abdominal pain, absence of menses, and irregular vaginal bleeding. The pain may present as sharp and focal or dull and generalized. On evaluation, the patient will have a positive urine pregnancy test, and physical exam may elicit abdominal tenderness with or without rebound or guarding and often will have blood in vaginal vault. In the setting of a ruptured ectopic pregnancy, the patient may present hemodynamically unstable, with tachycardia, hypotension, and peritonitis with severe pain from hemoperitoneum.

Clinical diagnosis

History

- The clinician should ask about last menstrual period and menstrual history, history of pelvic infections, contraception, and onset and severity of symptoms.

Physical examination

- Vital signs should be obtained immediately to evaluate for hemodynamic instability in the case of a ruptured ectopic pregnancy.
- A thorough abdominal exam should be performed evaluating for rebound tenderness and guarding, as well as signs of peritonitis.
- A bimanual pelvic exam should palpate for adnexal masses with attention to eliciting adnexal tenderness.
- On speculum exam, the presence of vaginal bleeding should be noted.

Disease severity classification

- Ectopic pregnancies account for 6% of all maternal deaths, and are the most common cause of maternal death in the first trimester (12 weeks) of pregnancy.

Laboratory diagnosis

List of diagnostic tests

- The measurement of serial serum β-hCG, combined with transvaginal ultrasound, is the key to evaluating for ectopic pregnancy. When working up a patient for pregnancy of unknown location, trending HCG levels can help determine if a pregnancy is a normal intrauterine pregnancy or an abnormal pregnancy. Complete blood count (CBC) to evaluate blood loss.
- Serum progesterone in early gestation can help differentiate a normal intrauterine pregnancy from an abnormal pregnancy.
- Type and screen should be ordered to assess Rh status and the need for anti-D immune globulin administration for women who are Rh negative.
- Renal and liver function tests to assess for contraindications to methotrexate.

List of imaging techniques
- Transvaginal ultrasound should be performed on all patients presenting with symptoms of ectopic pregnancy. If findings diagnostic of an intrauterine pregnancy (IUP) are seen, an ectopic can be ruled out. If evidence of a pregnancy is seen in an ectopic site such as the adnexa or cervix, the diagnosis of ectopic is made. If no definitive IUP or ectopic pregnancy are seen, the findings must be correlated with serial β-hCG.
- The "discriminatory zone" refers to the β-hCG level at which an IUP is reliably seen using transvaginal sonography. Abdominal sonography is significantly less sensitive, and is therefore NOT recommended. Various centers use levels ranging from 1500–3000 mIU/mL. Use of a lower value leads to fewer missed ectopic pregnancies but more IUPs falsely diagnosed as ectopics, whereas use of a greater value has opposite effects. Authorities agree that β-hCG levels are best used as a proxy for gestational age when it is uncertain. When known with certainty, viable IUPs are always seen by 5 weeks and 5 days of gestation. Of note, multiple gestations will have β-hCG values in the "discriminatory zone" at earlier gestational ages when it is too early to visualize the normal multiple IUPs. For this reason, gestational age is better used for women who have undergone fertility treatments.

Potential pitfalls/common errors made regarding diagnosis of disease
- Common errors include a rush to treatment for suspected ectopic pregnancy based upon a single β-hCG level and sonogram in the stable patient. Most authorities agree there is no reason to treat with methotrexate on the first visit. The unstable patient requires immediate definitive surgical management, and the stable patient should be treated more conservatively to avoid misdiagnosis. Patience will often result in a more clear diagnosis, which is of course vital to avoid incorrectly interrupting a desired pregnancy.
- A large percentage (up to 50%) of pregnancies of unknown location will in fact be failed IUPs. Many authorities suggest dilation and curettage or other tissue diagnosis (to establish definitively whether the pregnancy was located in the uterus) prior to methotrexate treatment. This approach avoids inadvertent unnecessary treatment of IUPs with medical management for suspected ectopic pregnancy.
- Inadvertent treatment of IUP with methotrexate can result in miscarriage or severe fetal abnormalities, and is responsible for over $20 million in awards to date.

Treatment
Treatment rationale
- Treatment of an unruptured ectopic pregnancy can be medical or surgical, depending on multiple factors such as desired future fertility, size of the ectopic pregnancy, and location.
- If an ectopic pregnancy ruptures, it requires immediate surgical management.
- Surgical management may include salpingectomy or salpingostomy if the pregnancy is within the fallopian tube.
- Medical management with methotrexate can be considered if patient is stable and compliant with follow-up.
  - Methotrexate is most successful in unruptured, hemodynamically stable patients with a β-hCG of <5000, a gestational sac measuring <4 cm, and no fetal cardiac activity seen on ultrasound.

Table of treatment
- Medical management with methotrexate, a folic acid antagonist, is an option for approximately one-third of all patients with ectopic pregnancies. Single and multidose regimens can be used.
  - The standard single-dose treatment is 50 mg/m^2 with an additional dose given on day 7 from administration if an appropriate decline in β-hCG is not seen.
  - The multidose regimen is given with a leucovorin rescue as follows: methotrexate (1 mg/kg per day) on Days 1, 3, 5, and 7, and oral leucovorin (0.1 mg/kg) on Days 2, 4, 6, and 8.

- Surgical management options include salpingectomy and salpingostomy for tubal ectopic pregnancies. For interstitial pregnancies, cornuostomy vs cornual resection can be performed.

Treatment	Comments
Conservative	Expectant management can be considered only in an ectopic with low, down-trending levels of β-hCG
Medical Methotrexate 50 mg/m² (single dose) or 1 mg/kg per day on days 1, 3, 5, and 7 (multidose) See Algorithm 29.2 for methotrexate protocol.)	Clinical pearls • Patients should be counseled on side effects, most commonly GI upset. • Abdominal pain may worsen with methotrexate, as ectopic aborts through fallopian tube. • For single-dose MTX, β-hCG should be monitored on day 4 and 7, and a 15% drop in the value (D4-D7) indicates treatment is working
Surgical • Salpingostomy • Salpingectomy	Salpingostomy is preferred for smaller unruptured ectopics in women desiring future fertility; salpingectomy is preferred for larger, actively bleeding ectopics or in women NOT desiring future fertility.

Algorithm 29.2 Two-dose methotrexate protocol

Day 1	First dose IM injection of MTX 50/m², draw serum β-hCG.
Day 4	Second dose IM injection of MTX 50/m².
Day 7	Draw serum hCG. If > 15% decrease from Day 1, follow β-hCG levels weekly. If < 15% decrease, administer third dose MTX 50/m².
Day 11	Draw serum hCG. If > 15% decrease from Day 1, follow β-hCG levels weekly. If < 15% decrease, administer fourth dose MTX 50/m².
Day 14	Draw serum hCG. If > 15% decrease from Day 1, follow β-hCG levels weekly. If < 15% decrease, advise surgical management.

β-hCG, quantitative beta subunit of human chorionic gonadotropin; MTX, methotrexate; IM, intramuscular

Adapted from: Alur-Gupta S, Cooney LG, Senapati S, et al. Two-dose versus single-dose methotrexate for treatment of ectopic pregnancy: a meta-analysis. *Am J Obstet Gynecol* 2019 Jan 7; pii: S0002-9378(19)30004-3. doi: 10.1016/j.ajog.2019.01.002. [Epub ahead of print]

Prevention/management of complications

- Methotrexate (single and multiple dose) has been reported to cause stomatitis, gastroenteritis, leukopenia, thrombocytopenia, pneumonitis and alopecia. Typically, a CMP and CBC with a platelet count are checked prior to therapy to avoid administration in a patient with liver or renal disease.

CLINICAL PEARLS
- Heterotopic pregnancies (coexistence of both IUP and ectopic pregnancies) occur rarely (1/4–10 000), but relatively commonly after IVF (1/100).
- Although the overall chances of pregnancy are greatly reduced by tubal ligation or use of an IUD, when women using these contraceptive methods become pregnant up to 50% of these pregnancies are ectopic.

Special populations
- For women developing an ectopic pregnancy after failed tubal sterilization, complete bilateral salpingectomy may be indicated.

Prognosis

> **BOTTOM LINE/CLINICAL PEARLS**
> - With careful follow-up care, both medical and surgical management can lead to excellent outcomes.
> - After having an ectopic pregnancy, a woman must always be vigilant in future pregnancies, as prior ectopic pregnancy is the major risk factor.
> - Other groups requiring a higher index of suspicion included contraceptive failures (tubal ligation or IUD) and infertile women (whether they conceived with or without IVF).

Follow-up tests and monitoring
- Persistent trophoblast tissue (persistent ectopic) may result from incomplete removal or from extrusion of pregnancy tissue out the end of the tube prior to surgery with implantation at another ectopic site (e.g. omentum). This occurs in approximately 1% of salpingectomy cases and 10% (5–20%) of salpingostomy cases. Serial β-hCG levels (usually weekly) until negative are recommended after surgical therapy.

Reading list

Alur-Gupta S, Cooney LG, Senapati S, et al. Two-dose versus single-dose methotrexate for treatment of ectopic pregnancy: a meta-analysis. *Am J Obstet Gynecol* 2019 Jan 7;pii: S0002-9378(19)30004-3. doi: 10.1016/j.ajog.2019.01.002. [Epub ahead of print]

Barnhart KT. Ectopic pregnancy. *N Engl J Med* 2009;361:379-87.

Barnhart KT. Early pregnancy failure: beware of the pitfalls of modern management. *Fertil Steril* 2012;98:1061-5.

Barnhart KT. Differences in serum human chorionic gonadotropin rise in early pregnancy by race and value at presentation. *Obstet Gynecol* 2016 Sep;128(3):504-11.

Centers for Disease Control and Prevention. Ectopic pregnancy – United States, 1990-1992. *MMWR Morb Mortal Wkly Rep* 1995;44(3):46.

Chung K, Chandavarkar U, Opper N, et al. Reevaluating the role of dilatation and curettage in the diagnosis of pregnancy of unknown location. *Fertil Steril* 2011;96:659-62.

Gracia CR, Brown, HA, Barnhart KT. Prophylactic methotrexate after linear salpingostomy: a decision analysis. *Fertil Steril* 2001;76:1191-5.

Practice Committee of the American College of Obstetricians and Gynecologists. ACOG Practice bulletin no. 193: Tubal ectopic pregnancy. *Obstet Gynecol* 2018 Mar;131(3):e91-e103.

Practice Committee of the American Society for Reproductive Medicine. Medical treatment of ectopic pregnancy: a committee opinion. *Fertil Steril* 2013;100:638-44.

Suggested websites

American Pregnancy Association. http://americanpregnancy.org/pregnancy-complications/ectopic-pregnancy/

WebMD. http://www.webmd.com/baby/guide/pregnancy-ectopic-pregnancy#1

MedicineNet. http://www.medicinenet.com/ectopic_pregnancy/article.htm

Guidelines
National society guidelines

Title	Source	Date/full reference
Medical treatment of ectopic pregnancy	Practice Committee, ASRM	2013 *Fertil Steril* 2013 Sep;100(3):638-44.
Tubal ectopic pregnancy: ACOG practice bulletin no. 193	Practice Committee of the American College of Obstetricians and Gynecologists	*Obstet Gynecol* 2018 Mar;131(3):e91-103.

Evidence

Type of evidence	Title and comment	Date/full reference
Meta-analysis	Two-dose versus single-dose methotrexate for treatment of ectopic pregnancy: a meta-analysis. Comment: This analysis includes 7 RCTs including 1173 subjects randomized to 2 vs 1 injection protocols; two-dose protocol proved superior.	*Am J Obstet Gynecol* 2019 Jan 7; pii: S0002-9378(19)30004-3. doi: 10.1016/ j.ajog.2019.01.002. [Epub ahead of print]

Additional material for this chapter can be found online at:
www.wiley.com/go/sperling/mountsinai/obstetricsandgynecology

This includes a case study, multiple choice questions, advice for patients, and ICD codes.

CHAPTER 30

Osteoporosis

Holly C. Loudon
Department of Obstetrics, Gynecology and Reproductive Science, Icahn School of Medicine at Mount Sinai, New York, NY

OVERALL BOTTOM LINE
- Osteoporosis-related fractures are a significant cause of morbidity and mortality.
- Women have a 5-fold greater prevalence of osteoporosis compared to men and sustain 80% of all hip fractures.
- Genetics is the main determinant of peak bone mass and bone quality.
- The most rapid bone loss in women occurs during menopause due to the marked decline in estrogen levels.
- Bone health, including calcium and vitamin D intake and exercise, should be addressed in all age groups.
- Formal screening for osteoporosis in women should begin at age 65, unless additional risk factors exist.

Background

Definition of disease

- Osteoporosis is a disease that includes loss of bone mass, degradation of bone microarchitecture, decreased bone quality, and a resulting increased risk of bone fracture.
- DXA (DEXA, dual energy X-ray absorptiometry) is the best technique available to routinely assess bone mineral density in postmenopausal women. The DXA reports both T scores and Z scores.
- Osteoporosis is defined as a T score of less than or equal to -2.5, and low bone mass is defined as a T score of less than -1 to greater than -2.5.
- The T score is produced by comparing the patient's bone mineral density to the mean bone mineral density of a young healthy cohort that is the same sex as the patient.
- The Z score compares the patient's bone mineral density to the mean for their age and sex.

Incidence/prevalence

- Worldwide, osteoporosis causes more than 8.9 million fractures annually and affects 200 million women.
- The risk of osteoporosis increases with age and affects one-fifth of women aged 70, two-fifths of women aged 80, and two-thirds of women aged 90.

Economic impact

- In 2005 the cost for the direct care of the estimated 2 million osteoporosis-related fractures in the United States was projected to be $17 billion. Hip fractures comprised approximately 72% of that cost.

Etiology

- 90% of bone mass is acquired during childhood and adolescence. This peak bone mass is believed to contribute to risk for osteoporosis later in life.

Mount Sinai Expert Guides: Obstetrics and Gynecology, First Edition. Edited by Rhoda Sperling.
Companion Website: www.wiley.com/go/sperling/mountsinai/obstetricsandgynecology

- Menopause and the associated marked decline in estrogen cause a period of rapid bone loss in women, beginning about 1 year before menopause and continuing for about 3 years. The end result is a loss of 6–7% of bone.
- Other causes of hypoestrogenism are also associated with loss of bone mineral density and include anorexia nervosa, lactation, hypogonadism, and medications such as depot-medroxyprogresterone acetate (DMPA), gonadotropin-releasing hormone antagonists, and aromatase inhibitors.

Pathology/pathogenesis

- Peak bone mass is primarily determined by heritable factors but can also be influenced by lifestyle, health, and environmental factors.
- Final peak bone mass occurs by 19–20 years of age.
- Beginning at approximately age 30, there is a net loss of bone mineral density.
- Remodeling and repair of bone occurs through resorption, which is controlled by osteoclasts, and bone formation, which is controlled by osteoblasts.
- During times of relative hypoestrogenism, bone physiology is dominated by bone resorption and osteo-clast activity, with a resultant loss in bone mineral density.
- Throughout life, weight bearing exercise, resistance exercise, and aerobic exercise have been shown to be beneficial for spine bone mineral density. Walking has been shown to be beneficial for hip bone mineral density.
- Vitamin D and calcium are important for bone health. Vitamin D deficiency results in poorly mineralized bone that is more prone to fracture, and prolonged calcium deficiency results in osteoporosis.

Predictive/risk factors

- Postmenopausal women younger than 65 should be screened for osteoporosis if they have an elevated FRAX score (http://www.sheffield.ac.uk/FRAX/). Alternatively, screening should be considered for postmenopausal women younger than 65 with any of the following risk factors:

Medical history of fragility fracture
Body weight < 127 pounds
Parent with hip fracture
Smoker (current)
Alcohol consumption ≥ 3 drinks/day
Rheumatoid arthritis
Other medical causes of bone loss (medications or diseases)

Prevention

> **BOTTOM LINE/CLINICAL PEARLS**
> - Weight-bearing exercise and adequate calcium and vitamin D intake help prevent osteoporosis.
> - Reducing the risk of falls through lifestyle and environmental modification can help prevent osteoporosis-related fractures.

Screening

- **Dual-energy X-ray absorptiometry (DXA)** of the lumbar spine and hip is the recommended method of diagnosing osteoporosis. When this method is used, the World Health Organization's (WHO) diagnostic criteria using T score can be applied.

- **Peripheral DXA** can be used at the heel, finger, or wrist to determine fracture risk, but the WHO classification does not apply and this method cannot be used to monitor treatment.
- **Quantitative ultrasound densitometry** of the heel, patella, or tibia provides a quantitative measurement of bone, but the WHO classification does not apply and this method cannot be used to monitor treatment.
- **Quantitative computed tomography** can measure bone mineral density; however, this method is not typically used because it results in a much greater radiation exposure than other screening methods.

Primary prevention
- Weight-bearing exercise
- Adequate vitamin D intake. The Institute of Medicine (IOM) recommends 600 international units daily for females ages 9–70, and 800 international units daily for women 71 and older.
- Adequate calcium intake. The IOM recommends a daily allowance of 1000 mg for women ages 19–50, and 1200 mg for women ages 51 and older.
- There is a possible association between calcium supplementation and coronary artery calcification/coronary artery events. Therefore, dietary sources of calcium are currently considered to be safer than supplements.

Secondary prevention
- Prevention of falls through environmental modification can reduce the risk of fractures. Fall prevention should include the use of adequate lighting; removal of loose rugs, cords, and clutter; avoidance of the need to use a stepstool to reach stored items; safety grab bars and nonskid strips in the bathtub/shower; handrails and nonskid treads on stairs.

Diagnosis
- A clinical diagnosis of osteoporosis can be made when there is a low-trauma fracture in an at-risk woman. Imaging in this setting is not necessary. Low-trauma fractures can be diagnosed when a fracture occurs in a situation that would not typically cause a fracture (e.g. a short fall from a standing position).
- A T score of less than or equal to −2.5 at the femoral neck *or* hip *or* lumbar spine establishes the diagnosis of osteoporosis.
- A T score of less than −1 but greater than −2.5 at the femoral neck *or* hip *or* lumbar spine establishes the diagnosis of low bone mass (formerly called osteopenia).
- See Algorithm 30.1.

Typical presentation
- Patients are most commonly diagnosed on routine screening with DXA; however, some patients are diagnosed at the time of a fragility fracture that is not otherwise explained.

Clinical diagnosis
History
- The most important determinant of osteoporosis in postmenopausal women is age. Therefore, all women 65 years and older should be screened for osteoporosis.
- In women younger than 65, additional risk factors should be identified and used to guide earlier screening with DXA. Common risk factors include:
  - Smoking
  - Alcohol consumption of 3 or more drinks/day
  - Inadequate physical activity
  - Obesity
  - Prior fracture as an adult

Algorithm 30.1 Diagnostic and management algorithm for osteoporosis in women

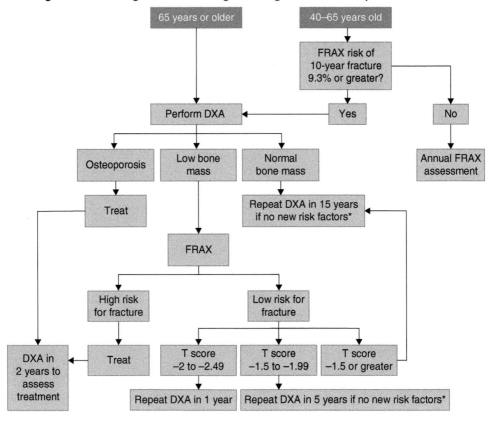

*assess annually for new risk factors using FRAX

- Hypogonadal states
- Diseases or medications associated with osteoporosis (see below)
- In women younger than 65, the fracture risk assessment tool (FRAX) can also be used to determine which women should undergo earlier screening with DXA. In women FRAX is validated for use starting at age 40; it can be used only in people who are not taking medications to treat osteoporosis. When the FRAX tool shows a 10-year risk of major osteoporotic fracture of 9.3%, women should be screened with DXA. This cutoff is used because it is the risk of fracture in a 65-year-old Caucasian woman with no risk factors.

The fracture risk assessment tool (FRAX)

- http://www.sheffield.ac.uk/FRAX/
- The FRAX tool was developed in collaboration with the World Health Organization and can be used to predict the risk of osteoporotic fracture in the next 10 years. The two main uses for FRAX are to determine which patients with low bone mass should receive treatment and which patients under age 65 with additional risk factors should be screened for osteoporosis.
- When to treat a patient with low bone mass: when the 10-year risk of hip fracture is 3% or greater, or 10-year risk of major osteoporotic fracture is 20% or greater.
- When to screen women < 65 years of age for osteoporosis: when the risk of a major osteoporotic fracture in the next 10 years is 9.3% or greater.

- Risk factors used in FRAX calculation:
  - Age
  - Sex
  - Body mass index
  - Previous fragility fracture
  - Hip fracture in a parent
  - Smoking (current)
  - Corticosteroid use (5 mg or more of prednisolone daily x 3 months)
  - Alcohol use (3 or more drinks daily)
  - Rheumatoid arthritis
  - Other secondary causes of osteoporosis

Laboratory diagnosis
- There are no recommended laboratory tests for osteoporosis.
- The Institute of Medicine recommends a serum vitamin D level of 20 ng/mL. However, routine screening for vitamin D levels is not recommended. Patients should be advised on recommended daily allowance of vitamin D.
- Bone turnover markers are not recommended because they cannot be used to diagnose osteoporosis. These markers are byproducts of bone resorption and include deoxypyridinoline, N-telopeptides, and C-telopeptides.

List of imaging techniques
- Dual X-ray absorptiometry is the recommended method of diagnosing osteoporosis.
- Peripheral DXA is a useful diagnostic method because it is affordable and therefore can be implemented in a primary care or ob/gyn office setting. This method cannot be used to monitor treatment once osteoporosis is diagnosed.
- Quantitative ultrasound densitometry is an uncommonly used method that has the same limitations as peripheral DXA.

Potential pitfalls/common errors made regarding diagnosis of disease
- Before starting treatment, consideration should be given for **secondary causes of osteoporosis**, which may require treatment. In particular, fracture in a young postmenopausal woman or a low T score (i.e. bone mineral density lower than expected for a given age) should raise suspicion of a secondary cause.
- **Diseases that can cause or contribute to osteoporosis and fractures include** rheumatic and autoimmune diseases; endocrine, hematologic, and gastrointestinal disorders; hypogonadal states.
- **Lifestyle factors that can cause or contribute to osteoporosis and fractures include** calcium and vitamin D deficiencies; excess vitamin A or excess aluminum (antacids); high caffeine, salt, or alcohol intake; smoking; physical inactivity or immobilization; thinness; falling.
- **Medications that can cause or contribute to osteoporosis and fractures include** heparin, anticonvulsants, aromatase inhibitors, barbiturates, chemotherapeutic agents, cyclosporine A, tacrolimus, depot-medroxyprogesterone acetate, glucocorticoids, gonadotropin-releasing hormone agonists, lithium.

Treatment
Treatment rationale
- Bisphosphonates are considered first-line therapy and reduce vertebral fractures by 35–65%. Because there is a risk of atypical fractures and osteonecrosis of the jaw, it is not known whether there should be a maximum duration of therapy. Currently, there is a trend to interrupt use after 5–10 years.
- Selective estrogen-receptor modulators (SERMs) are recommended for patients with contraindications to bisphosphonates and have been shown to reduce vertebral fractures. SERMs may be a good choice

for younger postmenopausal women because they reduce the risk of invasive breast cancer in post-menopausal women who are at both average and high risk for breast cancer. SERMs increase the risk of venous thromboembolism and death from stroke but do not increase the risk of stroke. Raloxifene is the most commonly used drug in this class. Using raloxifene in early menopause, then switching to a bis-phosphonate after 5–10 years provides the benefit of a reduction in breast cancer in an age group that has a relatively lower risk of thromboembolic events, while also limiting exposure to bisphosphonates. Although the SERM tamoxifen has shown to improve bone density, it is not approved for osteoporosis treatment.

- Denosumab is a human monoclonal antibody that binds to and inhibits the receptor activator of nuclear factor kB (RANK) ligand, which promotes proliferation and differentiation of osteoclasts. This drug is administered subcutaneously every 6 months. It is approved for postmenopausal women with osteo-porosis who are at high risk for fractures. Denosumab reduces vertebral fractures by 68% and hip fractures by 40%.
- Hormone therapy: both estrogen and combined estrogen/progesterone therapy reduce hip and vertebral fractures by 33–36% and are approved for the prevention of osteoporosis. Approval as a treatment for osteoporosis was not obtained because the study design of the Women's Health Initiative did not meet Food and Drug Administration (FDA) requirements for treatment approval. Currently, the only FDA approved primary use for hormone therapy is the treatment of hot flashes related to menopause. Therefore, women who are already on hormone therapy for hot flashes can be considered to have acceptable treatment or preventive therapy for osteoporosis.
- Salmon calcitonin (nasal spray or subcutaneous injection) is less effective for fracture reduction and is not effective in early menopause. It should be used only for women with less severe disease who cannot tolerate other treatments.
- Recombinant human parathyroid hormone (teriparatide) is given as a daily subcutaneous injection and is reserved for women with severe osteoporosis or prior fractures. Use is restricted to 2 years because of the increased risk of osteosarcoma in laboratory rats undergoing high-dose treatment.

Table of treatment

Medications	Contraindications
Bisphosphonates: • Alendronate (Fosamax) • Risedronate (Actonel) • Risedronate (Atelvia) • Ibandronate (Boniva) • Zoledronic acid (Reclast)	• Inability to stand/sit upright for 30 minutes (except zoledronic acid) • Abnormalities of esophagus • Hypocalcemia • Hypersensitivity to the drug • Avoid oral alendronate if risk of aspiration is elevated • For zoledronic acid only: creatinine clearance < 35 mL/min or acute renal impairment
Selective estrogen receptor modulators: • Raloxifene (Evista)	• Venous thromboembolism • Women who may become pregnant or who are breastfeeding
Calcitonin—salmon: • Fortical • Miacalcin	• Allergy to salmon calcitonin or synthetic salmon calcitonin
Parathyroid hormone: • Teriparatide (recombinant human PTH 1-34, Forteo)	• Hypersensitivity to the drug • Anaphylaxis and angioedema have occurred • Restricted to 2 years of use because of the risk of osteosarcoma

(*Continued*)

Medications	Contraindications
RANK ligand inhibitor: • Denosumab (Prolia)	• Hypocalcemia
Hormone therapy (approved for prevention only): • Conjugated estrogen tablets (Premarin) • Estropipate tablets (Ogen) • 17β-estradiol patch (Alora, Climara, Menostar, Vivelle, Vivelle-Dot, Estradot, Estraderm) • 17β-estradiol cream (Estrace) • Conjugated estrogen + medroxyprogesterone acetate tablets (Premphase, Prempro) • Ethinyl estradiol + norethindrone acetate tablets (femhrt) • 17β-estradiol + norethindrone acetate tablets (Activella) • 17β-estradiol + norgestimate tablets (Prefest) • 17β-estradiol + levonorgestrel patch (Climara Pro)	• Undiagnosed vaginal bleeding • Breast cancer (known or suspected) • Estrogen-dependent malignancy (known or suspected) • Venous thromboembolism, active or past • Arterial thromboembolic disease (e.g. stroke, myocardial infarction) within the last 1 year • Liver dysfunction • Thrombophilic disorders (e.g. protein C, protein S, antithrombin deficiency) • Hypersensitivity to the drug • Pregnancy, known or suspected

Prevention/management of complications

• Bisphosphonates have been associated with osteonecrosis of the jaw and atypical fractures of the femoral shaft. The cases have been rare and the actual risk is difficult to quantify. Osteonecrosis is most commonly seen at the time of dental extraction in those being treated with high doses of IV bisphosphonates as part of supportive cancer therapy. In such patients consideration can be given to stopping the bisphosphonate at the time of dental procedures although there is no requirement to do so.

• Bisphosphonates can cause esophageal irritation and ulceration.

• Zolendronate, a bisphosphonate administered by infusion every 1–2 years, has been associated with renal failure in patients with compromised renal function. Renal function should be assessed prior to initiating this treatment.

• Denosumab is associated with a higher rate of infections requiring hospitalization, so its use should be reserved for women who are at high risk of fracture and have failed other treatments.

• Because of raloxifene's association with venous thrombosis, it should not be used in women with a history of venous thromboembolism. Because it is associated with an increased risk of death from stroke, its risks and benefits should be weighed carefully in setting of a stroke history. Raloxifene causes vasomotor symptoms, particularly in women who are earlier in menopause, and this side effect may limit its acceptability.

CLINICAL PEARLS
• Bone density screening in women, ideally with DXA, should begin at age 65.
• The FRAX tool can identify postmenopausal women who should be screened prior to age 65.
• The FRAX tool can be used to guide treatment in women with low bone mass.
• Treatment is recommended for women with a T score of −2.5 or less, a low trauma fracture, or a T score from −1 to −2.5 who also have a FRAX score greater than or equal to 3% for risk of a hip fracture, or 20% for risk of a major osteoporotic fracture in the next 10 years.
• The FRAX tool should be used annually to assess all women 65 and over for new risk factors. This includes women who are already being treated for osteoporosis or low bone mass.

Special populations
Others
- Cautions related to comorbidities and medication selection are described in the Table of Treatment and in Prevention/Management of Complications.

Prognosis

> **CLINICAL PEARLS**
> - In women > 80 years old who have had a hip fracture, only 56% could walk independently after 1 year.
> - 3–6% of women die of complications during hospitalization for hip fracture. These outcomes worsen with age and comorbidities.

Prognosis for treated patients
- After initiation of treatment, a DXA should be repeated in 2 years to assess the effect of treatment.
  - If the bone mineral density is the same or improved, this is considered a treatment success, and another DXA is not necessary unless new risk factors are identified.
  - If the bone mineral density has worsened, then treatment compliance should be assessed and secondary causes of bone loss should be considered. The DXA report should specify whether the patient's bone loss is considered to be real, that is, the bone loss is greater than the margin of error for that office's DXA machine.

Follow-up tests and monitoring
- After initiation of treatment, a DXA should be repeated in 2 years as described in Prognosis for Treated Patients.
- In women who have normal bone mass (normal T score) a DXA should be repeated in 15 years, unless new risk factors are identified.
- In a woman with low bone mass and a FRAX result indicating a low risk of fracture:
  - If the T score is −1.5 or greater, DXA should be repeated in 15 years.
  - If the T score is between −1.5 and −1.99, DXA should be repeated in 5 years.
  - If the T score is between −2.0 and −2.49 a DXA should be repeated in 1 year.
  - The FRAX tool should be used annually and DXA intervals should be modified, if new risk factors result in an increased fracture risk.
- In a woman with low bone mass and a FRAX result indicating a high risk of fracture, treatment should be recommended.

Reading list
American College of Obstetricians and Gynecologists. Osteoporosis: practice bulletin no. 129. *Obstet Gynecol* 2012;120:718-34. Reaffirmed 2016.

Boonen S, Autier P, Barette M, et al. Functional outcome and quality of life following hip fracture in elderly women; a prospective controlled study. *Osteoporos Int* 2004;15:87-94.

Cooper C, Atkinson EJ, Jacobsen SJ, et al. Population-based study of survival after osteoporotic fractures. *Am J Epidemiol* 1993;137:1001-5.

Kanis JA, Hans D, Cooper C et al., Interpretation and use of FRAX in clinical practice. Task Force of the FRAX Initiative. *Osteoporosis Int* 2011;22:2395-411.

National Osteoporosis Foundation. *Clinician's guide to prevention and treatment of osteoporosis*. Washington, DC: NOF; 2010.

Suggested websites
International Osteoporosis Foundation. https://www.iofbonehealth.org/facts-statistics
Fracture Risk Assessment Tool. http://www.sheffield.ac.uk/FRAX

Guidelines
National society guidelines

Title	Source	Date/full reference or URL
Clinician's guide to prevention and treatment of osteoporosis	National Osteoporosis Foundation	2014 The National Osteoporosis Foundation (NOF) clinician's guide to prevention and treatment of osteoporosis 2014. *Osteoporos Int* 2014;25(10):2359–81. doi: 10.1007/s00198-014-2794-2 http://link.springer.com/article/10.1007%2Fs00198-014-2794-2
Clinical practice guidelines for the diagnosis and treatment of postmenopausal osteoporosis	American Association of Clinical Endocrinologists and American College of Endocrinology	2016 https://www.aace.com/disease-state-resources/reproductive-and-gonad/clinical-practice-guidelines/aace-clinical-practice
Osteoporosis to prevent fractures: screening	US Preventive Services Task Force	2018 https://www.uspreventiveservicestaskforce.org/Page/Document/UpdateSummaryFinal/osteoporosis-screening1?ds=1&s=o
Management of osteoporosis in postmenopausal women: Position statement of The North American Menopause Society	The North American Menopause Society	2010 https://www.menopause.org/docs/default-document-library/psosteo10.pdf?sfvrsn=2
2010 Recommendations for the prevention and treatment of glucocorticoid-induced osteoporosis	American College of Rheumatology	2010 Grossman JM, Gordon R, Ranganath VK, et al. American College of Rheumatology 2010 recommendations for the prevention and treatment of glucocorticoid-induced osteoporosis. *Arthritis Care Res* 2010;62:1515-26. doi: 0.1002/acr.20295

Evidence

Type of evidence	Title and comment	Date/full reference
Randomized controlled trial	Calcium supplements with or without vitamin D and risk of cardiovascular events: reanalysis of the Women's Health Initiative limited access dataset and meta-analysis. Comment: There is a statistically significant increased risk of cardiovascular events in women who were not using calcium supplements at the start of the study, who were then randomized to calcium supplementation.	2011 Bolland MJ, Grey A, Avenell A, et al. *BMJ* 2011;342:d2040. (Level III)
Meta-analysis	The use of clinical risk factors enhances the performance of BMD in the prediction of hip and osteoporotic fractures in men and women. Comment: The performance characteristics of clinical risk factors for osteoporosis with and without BMD were validated in 11 independent population-based cohorts. The models developed allow for fracture risk prediction using clinical risk factors.	2007 Kanis JA, Oden A, Johnell O, et al. *Osteoporos Int* 2007 Aug;18(8):1033-46. https://www.ncbi.nlm.nih.gov/pubmed/17323110#

(Continued)

(*Continued*)

Type of evidence	Title and comment	Date/full reference
Secondary analysis of trial data using mixed models	Value of monitoring of bone mineral density after starting bisphosphonate treatment: secondary analysis of trial data. Comment: After bisphosphonate initiation, if DXA is unchanged or improved at 2 years then repeat DXA is not warranted in the absence of new risk factors.	2009. Bell KJ, Hayen A, Macaskill P, et al. *BMJ* 2009;338:b2266. (Level I)

Additional material for this chapter can be found online at:
www.wiley.com/go/sperling/mountsinai/obstetricsandgynecology

This includes advice for patients and ICD codes.

CHAPTER 31

Genital Ulcer Disease

Omara Afzal

Department of Obstetrics, Gynecology and Reproductive Science, Icahn School of Medicine at Mount Sinai, New York, NY

OVERALL BOTTOM LINE
- Genital ulcers can result from infectious as well as noninfectious causes. There are five sexually transmitted infection that can most commonly result in genital ulcer disease: Herpes simplex virus, syphilis, chancroid, lymphogranuloma venereum, and granuloma inguinale.
- Evaluation of a patient with genital ulcers should assess for presence of a sexually transmitted infection (STI) and history regarding sexual risk behaviors, geographic location, and pertinent signs and symptoms.
- Empiric therapy may be beneficial to avoid delay of treatment and risks of STI transmission.

Background
Definition of disease
- An open sore on external or internal surfaces of genitalia, caused by a break in the skin or mucous membranes

Incidence/prevalence
- Dependent on etiology, with most common being sexually transmitted pathogens of herpes simplex virus and primary syphilis

Etiology
- Infectious – sexually transmitted pathogens
  - Herpes simplex virus types I and II (HSV-1 and HSV-2)
  - *Treponoma pallidum* (causative agent of syphilis)
  - *Haemophilus ducreyi* (causative agent of chancroid)
  - *Chlamydia trachomatis* serovars L1-3 (causative agent of lymphogranuloma venereum, LGV)
  - *Klebsiella granulomatis* (causative agent of granuloma inguinale, also known as "donovanosis")
  - Primary infection with HIV
- Infectious – nonsexually acquired:
  - Nonsexually acquired acute genital ulceration (NAGU) – uncommon
- Noninfectious:
  - Fixed drug reaction – unusual, with use of certain drug groups
  - Behcet's syndrome – clinical manifestations believed to be due to vasculitis
  - Neoplasm
  - Trauma

Pathology/pathogenesis
- Histopathologic findings of ulcerations are usually nonspecific and include necrosis of the epithelium.

Mount Sinai Expert Guides: Obstetrics and Gynecology, First Edition. Edited by Rhoda Sperling.
© 2020 John Wiley & Sons Ltd. Published 2020 by John Wiley & Sons Ltd.
Companion Website: www.wiley.com/go/sperling/mountsinai/obstetricsandgynecology

Predictive/risk factors

- Major risk factor of sexually transmitted etiologies is recent history of unprotected sexual contact.
- Geographic location may be a risk factor for pathogens endemic in specific areas.

Prevention

> **BOTTOM LINE/CLINICAL PEARLS**
> - Preventative measures for sexually transmitted etiologies of genital ulcers include protected sexual contact. Early diagnosis and treatment may decrease transmission and spread of disease.

Screening

- History – recent history of unprotected sex or no recent history of unprotected sex

Primary prevention

- Preventative methods to avoid sexually transmitted infections – protected sexual encounters with condoms

Secondary prevention

- Sexual contacts of patients who are diagnosed with an STI should be notified, screened, and treated depending on timing of exposure to decrease transmission, reinfection, and spread of disease.

Diagnosis

> **BOTTOM LINE/CLINICAL PEARLS**
> - History – sexual history and risk behaviors, geographic locations, and pertinent signs and symptoms (painful versus painless ulcers, presence of lymphadenopathy, constitutional symptoms)
> - Exam findings – ulcerative lesions in vulvar/vaginal area, multiple versus single ulcers, presence or absence of lymphadenopathy, concomitant cervical discharge, thrush, or hepatomegaly
> - Investigations – diagnostic testing for HSV by polymerase chain reaction (PCR) or viral culture of ulcer, serologic screening for syphilis with a nontreponomal test (RPR), specialized cultures if available
> - Investigations may be based on history on physical especially in cases of noninfectious causes.

Differential diagnosis

Differential diagnosis	Features
Herpes simplex virus	One or more grouped vesicles on an erythematous base, subsequently open resulting in shallow ulcerations.
Chancroid	Ulcers begin as papules that go on to ulcerate; deep and ragged with a purulent yellow-gray base and an undermined violaceous border.
Syphilis (primary)	Single, indurated, well-circumscribed painless ulcer. Can also be multiple, soft, nonindurated, irregular, and occasionally painful lesions.
LGV	Begins as a single papule or shallow ulcer.
Granuloma inguinale	One or more nodular lesions that ulcerate. Ulcers slowly enlarge, are often friable and have raised rolled margins. "Kissing" lesions may occur from autoinoculation on adjacent skin.
Acute genital ulceration	Sudden onset of intensely painful large ulcers (>1 cm) and deep, with a red-violaceous border and necrotic base covered with grayish exudate, may be partially symmetric in appearance ("kissing").

(*Continued*)

Differential diagnosis	Features
Bechet's syndrome	Rare, multisystem inflammatory disease of unknown etiology, painful and deep genital and oral ulcerations and uveitis.
Fixed drug reaction	Similar presentation to herpes but lack of response to antivirals, negative HSV culture, and recent medication use should raise suspicion.

Typical presentation
- Present with genital ulcers, may be acute or chronic, single or multiple, with or without pain and discharge, or other associated symptomatology.

Clinical diagnosis
History
- Sexual history and risk behaviors, where the patient (or sexual contacts) reside or travel (certain pathogens may be more common in specific geographic areas), and pertinent signs and symptoms (painful versus painless ulcers, presence of lymphadenopathy, constitutional symptoms).
- Nonsexually acquired acute genital ulceration (NAGU) – rare, immune response to recent infection such as Epstein-Barr virus (EBV), mycoplasma, and Lyme disease, typically occurring in sexually inactive adolescent girls or young women and may be preceded by influenza-like symptoms.
- Fixed drug reaction – recent use of over-the-counter or otherwise drug groups, such as antibacterial agents, nonsteroidal anti-inflammatory drugs, antifungal agents, psychotropic agents, proton pump inhibitors, calcium channel blockers, and angiotensin-converting enzyme inhibitors.
- Traumatic lesions usually resulting from forced or aggressive sexual intercourse, often presenting as abrasions.

Physical examination
- Ulcerative lesions in vulvar/vaginal area, multiple versus single ulcers, presence or absence of lymphadenopathy, concomitant cervical discharge, thrush or hepatomegaly.
- Tender lymph nodes are often present in patients with HSV, chancroid, and LGV; the latter two may also have matting or suppuration of the lymph nodes or development of "buboe" (unilateral painful inguinal lymph nodes).
- Rubbery, nontender nodes are often seen in late primary syphilis.
- Patients without risk factors for an STI should be evaluated for evidence of autoimmune disease (such as oral ulcers, which may be seen in Behcet's syndrome).
- Acute genital ulceration is a clinical diagnosis and one of exclusion, based upon history (absence of recent sexual contact), age, severity, and physical exam.

Laboratory diagnosis
List of diagnostic tests
- HSV – PCR or viral culture of ulcer
- Syphilis – serologic screening with a nontreponomal test (RPR) and/or treponomal test (*T. pallidum* enzyme immunoassay), may be performed as stepwise testing
- LGV – serologic testing may be helpful
- Granuloma inguinale – biopsy specimen looking for Donovan bodies
- Chancroid – specialized cultures
- Acute genital ulceration – should include serology testing for EBV antibodies to identify acute infection

List of imaging techniques
- Imaging techniques generally do not aid in diagnosis of genital ulcers.

Potential pitfalls/common errors made regarding diagnosis of disease

- Examining number of lesions will aid in differential but can lead to misdiagnosis if used alone without diagnostic testing. Each infectious cause may occasionally present in a different manner. For example, genital herpes may present as a single ulcer or a fissure, or multiple syphilitic chancres may be misdiagnosed as HSV.
- In most clinical settings, there are no reliable point-of-care diagnostic tests; additionally many ulcers may not have specific etiology identified.

Treatment

Treatment rationale

- Empiric treatment may be initiated as diagnostic tests may take time to result, especially when there is a known exposure to a STI, genital ulcers suggestive of HSV, or patients who are at high risk for syphilis.
- Empiric treatment should be based on most likely diagnosis based upon patients history of exposure to an STI as well as physical exam, using knowledge of local epidemiology of possible etiologic agents.
  - Single, painless lesions – empiric treatment for primary syphilis with penicillin G benzathine (2.4 million units), administered intramuscular.
  - Single, painless lesions with significant inguinal lymphadenopathy – empiric treatment for LGV is reasonable, especially if in endemic area, with doxycycline 100 mg twice daily for 21 days.
  - Multiple painful lesions – suspect HSV and should receive antiviral therapy.
  - Atypical presentations may lead to diagnostic uncertainty; it is reasonable to treat empirically for HSV and syphilis due to their greater prevalence.

When to hospitalize

- Ulcers not amenable to outpatient therapy, requiring intravenous antibiotics, or with severe associated constitutional symptoms may require hospitalization.

Table of treatment

Treatment	Comments
Conservative	For noninfectious causes, generally supportive treatment with local hygiene and wound care as well as pain control is necessary. For infectious etiologies, patients should be advised to refrain from sexual activity while awaiting test results; counseling regarding partner testing and condom use to decrease transmission.
Medical Syphilis – penicillin G benzathine (2.4 million units) LGV – doxycycline 100 mg twice daily for 21 days Granuloma inguinale – azithromycin 1 g weekly or 500 mg daily for 3 weeks. HSV – acyclovir 400 mg three times daily or valacyclovir 1000 mg twice daily; both for 7–10 days Chancroid – azithromycin 1 gm or ceftriaxone 250 mg IM	

Prevention/management of complications

- Follow-up should be arranged within 1 week of initial visit to assess clinical response to therapy and review results of diagnostic testing. If ulcerative lesions continue or other symptoms develop, more testing may be required.
- Sexual contacts of patients who are diagnosed with an STI should be notified, screened, and treated if needed. This is key to decreasing transmission.

CLINICAL PEARLS
- Due to lack of point-of-care testing, diagnostic tests are performed that may take time; however, treatment should not be delayed and it is reasonable to initiate empiric therapy.
- Patient with genital ulcers should receive empiric therapy if they have a known exposure to an STI, ulcers suggestive of HSV, and patients at high risk for syphilis.
- Treatment of choice depends on patient's history of exposure to a specific STI and the clinical assessment.

Special populations
Pregnancy
- If an infectious etiology is identified, care must be taken to use antibiotics that are safe in pregnancy.

Children
- Sexually transmitted infectious etiologies should raise suspicion and evaluation for sexual abuse in children.

Elderly
- Care should be taken for evaluation of noninfectious etiologies as well especially in elderly or otherwise limited mobility patients, such as bedsores, compression ulcers, skin ulceration from erosive disease or irritation, and neoplasm-associated ulcers.

Prognosis

BOTTOM LINE/CLINICAL PEARLS
- Early treatment and avoidance of reinfection with sexually transmitted etiologies leads to a good prognosis with completed treatment.
- Follow-up is necessary to ensure successful treatment, as inappropriate treatment may lead to persistence of disease with risks of transmission.

Follow-up tests and monitoring
- Follow-up should be arranged within 1 week of initial visit to assess clinical response to therapy and review results of diagnostic testing. If ulcerative lesions continue or other symptoms develop, more testing may be required.

Reading list
Suggested websites
National STD Curriculum, University of Wisconsin. www.std.uw.edu
Centers for Disease Control and Prevention. http://www.cdc.gov/std

Guidelines
National society guidelines

Title	Source	Date/URL
2015 sexually transmitted diseases treatment guidelines	Centers for Disease Control and Prevention	https://www.cdc.gov/std/tg2015

Additional material for this chapter can be found online at:
www.wiley.com/go/sperling/mountsinai/obstetricsandgynecology

This includes ICD codes.

CHAPTER 32

Vulvodynia

Suzanne S. Fenske

Department of Obstetrics, Gynecology and Reproductive Science, Icahn School of Medicine at Mount Sinai, New York, NY

OVERALL BOTTOM LINE

- Vulvodynia is idiopathic, chronic vulvar pain of at least 3 months duration.
- Vulvodynia likely represents several different disorders.
- Vulvodynia is classified based on whether the pain is general or localized, provoked or spontaneous, primary or secondary and intermittent, persistent, constant, immediate, or delayed.
- It is a clinical diagnosis made with a thorough history and extensive physical examination.
- A lack of research evaluating treatment options has led to a "trial and error" approach.
- Treatment for vulvodynia begins with conservative options such as cognitive-behavioral therapy and physical therapy with stepwise progression to topical medications and systemic medications and finally vestibulectomy.

Background

Definition of disease

- Vulvodynia is idiopathic, chronic vulvar pain of at least 3 months duration.

Disease classification

- In 2015, the International Society for the Study of Vulvovaginal Disease (ISSVD), the International Society for the Study of Women's Sexual Health (ISSWSH), and the International Pelvic Pain Society (IPPS) revised the terminology and classification of vulvar pain. Vulvodynia can be localized (such as vestibulodynia) or generalized or mixed, provoked or spontaneous or mixed, primary or secondary and intermittent, persistent, constant, immediate, or delayed.

Incidence/prevalence

- 3 to 16% of women report a history of vulvar pain lasting at least 3 months.
- 4 to 7% report current symptoms of vulvar pain lasting at least 3 months.

Etiology

- The etiology of vulvodynia remains unknown.

Pathology/pathogenesis

- The pathogenesis of vulvodynia is unknown.
- One theory of a possible cause of vulvodynia suggests that estrogen affects sensory discrimination and pain sensitivity. When estrogen levels change over time, vulvar nerve sensitivity and sensory nociceptors may change. This can explain why it affects women at menopause and for some women on oral contraceptive pills.

Mount Sinai Expert Guides: Obstetrics and Gynecology, First Edition. Edited by Rhoda Sperling.
© 2020 John Wiley & Sons Ltd. Published 2020 by John Wiley & Sons Ltd.
Companion Website: www.wiley.com/go/sperling/mountsinai/obstetricsandgynecology

- Vulvodynia represents neuropathic pain. Another possible cause of vulvodynia is an insult to the tissue resulting in persistent neuropathic pain due to perceived persistent insult.
- Another possible cause of vulvodynia is pelvic floor muscle dysfunction. Inflammatory mediators are locally released when muscle fiber trauma occurs. This leads to muscle hyperalgesia and peripheral sensitization. With prolonged stimuli, central sensitization occurs. Central sensitization causes normally non-noxious stimuli to be perceived as painful.

Prevention

> **BOTTOM LINE/CLINICAL PEARLS**
> - No interventions have been demonstrated to prevent the development of the disease.

Screening
- There is no routine screening for vulvodynia.

Primary prevention
- There are no known interventions or treatments that prevent the first occurrence of vulvodynia.

Secondary prevention
- It is currently believed that vulvodynia is a larger category in which multiple diseases of different pathogenesis are lumped together.
- Given that vulvodynia likely incorporates multiple different diseases, it is difficult to discuss reoccurrence and prevention of reoccurrence. In some patients, vulvodynia remains a chronic problem that waxes and wanes. In other patients, vulvodynia does not recur.
- To avoid reoccurrence, it is imperative that the correct diagnosis and theorized pathogenesis is made.

Diagnosis

> **BOTTOM LINE/CLINICAL PEARLS**
> - Diagnosis of vulvodynia is suspected when a patient has a history of vulvar pain of 3 months duration and inflammatory, infectious and neoplastic etiology has been ruled out.
> - Suspicion of vulvodynia is further supported when physical examination reveals a positive cotton-swab test.
> - There is no imaging or laboratory tests to confirm a diagnosis of vulvodynia; however, negative testing for inflammation, infection, neoplasia, etc., supports the diagnosis of vulvodynia.

Differential diagnosis

Differential diagnosis	Features
Infectious etiology	- Physical findings consistent with infectious etiology would be present such as ulcers, vaginal discharge, edema, erythema. - Laboratory testing for infectious etiology would be conclusive.
Inflammatory dermatologic etiology	- Examples of this would be lichen sclerosus, allergic or contact dermatitis, lichen planus, vulvar intraepithelial neoplasia, etc. - Skin examination and biopsies would confirm inflammatory etiology.

(Continued)

(Continued)

Differential diagnosis	Features
Anatomic etiology	• Clitoral priapism is a rare cause of vulvar pain. • This diagnosis would be made on examination and findings of an edematous, tender clitoris.
Malignancy	• Most patients present with vulvar plaque, ulcer, or mass. • Vulvar biopsy is conclusive.
Postherpetic neuralgia	• History would demonstrate a recent herpetic outbreak and examination would demonstrate pain along dermatome.

Typical presentation

• Patients with generalized vulvodynia usually present to the office with complaints of generalized, diffuse pain that can be described as a raw sensation or burning or like a constant yeast infection. Patients with localized vulvodynia like vestibulodynia will often present with complaints of dyspareunia. Patients with vestibulodynia will report insertional pain. They will often report that they are unable to insert a tampon as well. The pain is often described as burning or sharp pain like knives. Patients will often report that they experience discomfort with light touch as well and are unable to wear tight pants or underwear.

Clinical diagnosis

History

• It is important to understand pain characteristics, such as time since onset, temporal pattern, duration, location, quality, elicitors, and whether pain is primary or secondary.
• Obtain history of any trauma, surgery, etc.
• Perform an extensive review of systems with emphasis on gastrointestinal and urologic symptoms.
• Obtain detailed sexual history focusing on desire, arousal, orgasm, frequency of satisfaction with sex, history of sexual distress as well as history of sexual abuse.
• Evaluate the dynamics of current relationship and ascertain how the current symptoms are being managed.
• Obtain a history of all previous treatments and outcomes.

Physical examination

• Initially the medial thigh, buttocks, and mons pubis should be palpated with cotton swab.
• Then, the labia majora, clitoral prepuce, perineum, and intralabial sulci should be palpated with cotton swab.
• Subsequently the labia minora should be gently palpated with cotton swab.
• The cotton swab should be used to palpate the vestibule gently at five locations: at the ostia of the Skene glands, at the ostia of the Bartholin glands and at 6 o'clock.
• Following the cotton-swab test, a single digit should be inserted into the vagina and the pelvic floor muscles should be examined for pain on palpation and hypertonicity.
• A speculum examination should be performed to assess for discharge, atrophy, erosions, ulcerations, and erythema.
• A bimanual examination is performed to assess the uterus and adnexa.
• Finally, a rectovaginal examination should be performed to assess the rectovaginal septum and posterior cul-de-sac.

Laboratory diagnosis

List of diagnostic tests

- Vaginal discharge should be examined by wet prep of the vaginal secretions with potassium hydroxide (KOH) and saline and pH testing of the vaginal vault.
- Vaginal discharge should be cultured for sexually transmitted infections, candidiasis, and bacterial vaginosis.
- Vulvar or vaginal biopsy sample should be obtained if there are specific findings at visual inspection or colposcopic inspection.
- Ultrasonographic imaging should be obtained if bimanual examination reveals an enlarged uterus or adnexal mass.

Potential pitfalls/common errors made regarding diagnosis of disease

- One commonly encountered error in diagnosis is the overdiagnosis of vulvodynia as due to infectious etiology. Physicians will often empirically treat for infection rather than considering vulvodynia as a diagnosis.
- Another commonly encountered error in diagnosis is the missed diagnosis of vestibulodynia and overdiagnosis of dyspareunia being vaginismus.

Treatment

Treatment rationale

- Typical treatment plan begins with noninvasive treatment options such as psychological interventions and pelvic floor physical therapy.
- Second line of treatment is medical. Medical treatment options can be topical as well as systemic. Local anesthetic is a topical treatment option that works to achieve long-lasting desensitization of the vestibular nerves. Capsaicin is another topical treatment option that produces a long-lasting desensitization to burning and pain after initial hyperesthesia. Topical treatment with estrogen and testosterone has been successfully in used in patients in whom the initiation of combined oral contraceptive pills was associated with symptoms. There is questionable support to using systemic anticonvulsant therapy; however, recommendation of this treatment is pending a randomized controlled trial.
- Vulvar vestibulectomy is third-line treatment. This procedure consists of excision of a semicircular segment of tissue involving the mucosa of the posterior vulvar vestibule and posterior hymenal ring.

Table of treatment

Treatment	Comment
Conservative • Cognitive-behavioral therapy • Pelvic floor physical therapy • Electromyographic biofeedback	Conservative treatment options are the recommended initial treatment options for all patients.
Medical • Local anesthetic • Capsaicin • Botulinum type A • Topical hormonal treatment	Although extremely rare, distant spread of botulinum toxin beyond the side of injection has been reported and resulted in dysphagia and breathing difficulties. Capsaicin causes hyperesthesia on initial exposure and, therefore, is not well tolerated.
Surgical • Vestibulectomy	Vestibulectomy is an option for patients with vestibulodynia. For those with intractable pain, vestibulectomy is an appropriate next step after unsuccessful medical treatment.
Complementary • Acupuncture • Hypnotherapy	Two uncontrolled prospective pilot studies showed that participants reported improvement in pain and sexuality after taking part in acupuncture and hypnotherapy. Prior to recommending these as treatment options, additional studies are recommended.

CLINICAL PEARLS
- Treatment of vulvodynia can be a slow process and there is no set algorithm that can be applied to all patients.
- If the etiology is thought to be due to lack of estrogen and testosterone, then repletion of hormones with topical estradiol and testosterone and avoidance of oral contraceptive pills has successful outcome.
- If the etiology is thought to be due to sensitization, then treatment aimed at desensitization is successful.

Prognosis

BOTTOM LINE/CLINICAL PEARLS
- Vulvodynia has many possible medical treatments, but very few controlled trials have been performed to verify the efficacy of these treatments.
- Treatment is usually based on "trial and error."
- Surgical management of vestibulodynia results in success rates of 60 to 90%.

Reading list

Borenstein J, Goldstein AT, Stockdale CK, et al. 2015 ISSVD, ISSWSH and IPPS consensus terminology and classification of persistent vulvar pain and vulvodynia. *Obstet Gynecol* 2016;127:745.

Burrows LJ, Goldstein AT. The treatment of vestibulodynia with topical estradiol and testosterone. *Sex Med* 2013;1:30.

Edwards L. Vulvodynia. *Clin Obstet Gynecol* 2015;58:143.

Goldstein AT, Pukall CF, Brown C, et al. Vulvodynia: assessment and treatment. *J Sex Med* 2016;13:572-90.

Haefner HK, Collins ME, Davis GD et al. The vulvodynia guideline. *J Low Genit Tract Dis* 2005;9(1):40-51.

Kliethermes CJ, Shah M, Hoffstetter S, et al. Effect of vestibulectomy for intractable vulvodynia. *J Minim Invasive Gynecol* 2016;23(7):1152-57.

Steinberg AC, Oyama IA, Rejba AE, et al. Capsaicin for the treatment of vulvar vestibulitis. *Am J Obstet Gynecol* 2005;192:1549-53.

Guidelines
National society guidelines

Title	Source	Date/full reference or URL
2015 ISSVD, ISSWSH, IPPS consensus terminology and classification of persistent vulvar pain	ISSVD, ISSWSH, IPPS Comment: Definition is vulvar pain lasting at least 3 months without clear cause which may have associated factors. Vulvar pain can be due to infectious, inflammatory, neoplastic, neurologic, trauma, iatrogenic and hormonal etiologies.	*Obstet Gynecol* 2016 Apr;127(4):745-51.
The vulvodynia guideline	National Vulvodynia Association Vulvodynia has many possible treatments, but very few controlled trials have been performed to verify treatment options.	2005 https://www.nva.org/wp-content/uploads/2015/01/Haefner-Vulvodynia-Guideline-2005.pdf

PART 3

Reproductive Endocrinology

CHAPTER 33

Evaluation of the Infertile Couple

Taraneh Gharib Nazem, Devora Aharon, and Alan B. Copperman
Reproductive Medicine Associates of New York; Division of Reproductive Endocrinology and Infertility, Icahn School of Medicine at Mount Sinai, New York, NY

Background
Definition
- Infertility is defined as the inability to achieve a successful pregnancy after 12 months or more of regular unprotected intercourse, or after 6 months among women over 35 years of age.
- Cycle fecundability is the probability of achieving pregnancy in one menstrual cycle.
- Cycle fecundity is the likelihood that any one cycle will result in a live birth.

Impact
Incidence
- Fecundability for healthy young couples is estimated to be 0.25, meaning there is a 75% chance of failure to conceive in one cycle. However, this rate declines with each consecutive unsuccessful cycle and can reach 0.03 by 12 months.
- Infertility prevalence rises with age. Data show fertility peaks at ages 20–24 years, and then decreases to 4–8% from ages 25–29, 15–19% from ages 30–34, 26-46% from ages 35–39, and to as much as 95% by ages 40–45. The rate of miscarriage rises with increasing age, and success rates achieved with artificial reproductive technologies (ART) decline with aging.
- The overall prevalence of infertility has remained stable at approximately 12% over the past five decades.
- The percentage of women receiving evaluation or treatment for infertility has increased over time. In 1982, 6.6 million (9%) women reported ever receiving infertility services. This number peaked at 9.3 million (15%) in 1995 but has since remained steady at 7.3 million (12%) from 2002 to 2010.

Economic impact
- In the United States, total expenditure on infertility services is estimated to be $2–3 billion per year.
- Insurance coverage for infertility treatment in the US is not uniform and is influenced by employers and state mandates.
- Out-of-pocket expenses for infertility services are variable and may be costly.

Social impact
- Infertility causes distress and anxiety for patients.
- Due to the introduction of in vitro fertilization and other ART to women of advanced age planning pregnancies, to changes in family structures (LGBTQIA patients and single women), and to greater awareness and media attention of fertility services, evaluation and treatment for infertility have become more targeted over the last 30 years.

Mount Sinai Expert Guides: Obstetrics and Gynecology, First Edition. Edited by Rhoda Sperling.
© 2020 John Wiley & Sons Ltd. Published 2020 by John Wiley & Sons Ltd.
Companion Website: www.wiley.com/go/sperling/mountsinai/obstetricsandgynecology

Etiology
- There are many different factors, both known and unknown, that affect the human reproductive system.

Pathology/pathogenesis
Normal fertility
- Pregnancy results from the successful completion of a complex series of physiological events involving the male and female that culminates in embryo implantation.
- At baseline, human reproduction requires ovulation, the production of a competent oocyte, adequate sperm, proximity of the sperm and oocyte in the female reproductive tract, transport of the embryo to the uterine cavity, and implantation in the endometrium.
- Interruption of any component of this process will result in a decline in fertility.

Physiology of maternal aging
- Maternal age is the single most important factor that influences chance of conception.
- Women are endowed with the highest number of germ cells in utero, with 6–7 million oocytes at 20 weeks gestation. Thereafter, the number of oocytes present in primordial follicles declines through a process of atresia. At birth, the number of follicles is estimated to be 1–2 million; by puberty, 300 000; and by menopause, less than 1000 remain. Over the span of a woman's reproductive life, about 400 oocytes will ovulate.
- The quality of oocytes also declines with age. An increase in meiotic nondisjunction results in a higher rate of oocyte and embryo aneuploidy. The actual cause of aneuploidy is poorly understood, but it is possible that mitotic spindle dysfunction or loss of adhesion between sister chromosomes might be contributory.
- The risk of aneuploidy increases with advancing age, reaching almost 100% by age 45. Chromosomal abnormalities account for 70–80% of first trimester losses.

Paternal aging
- Increasing male age has been associated with decreases in semen volume, sperm motility, and morphologically normal sperm.
- Men experience decreased gonadal function with advancing age. Testosterone production starts to decline around age 40.
- Evidence shows that pregnancy rates decline and time to conception rises with paternal aging. Decline in male fertility begins in the early 40s, but this change is subtle and in many cases may be insignificant, especially in contrast to the precipitous age-related decline seen in women.

Causes of infertility

Ovarian/ovulatory disorders	Hypothalamic dysfunction – Weight/body composition – Stress – Strenuous exercise – Infiltrative disease (e.g. lymphoma, histiocytosis) Pituitary disease – Prolactinoma – Empty sella syndrome – Sheehan syndrome – Cushing disease – Acromegaly – Other pituitary tumors – Thyroid disease

	Ovarian dysfunction – Ovarian failure (aging, exogenous treatment, genetic disorders (e.g. Turner's syndrome, Fragile X premutation) – Ovarian hyperandrogenism (e.g. polycystic ovarian syndrome [PCOS])
Tubal/peritoneal	Infectious – Pelvic inflammatory disease Structural – Tubal ligation/sterilization procedure – Ectopic pregnancy – Peritubal adhesive disease (e.g. history of ruptured appendix) Intrauterine device (e.g. Dalkon Shield) Endometriosis
Uterine	Structural/inherited – Unicornuate/septate/bicornuate/didelphys uterus – Diethylstilbestrol (DES) exposure in utero Structural/acquired – Leiomyoma – Endometrial polyp – Uterine synechiae (e.g. Asherman's syndrome)
Cervical	Structural – Loop electrosurgical excision procedure (LEEP) or coninization of cervix – Trauma – Cervical stenosis
Male factor	Structural – History of inguinal hernia – Varicocele, spermatocele – Testicular masses – Absence or obstruction of vas deferens – Epididydmal obstruction or dysfunction – Cryptorchidism – Ejaculatory dysfunction – Vasectomy Infectious – Sexually transmitted infections – Viral orchitis – Testicular atrophy due to viral illness Chronic diseases – Renal disease – Thyroid dysfunction – Diabetes mellitus – Malignancy – Sickle cell disease – Malnourishment Hypothalamic-pituitary disorders – Kallman syndrome – Tumors (e.g. craniopharyngioma, macroadenoma) – Hyperprolactinemia – Obesity

(Continued)

(*Continued*)

	Primary gonadal disorders – Y chromosome microdeletion – Klinefelter's syndrome
	Disorders of sperm transport – Kartagener syndrome (primary ciliary dyskinesia)
	Medications (e.g. steroid use, chemotherapy agents, antihypertensives, sulfasalazine, etc.)
Unexplained	
Other	Autoimmune disease Lifestyle factors (e.g. smoking) Occupational hazards – Chemical exposures – Insecticides, pesticides – Lead – Organic solvents – Radiation

Diagnosis

BOTTOM LINE/CLINICAL PEARLS
- The first step in determining the cause of infertility is to obtain a thorough history and physical exam.
- Diagnostic testing should focus on confirming tubal patency and evaluating the female reproductive tract, including the uterine cavity.
- Ovulation competency should be established either by history or laboratory evaluation.
- Ovarian reserve testing should be considered particularly in women > 35 years of age.
- A semen analysis should be obtained.
- A specific etiology may not be determined and a diagnosis of "unexplained infertility" may be made in some cases.

Differential diagnosis

Diagnosis	Frequency
Very common (>20%)	
Ovulatory dysfunction	20–40%
Tubal and peritoneal pathology	30–40%
Male factors	30–40%
Common (6–20%)	
Unexplained	10–20%
Uncommon (1–5%)	
Endometriosis	5%
Cervical factors	3%
Rare (<1%)	
Uterine anomalies	<1%

Algorithm 33.1 Diagnostic algorithm for infertility

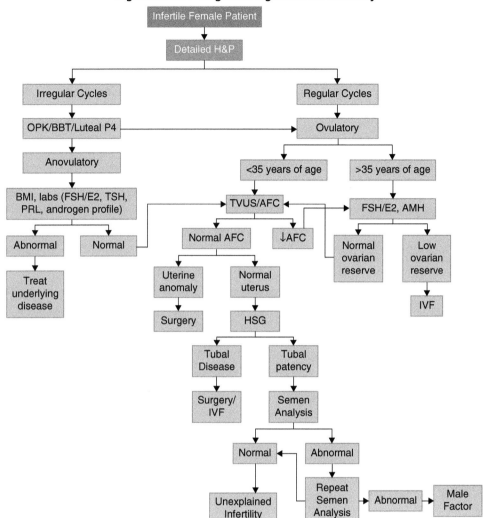

Clinical diagnosis
- Evaluation of infertility is recommended after 12 months of unprotected intercourse; however, for women over the age of 35, a workup may be initiated by 6 months.
- Earlier evaluation of infertility is also recommended in cases of oligomenorrhea or amenorrhea, known or suspected uterine/tubal/peritoneal disease, stage III–IV endometriosis, and known or suspected male subfertility.
- See Algorithm 33.1.

History
- A detailed history can guide the clinician toward the cause of infertility and is essential in the initial evaluation of a couple.
- A comprehensive medical, reproductive and family history should be obtained. Relevant history should also include the following:
  - Infertility history: duration of infertility, results of prior evaluation/treatments, coital frequency, sexual function

- Menstrual history: age of menarche, cycle length, and characteristics
- Pregnancy history: gravidity, parity, previous pregnancy outcomes, complications
- Gynecologic history: contraception use, history of sexually transmitted infections, pelvic inflammatory disease, abnormal Pap smears, and related medical or surgical treatments
- Symptoms of targeted diseases: pelvic/abdominal pain, dyspareunia, dyschezia, thyroid disease, galactorrhea, hirsutism
- Past medical history with specific attention to thyroid problems and hyperandrogenism
- Past surgeries (gynecologic or abdominal)
- Current medications and allergies
- Family history including birth defects, developmental delay, early menopause, reproductive issues
- Social history: tobacco, alcohol, recreational drug use, toxic behaviors
- Occupational history, hazardous exposures
- Relevant history of male partner

Physical examination
- Assessment of weight, height, body mass index (BMI), and vital signs, including blood pressure and pulse
- Thyroid size, presence of thyroid nodules
- Breast exam including palpation for masses, expression of nipple secretion, Tanner staging
- Signs of androgen excess (hair thickness, growth pattern, acne)
- Anatomical assessment of the clitoris, hymenal ring, vagina, and cervix
- Pelvic exam to determine uterine orientation, size, and mobility, adnexal masses or tenderness, and uterosacral or cul-de-sac nodularity, tenderness, or masses

Laboratory diagnosis
List of diagnostic tests
- Evaluation of ovarian reserve
  - Day 3 follicle stimulating hormone (FSH) with accompanying estradiol level is the most common test of ovarian reserve. Because FSH concentrations vary significantly throughout a cycle, serum FSH concentration is best obtained in the early follicular phase (cycle days 2–4). Estradiol by itself has little value as an ovarian reserve test but is necessary to interpret FSH level, as an elevated estradiol may suppress FSH levels by negative feedback. A woman is considered to have decreased ovarian reserve if basal FSH is > 13 mIU/mL.
  - Anti-Müllerian hormone (AMH) is produced by the granulosa cells of preantral and small antral follicles and is indicative of the remaining follicular pool. AMH is gonadotropin independent; therefore, there is little variability in levels throughout and between menstrual cycles. Normal levels of AMH range from 1 to 3 ng/mL. AMH <1 ng/mL is suggestive of reduced ovarian reserve; however, the result should be interpreted within the context of a woman's age.
  - Clomiphene Citrate Challenge Test (CCCT) is a provocative test to measure FSH. Clomiphene is an estrogen agonist/antagonist that binds to estrogen receptors in the hypothalamus and drives release of FSH and luteinizing hormone (LH) from the pituitary. CCCT involves administration of 100 mg of oral clomiphene citrate on cycle days 5–9 with measurement of FSH on day 3 and day 10 and estradiol on day 3. FSH concentrations are high in women with smaller follicular pools as they have less production of inhibin B and estradiol and less negative feedback on FSH production. Classically, if the day 10 FSH is >10 mIU/mL, then reduced ovarian reserve is diagnosed. This test is no longer widely used, as newer tests, such as AMH, are simpler and better correlated with ovarian reserve.
  - Inhibin B is secreted during the follicular phase of the menstrual cycle by granulosa cells of smaller antral follicles and therefore has been suggested to have value in determining ovarian reserve. However, because inhibin B varies widely throughout the menstrual cycle and in response to exogenous gonadotropin releasing hormone or FSH stimulation, it is not a reliable measure of ovarian reserve.

- Assessment of ovulatory function
  - Ovulation most likely occurs among women with regularly occurring menstrual cycles (25–35 days in length); however, if there is any uncertainty, there are several diagnostic tests that can be confirmatory.
  - A serum progesterone level > 3 ng/mL in the midluteal phase (18–24 days after onset of menses) is diagnostic of ovulation.
  - Ovulation predictor kits (OPKs) are commercially available for home use. OPKs measure urinary LH and can detect the LH surge, which occurs approximately 36 hours prior to ovulation. Women test their urine 1–2 days before the expected surge. False-positive results may occur with any condition associated with elevated LH levels such as polycystic ovarian syndrome (PCOS), primary ovarian insufficiency, or menopause.
  - Basal body temperature (BBT) is a simple, inexpensive option involving charting of a woman's temperature around the same time every day. A biphasic pattern in temperature is characteristic of ovulatory cycles. Temperature is usually less than 98°F before ovulation and greater than 98°F after ovulation due to the effect of progesterone, produced by the corpus luteum, on the temperature regulating center in the hypothalamus. Progesterone causes an increase in the basal temperature from 0.5° to 1.0°F in the luteal phase.
  - Endometrial biopsy can demonstrate histologic changes of the endometrium caused by progesterone after ovulation. Progesterone transforms the endometrium from a proliferative to secretory environment. In the absence of exogenous progesterone, a secretory endometrium is indicative of recent ovulation. Previously, endometrial biopsy was a basic screening tool for luteal phase defects, but now that less-invasive methods of determining ovulatory status are available it is not as commonly used.
  - Given the wide variety of causes of anovulation, several tests may be considered to determine the etiology.
    - Thyroid stimulating hormone (TSH) is the initial screening test for thyroid disease. Free T_4 levels should be checked if TSH is abnormal.
    - Prolactin levels are most accurate when performed in the morning during the follicular phase as they fluctuate throughout the day and tend to be higher in the luteal phase.
    - Day 3 FSH or AMH can determine if ovarian insufficiency is the cause of anovulation.
    - If a woman has signs of hyperandrogenism, additional testing is warranted including testosterone, dehydroepiandrosterone sulfate (DHEAS) and 17-hydroxyprogesterone (17-OHP) levels. 17-OHP levels should also be performed in the morning during the follicular phase as the corpus luteum produces 17-OHP. An elevated 17-OHP is indicative of congenital adrenal hyperplasia.
- Tubal factor infertility
  - Chlamydia antibody testing is a method of detecting antibodies to *Chlamydia trachomatis*, which has been associated with tubal pathology. This test has limited clinical utility and is not commonly performed.
- Cervical evaluation
  - The postcoital test (PCT), in which a sample of cervical mucus is obtained just before ovulation, is used to determine abnormalities with cervical mucus as well as to evaluate the number of sperm that have penetrated the mucus. PCT is neither sensitive nor specific for the diagnosis of infertility and is no longer commonly performed in the routine evaluation of infertility. It may be considered for couples in which a formal semen analysis is unable to be obtained.
- Male factor infertility
  - Semen analysis (SA) is the standard for evaluation of the male partner. The male partner should abstain from ejaculation 2–5 days prior to collection. Normal parameters for a semen analysis are volume 1.5–5 mL, sperm concentration > 20 million sperm/mL, motility > 50%, morphology > 4% normal forms (Kruger classification). If the initial SA is abnormal, a second confirmatory sample should be obtained.

List of imaging techniques
- Evaluation of ovarian reserve
  - Assessment of antral follicle count (AFC) by transvaginal ultrasound (TVUS) is an indirect but useful method of evaluating ovarian reserve. Performed in the early follicular phase, the sum of the antral follicles in both ovaries visualized on TVUS is calculated. Antral follicles are 2–10 mm in mean diameter. A low AFC is considered 3–6 total antral follicles.
- Uterine factor infertility
  - TVUS, 3D ultrasound, and magnetic resonance imaging (MRI) are all useful imaging techniques for the diagnosis of uterine pathology, including leiomyomas and congenital malformations, as well as ovarian pathology.
  - Saline-infusion sonograms (SIS), which involve instillation of saline into the uterine cavity during TVUS, evaluate the size and contour of the uterine cavity and are useful for detecting and delineating intrauterine pathology, including endometrial polyps, submucosal fibroids, and uterine synechiae.
  - Hysterosalpingogram (HSG) is a study in which a radio-opaque contrast is introduced into the uterine cavity and X-rays of the pelvis are obtained. HSG can define the size and shape of the uterine cavity while simultaneously assessing tubal patency. An HSG can identify developmental anomalies (unicornuate, septate, or bicornuate uterus) as well as acquired pathology (endometrial polyps, submucosal fibroids, uterine synechiae).
  - Hysteroscopy is the definitive method for diagnosis and treatment of intrauterine pathology; however, it is costly and invasive and should be reserved until after other imaging modalities have identified intrauterine pathology.
- Tubal factor infertility
  - HSG is the standard method to evaluate tubal patency. It is performed in the early follicular phase after the cessation of menstrual flow. It can document proximal or distal occlusion, demonstrate salpingitis isthmica nodosa, uncover structural deficiencies, and determine presence of fimbrial phimosis or peritubal adhesions. HSG may offer potential therapeutic benefit. Proposed mechanisms of action include release of intratubal mucus plugs, breakdown of adhesions, or tubal cilia stimulation.
  - SIS can also be used to determine tubal patency by injecting saline and identifying fluid in the cul-de-sac on ultrasound. This test is limited by the inability to determine unilateral or bilateral patency.
  - Laparoscopy with chromotubation is another option; however, rarely is this a first-line screening test, especially when laparoscopy is not otherwise indicated. For chromotubation, dilute methylene blue or indigo carmine dye is injected through the cervix and spillage through the fallopian tubes is directly visualized on laparoscopy. The procedure additionally allows for correction of causes of tubal disease such as fimbrial phimosis or peritubal adhesions.

Potential pitfalls/common errors made regarding diagnosis of disease
- One of the common pitfalls in the workup of the infertile couple is failure to completely work up the male patient. Prior history of children from the male partner does not preclude the need for a semen analysis. A full history and targeted testing of the male patient is an essential component of the diagnostic workup.
- Often, providers will utilize the hysterosalpingogram as a method of assessing both the fallopian tubes and uterus; however, there are limitations to the HSG, particularly concerning congenital uterine anomalies. If there is a high suspicion for uterine malformation, 3D ultrasound or MRI is warranted.

Reading list
Broekmans FJ, Kwee J, Hendriks DJ, et al. A systematic review of tests predicting ovarian reserve and IVF outcome. *Hum Reprod Update* 2006;12(6):685-718.

Broekmans FJ, de Ziegler D, Howles CM, et al. The antral follicle count: practical recommendations for better standardization. *Fertil Steril* 2010;94:1044.

Chandra A, Copen CE, Stephen EH. Infertility service use in the United States: Data from the National Survey of Family Growth, 1982–2010. *Natl Health Stat Report* 2014 Jan 22;(73):1-20.

Fritz, M, Speroff L. *Clinical gynecologic endocrinology and infertility.* Baltimore: Williams & Wilkins; 2011.

Infertility workup for the women's health specialist. ACOG committee opinion no. 781. *Obstet Gynecol* 2019;130(6):e377-84.

Luttjeboer F, Harada T, Hughes E, et al. Tubal flushing for subfertility. *Cochrane Database Syst Rev* 2007 Jul 18;(3):CD003718.

Practice Committee of the American Society for Reproductive Medicine. Diagnostic evaluation of the infertile female: a committee opinion. *Fertil Steril* 2012;(98):302-7.

Practice Committee of the American Society for Reproductive Medicine. Definitions of infertility and recurrent pregnancy loss: a committee opinion. *Fertil Steril* 2013;(99):63.

Practice Committee of the American Society for Reproductive Medicine. Diagnostic evaluation of the infertile male: a committee opinion. *Fertil Steril* 2015;(103):18-25.

Practice Committee of the American Society for Reproductive Medicine. Testing and interpreting measures of ovarian reserve: a committee opinion. *Fertil Steril* 2015;(103):9-17.

Practice Committee of the American Society for Reproductive Medicine in collaboration with the Society for Reproductive Endocrinology and Infertility. Optimizing natural fertility: a committee opinion. *Fertil Steril* 2017;(107):52-58.

Seifer DB, Baker VL, Leader B. Age-specific serum anti-Müllerian hormone values for 17,120 women presenting to fertility centers within the United States. *Fertil Steril* 2011;95:747.

Strauss RL, Barbieri JF III, Yen SSC. *Yen & Jaffe's reproductive endocrinology: physiology, pathophysiology, and clinical management.* 7th ed. Philadelphia: Elsevier/Saunders; 2014.

World Health Organization. *Meeting to develop a global consensus on preconception care to reduce maternal and childhood mortality and morbidity.* Annex 3: Health Problems, Problem Behaviours and Risk Factors, Infertility/subfertility. Geneva: World Health Organization; 2013:46-9.

Suggested websites

American Society for Reproductive Medicine. www.asrm.org
RESOLVE: The National Infertility Association. www.resolve.org
European Society of Human Reproduction and Embryology. www.eshre.eu
World Health Organization. www.who.int

Guidelines
National society guidelines

Title	Source	Date/full reference
Diagnostic evaluation of the infertile female: a committee opinion	American Society for Reproductive Medicine	*Fertil Steril* 2015 Jun;103(6):e44-50.
Diagnostic evaluation of the infertile male: a committee opinion	American Society for Reproductive Medicine	*Fertil Steril* 2015 Mar;103(3):e18-25.
Management of women with premature ovarian insufficiency	European Society of Human Reproduction and Embryology	*Hum Reprod* 2016 May;31(5):926-37.
Guideline on the management of women with endometriosis	European Society of Human Reproduction and Embryology	*Hum Reprod* 2014 Mar;29(3):400-12.

Additional material for this chapter can be found online at:
www.wiley.com/go/sperling/mountsinai/obstetricsandgynecology

This includes a case study, multiple choice questions, advice for patients, and ICD codes.

CHAPTER 34

Ovulation Induction/ART/IVF/ICSI

Kathryn L. Shaia[1], Alan B. Copperman[2], and Eric Flisser[2]

[1] Duke Fertility Center, Division of Reproductive Endocrinology and Infertility, Department of Obstetrics and Gynecology, Duke University School of Medicine, Durham, NC

[2] Reproductive Medicine Associates of New York; Division of Reproductive Endocrinology and Infertility, Icahn School of Medicine at Mount Sinai, New York, NY

OVERALL BOTTOM LINE

- Ovulation induction is the process of stimulating the development and release of oocytes in anovulatory patients.
- Superovulation is the process of stimulating multifollicular development to improve fecundability in patients with infertility.
- Ovulation disorders occur in up to 25% of women. When a specific cause for anovulation can be identified, treatment of the underlying disorder, such as endocrine dysfunction like hypothyroidism and hyperprolactinemia, often restores normal fertility.
- After excluding intrinsic ovarian abnormalities (e.g. premature ovarian failure), various pharmacological compounds, either oral or injectable, are used to stimulate follicle development to induce oocyte maturation and ovulation.
- For most anovulatory women, no specific dysfunction can be identified. If simple methods fail to induce ovulation, advanced assisted reproductive technologies (ART) are frequently effective, the most common being in vitro fertilization (IVF).
- Assisted reproductive technologies encompass all techniques involving extracorporeal manipulation of oocytes and assisted fertilization, most commonly, IVF and intracytoplasmic sperm injection (ICSI).
- The use of donor gametes (sperm and oocytes) and, in some cases, gestational surrogates also play important roles in modern ART.
- ICSI, the injection of a sperm cell into the oocyte, can be used to overcome severe abnormalities of sperm production.
- ICSI is also utilized with IVF for other etiologies of infertility in the presence of normal semen parameters, such as previously documented failure of conventional fertilization.

Indications

Indications for ovulation induction and controlled ovarian hyperstimulation

- Hypothalamic-pituitary-ovarian axis dysfunction
  - Metabolic dysfunction
    - Excessive exercise
    - Eating disorders
    - Extreme weight loss
    - Extreme stress
    - Anovulation and oligoovulation
    - Polycystic ovary syndrome (PCOS)
  - Endocrine disorders
    - Hyperprolactinemia

Mount Sinai Expert Guides: Obstetrics and Gynecology, First Edition. Edited by Rhoda Sperling.
© 2020 John Wiley & Sons Ltd. Published 2020 by John Wiley & Sons Ltd.
Companion Website: www.wiley.com/go/sperling/mountsinai/obstetricsandgynecology

  - ■ Congenital adrenal hyperplasia
  - ■ Cushing disease or syndrome
  - ■ Acromegaly
  - ■ Thyroid dysfunction
  - ■ Sheehan syndrome
  - ■ Empty sella syndrome
  - ■ Panhypopituitarism
- Idiopathic (unexplained) infertility

Indications for IVF
- Absent, obstructed or severely damaged Fallopian tubes
- Severe male factor infertility
- Diminished ovarian reserve
- Recurrent ovulation induction or controlled ovarian hyperstimulation treatment failure
- Ovulatory dysfunction
- Idiopathic infertility
- Hypogonadotropic hypogonadism
- Recurrent intrauterine insemination failure
- Preimplantation genetic diagnosis (PGD)
- Fertility preservation

Procedure
Ovulation induction
- Oral ovulation induction agents stimulate increased gonadotropin secretion by decreasing negative feedback effects of estrogen on the pituitary.
- Follicle number, follicle growth, and the uterine lining are all monitored with transvaginal ultrasound in conjunction with serum estradiol levels.
- Serum estradiol levels can complement ultrasonography in evaluating the maturation and growth of the developing follicles because 200–400 pg/mL estradiol per mature follicle is expected.
- Monitoring serum estradiol can also be used to anticipate and avoid ovarian hyperstimulation syndrome (OHSS).
- Once follicles reach approximately 18 mm in diameter, ovulation may be induced.
- Ovulation is typically achieved via administration of human chorionic gonadotropin (hCG), gonadotropin-releasing hormone (GnRH) analogs, or both.

Clomiphene citrate
- Clomiphene citrate, a selective estrogen receptor modulator (SERM), has traditionally been the drug of choice for ovulation induction in anovulatory women.
- Clomiphene is administered orally for 5 days, typically beginning on the third to fifth day after the onset of a spontaneous or progestin-induced menses. In women with amenorrhea, treatment can begin immediately if pregnancy has been excluded.
- In successful treatment cycles, one or more follicles grow to maturity with a concomitant rise in serum estrogen levels that ultimately triggers a lutenizing hormone (LH) surge and ovulation.

Aromatase inhibitors
- Aromatase inhibitors can also induce ovulation by inhibiting the enzyme that catalyzes the rate-limiting step in estrogen production.
- These agents decrease circulating estrogen levels, resulting in a compensatory increase in pituitary gonadotropin secretion due to decreased feedback inhibition, thus stimulating follicle development.

- Letrozole (2.5–7.5 mg daily) and anastrozole (1 mg daily) in 5-day courses have been used in a similar manner to clomiphene treatment (e.g. cycle days 3–7).

Gonadotropins

- Recombinant and urinary extracts can be used directly to stimulate follicle development in patients with no response to clomiphene or letrozole, previous unsuccessful treatment with oral agents, pituitary insufficiency, or hypothalamic dysfunction.
- Because of an increased risk of side effects such as multiple gestation and ovarian hyperstimulation syndrome, gonadotropin use requires careful monitoring by ultrasonography and serum estradiol levels.
- Additionally, it is more time consuming for the patient and more expensive than the oral agents.
- Mimicking the effects of the LH surge, hCG, or GnRH agonists are used to trigger ovulation.

IVF

- Patients who fail ovulation induction or those who do not qualify for a trial of ovulation induction (e.g. absent or abnormal fallopian tubes) may proceed to IVF.
- IVF begins with controlled ovarian hyperstimulation (COH). Most methods of COH include utilizing a combination of gonadotropins and GnRH agonists or a combination of gonadotropins and GnRH antagonists.
- Follicle number, follicle growth, and the uterine lining are all monitored with transvaginal ultrasound in conjunction with serum estradiol levels.
- Multifollicle development improves the efficiency of IVF.
- Transvaginal oocyte retrieval is performed after adequate follicle development has been achieved.
- To collect oocytes, typically a needle is passed through the vaginal fornices into the ovaries using transvaginal ultrasound guidance. Aspirating follicular fluid draws the oocytes into a test tube (Figure 34.1).
- Following oocyte pickup, fertilization is achieved via conventional insemination or ICSI.

IVF Procedure

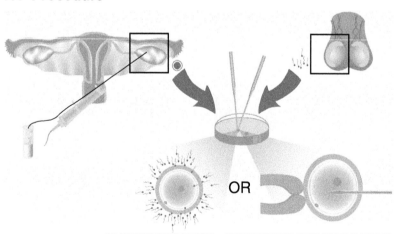

IVF (IN VITRO FERTILIZATION)   ICSI (INTRACYTOPLASMIC SPERM INJECTION)

Steps for in vitro fertilization:
1. Female is given hormone treatment to stimulate egg production
2. Eggs are retrieved transvaginally from female's uterus
3. Eggs are combined with sperm in a culture dish for fertilization
4. Fertilized eggs, or embryos, are placed in an incubator
5. Embryos are implanted in the female's uterus or stored for future transfer

Figure 34.1 Schematic representation and description of IVF procedure. Photo courtesy of Reproductive Medicine Associates of NY, 2017. See color version on website.

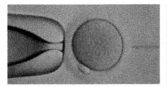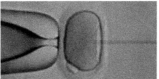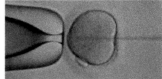

Figure 34.2 ICSI. An oocyte is stabilized by a holding pipette. The injection pipette contains a single sperm. The sperm is injected into the oocyte via the injection pipette penetrating the zona pellucida and plasma membrane. Photo credit: Richard Slifkin, © Reproductive Medicine Associates of New York, 2017.

- During the ICSI procedure, a single sperm is immobilized, drawn into a pipette, and injected into the oolemma (Figure 34.2).
- Fertilized embryos are typically cultured in incubators for 3 or 5 days. They are examined at intervals to assess development characteristics and to determine which embryos have arrested. After embryo culture, one or more embryos are returned to the patient's uterus.
- Supernumerary embryos may be cryopreserved for use in future IVF cycles.
- Professional guidelines exist for determining an appropriate number of embryos to transfer in order to enhance the likelihood of pregnancy and minimize the likelihood of multiple pregnancy and its potential complications.

Preimplantation genetic screening and/or diagnosis
- Preimplantation genetic testing can be used to diagnose embryos carrying genetic disease in patients known to be at risk in the form of preimplantation genetic diagnosis (PGD), whereas preimplantation genetic screening (PGS) can be employed to identify aneuploid embryos.
- For couples at risk of transmitting a specific genetic disease or abnormality to their offspring, IVF with PGD provides a means to identify and exclude affected embryos and thereby avoid that risk.
- PGD is applied to couples carrying autosomal dominant, autosomal recessive, sex-linked disorders, or balanced chromosomal translocations.
- Embryo biopsy is performed by creating a hole in the zona pellucida using a laser, acid Tyrode's solution, or a sharpened glass needle.
- Blastomeres are extracted using a small suction pipette.
- Genetic analysis is performed on a single blastomere, multiple trophectoderm cells, or on polar bodies, depending on the goal of the test being performed.
- Patients may use the results of preimplantation genetic testing to select an embryo for transfer that is euploid, and in the case of PGD, is lacking specific gene mutations.

Management of complications
Ectopic pregnancy
- Ectopic pregnancy occurs when embryo implantation occurs in an extrauterine location.
- Patients undergoing infertility treatment have higher rates of ectopic gestation, either from preexisting abnormal anatomic factors (Müllerian and tubal), from altered hormone environment that changes normal cell function, or from the presence of multiple embryos in the reproductive tract.
- Most ectopic pregnancies arise in the ampulla of the fallopian tube, although rarer cases involve the cornua, isthmus, or fimbria of the tube, the ovary, and other sites.
- Patients undergoing ART procedures have twice the risk of ectopic pregnancy as the general population (1–3% of all pregnancies from embryo transfer).
- Ectopic pregnancies are classically detected due to abdominal pain, delayed onset of menses, and irregular vaginal bleeding. However, early ultrasound may allow for diagnosis prior to the onset of symptoms.
- Medical and surgical management options exist for treatment of ectopic pregnancy.
- Unstable patients, patients with contraindications to medical management, patients unable to perform required follow-up, and patients with recurrent ectopic pregnancy are managed surgically, frequently using minimally invasive techniques.

Ovarian hyperstimulation syndrome (OHSS)

- Ovarian hyperstimulation syndrome is an uncommon but serious complication associated with ovarian stimulation.
- The syndrome is characterized by varying degrees of ovarian enlargement, ascites, hemoconcentration, hypercoagulability, and electrolyte imbalances.
- Patients with OHSS may present with abdominal distention, abdominal discomfort, and nausea. Severe OHSS can lead to serious and potentially fatal complications, including pleural effusion, acute renal insufficiency, and venous thromboembolism.
- Risk factors include PCOS, multifollicular development, and high serum estradiol levels.
- Treatment may require fluid replacement to maintain intravascular volume and other supportive care. Prophylactic anticoagulation may be indicated in some cases of severe OHSS.

Multiple gestation

- The incidence of a twin pregnancy is 8% (triplets, 0.5%) after use of clomiphene.
- Increasing numbers of embryos transferred during IVF therapy increases the probability of high order multiple pregnancy.
- Complications of multiple pregnancy include increased risk of miscarriage, premature contractions, premature labor and delivery, postpartum hemorrhage, transfusion, surgical delivery, fetal demise, gestational diabetes, hypertensive disorders of pregnancy, and permanent handicap to neonates.

Follow-up

- After successful embryo transfer, the patient will follow up to confirm an intrauterine pregnancy.
- Exogenous hormone supplementation is tapered to coincide with increasing placental production of progesterone.
- Patients may return to transfer previously cryopreserved embryos for subsequent pregnancies at a future date.

Algorithm 34.1 Simplified management/treatment algorithm[†]

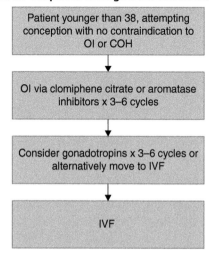

[†]Algorithms for management of infertility patients are heavily influenced and adapted to additional case-specific factors such as patient age, family building goals, and infertility diagnosis.

Miscellaneous
Time off from work
- Patients typically require at least 1 day off from work for oocyte retrieval. Ovarian stimulation and monitoring can typically be arranged to avoid significant disruption of daily obligations.

Nursing considerations
- Registered nurses are vital to the ART setting. They provide education, counseling, support, and nursing care to patients seeking assistance with conception.
- This role requires structured orientation to the clinical setting and demonstrated competence in the specialty.

Reading list
Fritz M, Speroff L. *Clinical gynecologic endocrinology and infertility*. Baltimore: Williams & Wilkins; 2011.

Fritz MA, Dodson WC, Meldrum D, et al. Infertility. In: *Precis, an update in obstetrics and gynecology: reproductive endocrinology*. 3rd ed. Washington, DC: American College of Obstetricians and Gynecologists; 2007, p. 161.

Hull MG, Glazener CM, Kelly NJ, et al. Population study of causes, treatment, and outcome of infertility. *Br Med J (Clin Res Ed)* 1985;291:1693.

Michalakis KG, DeCherney AH, Penzias AS. Chapter 57. Assisted reproductive technologies: in vitro fertilization & related techniques. In: DeCherney AH, Nathan L, Laufer N, et al., eds. *Current diagnosis & treatment: obstetrics & gynecology*. 11th ed. New York, NY: McGraw-Hill; 2013.

Practice Committee of the American Society for Reproductive Medicine. Effectiveness and treatment for unexplained infertility: a committee opinion. *Fertil Steril* 2006;86(5 Suppl 1):S111-4.

Practice Committees of the American Society for Reproductive Medicine; Society for Assisted Reproductive Technology. Intracytoplastic sperm injection (ICSI) for non-male factor infertility: a committee opinion. *Fertil Steril* 2012;98(6):1395-9.

Practice Committee of the American Society for Reproductive Medicine; Practice Committee of the Society for Assisted Reproductive Technology; Practice Committee of the Society of Reproductive Biology and Technology. Revised minimum standards for practices offering assisted reproductive technologies: a committee opinion. *Fertil Steril* 2014;102(3):682-6.

Practice Committee of Society for Assisted Reproductive Technology; Practice Committee of American Society for Reproductive Medicine. Preimplantation genetic testing: a committee opinion. *Fertil Steril* 2008; 90(5 Suppl):S136-43.

Practice Committee of Society for Assisted Reproductive Technology; Practice Committee of American Society for Reproductive Medicine. Guidance on the limits to the number of embryos to transfer: a committee opinion. *Fertil Steril* 2017;107(4):101-3.

Strauss RL, Barbieri JF III, Yen SSC. *Yen & Jaffe's reproductive endocrinology: physiology, pathophysiology, and clinical management*. Philadelphia: Elsevier/Saunders; 2014.

Suggested websites
American Society for Reproductive Medicine. www.asrm.org
RESOLVE: The National Infertility Association. www.resolve.org
European Society of Human Reproduction and Embryology. www.eshre.eu
World Health Organization. www.who.int

Additional material for this chapter can be found online at:
www.wiley.com/go/sperling/mountsinai/obstetricsandgynecology

This includes patient education materials, ICD codes, and SNOMED codes.
The following image is available in color: Figure 34.1.

CHAPTER 35

Polycystic Ovary Syndrome

Rashmi Kudesia[1] and Alan B. Copperman[2]
[1] Houston Methodist Hospital, CCRM Fertility, Houston, TX
[2] Reproductive Medicine Associates of New York; Division of Reproductive Endocrinology and Infertility, Icahn School of Medicine at Mount Sinai, New York, NY

OVERALL BOTTOM LINE

- Polycystic ovary syndrome (PCOS) is a multifaceted syndrome with gynecologic, endocrine, metabolic, and psychiatric sequelae.
- PCOS diagnosis is challenging in adolescence; however, the diagnosis should be considered and explained to the patient as early as possible.
- Most women with PCOS will be able to conceive and should receive fertility counseling to allow for appropriate utilization of contraception and ovulation induction treatment in accord with their reproductive life plan.
- Women with PCOS, even those at healthy weights, require enhanced screening for cardiometabolic disease.
- Early and ongoing intervention to prevent cardiometabolic disease and other PCOS-related comorbidities may result in normalization of health risks by the time of the menopausal transition.

Background
Definition of disease

- Polycystic ovary syndrome is most commonly defined by the Rotterdam criteria, requiring at least two of the following three signs/symptoms: (a) oligo- or anovulation, (b) clinical or biochemical evidence of hyperandrogenism, and (c) polycystic ovarian morphology (Figure 35.1).

Disease classification

- In addition to Rotterdam criteria, alternate classification systems include (a) National Institutes of Health (NIH) criteria: oligo- or anovulation with clinical or biochemical hyperandrogenism, and (b) Androgen Excess & PCOS (AEPCOS) Society criteria: clinical or biochemical hyperandrogenism with one or both of the remaining criteria, which include oligo- or anovulation and polycystic ovarian morphology.

Incidence/prevalence

- PCOS is the most common endocrine disorder in women.
- By Rotterdam criteria, prevalence may be as high as 15%; by NIH criteria, estimates range from 6–10% (Fauser et al. 2012).
- In infertile populations, PCOS prevalence varies highly by ethnicity and may be as much as 40% in highest risk infertile populations such as South Asians (Kudesia et al. 2017; Wang and Alvaro 2013; Zhao and Qiao 2013).

Mount Sinai Expert Guides: Obstetrics and Gynecology, First Edition. Edited by Rhoda Sperling.
© 2020 John Wiley & Sons Ltd. Published 2020 by John Wiley & Sons Ltd.
Companion Website: www.wiley.com/go/sperling/mountsinai/obstetricsandgynecology

Economic impact
- In the United States, the mean annual cost of evaluating and treating reproductive-aged women with PCOS has been estimated at $4.36 billion (Azziz et al. 2005).

Etiology
- The exact etiology of PCOS remains unknown.
- Familial associations are frequently observed, with metabolic sequelae noted in both female and male family members.
- Genome-wide association studies (GWAS) have identified possible candidate genes related to PCOS and its related comorbidities, but this work remains in early stages.

Pathology/pathogenesis
- The exact pathogenesis remains unknown but characteristic pathology includes elevated secretion and/or concentrations of luteinizing hormone (LH). In turn, elevated LH levels lead to excess activity of ovarian theca cells, favoring an androgenic, rather than estrogenic environment.
- An elevated anti-Müllerian hormone (AMH) level is frequently observed in women with PCOS, but it remains unclear whether AMH may be pathogenic or simply a manifestation of the syndrome.
- The androgenic ovarian environment leads to follicular atresia and failure of follicles to mature and ovulate, as well as other symptoms of hyperandrogenism, including hirsutism, acne, and androgenic alopecia (Figure 35.2).
- In association, PCOS women often demonstrate peripheral insulin resistance, which has been linked to serum hyperandrogenemia and ovarian hyperthecosis, though the exact mechanism(s) linking these aspects of the syndrome remain controversial.

Predictive/risk factors
- Precise odds ratios are not available for prediction of PCOS and likely vary between different patient populations. However, a number of risk factors have been identified and include:

Risk factor
Family history
Obesity
Type 1, type 2, and gestational diabetes mellitus

https://dx.doi.org/10.2147%2FCLEP.S37559

Prevention

> **BOTTOM LINE/CLINICAL PEARLS**
> - No interventions have been demonstrated to prevent the development of the disease.
> - Though lifestyle modification prior to conception has the theoretical potential for mitigating expression of PCOS phenotype in offspring due to healthier intrauterine fetal programming, this theory remains unproven as yet.

Screening
- The role of screening in PCOS is primarily for secondary prevention of associated comorbidities.
- Timely diagnosis would assist in secondary prevention, and could be enhanced by universal utilization of the menstrual cycle as a vital sign (American Academy of Pediatrics Committee on Adolescence 2006). This screening mechanism reinforces patient understanding of a normal menstrual cycle and helps alert providers to patients with irregular cycles, who may require evaluation for possible PCOS.

Secondary prevention

- Data suggest improved ovulation rates and obstetric outcomes with preconception lifestyle interventions (Legro et al. 2015).
- Lifestyle interventions can reduce symptomatology of disease, including body composition, hyperandrogenism, and insulin resistance (Moran et al. 2011).

Diagnosis

> **BOTTOM LINE/CLINICAL PEARLS**
> - Patients with PCOS will typically present with symptoms including: irregular menstrual cycles (sometimes including very heavy anovulatory bleeding), difficulty maintaining a healthy weight even at a young age, or excessive facial or body hair.
> - Exam findings may include hirsutism or androgenic hair distribution, overweight or obese body mass index (BMI), or abnormal weight distribution as measured by waist:hip ratio (WHR), and/or signs of insulin resistance, such as acanthosis nigricans.
> - Transvaginal ultrasound may demonstrate polycystic ovarian morphology in at least one ovary, defined as an ovarian volume of 10 cm^3 or greater, and/or a count of 12 or more preantral follicles (2–9 mm); with a high-resolution probe (transducer frequency ≥ 8 MHz), one may utilize stricter criteria of 25 or more preantral follicles.
> - Androgen testing should include at least total testosterone and dehydroepiandrosterone sulfate (DHEAS).
> - Fasting lipid profile and 2-hour glucose tolerance testing (GTT) may identify cardiometabolic dysfunction.

Differential diagnosis

Differential diagnosis	Features
Late-onset congenital adrenal hyperplasia	Will likely present with more severe hirsutism or virilization; will demonstrate elevated serum 17-hydroxyprogesterone (17-OHP) levels
Androgen-producing tumor	Will likely present with more severe hirsutism or virilization; serum androgen level(s) will be extremely elevated
Cushing's syndrome	May present with additional pathognomic stigmata of Cushing's; if tested, will have elevations in 24-hour urinary free cortisol, late-night serum cortisol, and/or a.m. cortisol after dexamethasone suppression
Primary ovarian insufficiency	May report other hypoestrogenic symptoms, such as vaginal dryness or hot flushes
Thyroid disease	Symptoms may reflect sluggish metabolism (weight gain, fatigue, dry skin, cold intolerance)
Hyperprolactinemia	May report galactorrhea
Structural pathology (polyps, fibroids)	Bleeding pattern may include postcoital spotting (polyp); bleeding may be accompanied by dysmenorrhea or abnormally heavy menstrual flow; saline-infusion ultrasound will identify intrauterine lesions

Typical presentation

- PCOS will typically present as the young postmenarcheal female who reports a long-standing history of irregular or absent periods. This pattern may be distressing to her because it appears abnormal; because the bleeds are unpredictable, heavy, and/or possibly disruptive to school or work; or because she is having difficulty conceiving. Some women will also report hirsutism, weight issues, or a history of mood disorders. In many instances, the PCOS patient will have previously been put on birth control to help regulate her menses or prevent formation or recurrence of ovarian cysts.

Clinical diagnosis
See Algorithm 35.1.

Algorithm 35.1 Diagnostic algorithm for PCOS
1. Full menstrual history and assessment of clinical hyperandrogenism
2. Obtain basic bloodwork (androgen panel, TSH, prolactin) and ovarian ultrasound
3a. If has cycles (unclear ovulatory), do day 3 bw and midluteal progesterone
3b. If amenorrheic, random hormone profile

History
- Age at menarche
- Menstrual pattern, including frequency, amount of bleeding, and changes over time
- Gynecologic history, including history of ovarian cysts
- Changes in weight, and if so, whether these correlate with any changes in menstrual pattern
- Recent medical diagnoses or metabolic screening
- Dietary and exercise habits
- Excessive facial or body hair, acne, or male-pattern baldness or hair distribution
- Symptoms of anxiety and/or depression
- Medication history, including prior utilization of birth control
- Family history of PCOS, infertility, and/or cardiometabolic disease

Physical examination
- A full physical examination is indicated, with specific attention to:
- Height and weight to evaluate body mass index
- Body fat distribution, looking for elevated waist:hip ratio
- Elevations in blood pressure or heart rate
- Signs of insulin resistance (acanthosis nigricans, skin tags)
- Presence and degree of hirsutism or virilization (Figure 35.2)
- Presence of any symptoms that might indicate an alternate diagnosis (e.g. Cushing's syndrome may be suggested by findings such as purple abdominal striae, buffalo hump, peripheral wasting, and so forth)

Disease severity classification
- Meeting the classic NIH criteria is associated with a more severe PCOS phenotype, and higher risk of cardiometabolic sequelae. Nonetheless, screening guidelines should be applied similarly to women regardless of which diagnostic criteria they meet.

Laboratory diagnosis
List of diagnostic tests
- Androgen panel (ideally performed by liquid chromatography-tandem mass spectrometry rather than immunoassay) should be performed on all women to rule out other virilizing etiologies. The panel should include total testosterone, DHEAS and 17-OHP (may be falsely elevated in luteal phase) at minimum; depending on available laboratory resources, could consider bioavailable testosterone and androstenedione.
- Hormonal profile (β-hCG [human chorionic gonadotropin], estradiol, follicle stimulating hormone/LH, progesterone) should be obtained on all women. The profile can be tested on days 2–3 if the patient reports even somewhat regular periods, or at random if she is amenorrheic or very irregular.
- Thyroid stimulating hormone (TSH) and prolactin should be tested on all women with irregular cycles to rule out these aberrations as primary etiology.

- A serum AMH level is not required for diagnosis but may assist in assessing the severity of disease, if extremely elevated compared to age-based norms.

List of imaging techniques
- Transvaginal ultrasound should be obtained with antral follicle count and measurement of ovarian volume (Figure 35.1).

Potential pitfalls/common errors made regarding diagnosis of disease
- Though PCOS is the most common etiology for ovulatory dysfunction, women with irregular cycles may be misdiagnosed with PCOS without a full evaluation or strictly meeting criteria.
- Lean women with PCOS may be missed because they do not present in a stereotypical fashion.
- Adolescents may be diagnosed prematurely or missed due to the overlap of pubertal and PCOS symptoms.

Treatment
Treatment rationale
- There are five main domains that may require treatment: irregular bleeding, hirsutism, weight, mood disorders, and infertility. Each should be assessed regularly. Not all domains will affect all patients, and primary concerns may shift over time.
- Irregular bleeding: assess the risk for endometrial disease and perform biopsy if indicated (Committee on Practice Bulletins—Gynecology 2013). Even a 5% weight loss may improve menstrual regularity. First-line treatment options include hormonal therapy, such as oral contraceptives (OCPs), or the Mirena intrauterine device.
- Hirsutism: Options include mechanical approaches (plucking, threading), hair removal procedures (electrolysis or laser hair removal), and medical (OCPs +/– anti-androgen therapy).
- Weight: Monitor weight, BMI, and WHR regularly; discuss nutrition consult and exercise regimen. Metabolic assessment should include a fasting lipid panel and 2-hour 75 g oral glucose tolerance test and/or hemoglobin A1c. Treat abnormal results as indicated, including referral to appropriate subspecialists (medical endocrinology, cardiology). Consider bariatric surgery for women with BMI > 40 or those with BMI > 35 and weight-associated comorbidities.
- Mood disorders: Screen for anxiety and depression; refer and treat as appropriate.
- Infertility: emphasize preconception health optimization. Once the patient is cleared for conception, first-line treatment includes ovulation induction with letrozole (preferred) or clomiphene citrate. Second-line treatments include escalation to injectable gonadotropins or ovarian diathermy, with in vitro fertilization as a third-line option (Thessaloniki 2008).
- See Algorithm 35.2.

Algorithm 35.2 Management/treatment algorithm for PCOS

1. Diagnosis made
2. Counsel regarding risks and lifestyle intervention, offer nutrition consultation
3. Trying to conceive?
   a. If yes – confirm appropriate preconception health and then proceed – letrozole first, if no response consider clomiphene citrate; second line: gonadotropins, ovarian drilling, IVF
   b. If no – evaluate for other complaints and treat as appropriate

Heavy irregular bleeding or long periods of unopposed estrogen? Consider endometrial biopsy
Contraindications to hormonal therapy?
If yes, consider Mirena
If no, consider OCPs or Mirena
If hirsutism, and OCPs insufficient, consider add anti-androgenic medication
If mood disorders, refer to mental health professional
If weight, refer to bariatric surgery

When to hospitalize
- The main reason for hospitalization required for PCOS would be severe ovarian hyperstimulation after fertility treatment with injectable gonadotropins.
- Signs of severe hyperstimulation include moderate-to-severe ascites, rapid weight gain, shortness of breath, nausea, and emesis.

Managing the hospitalized patient
- The management of severe hyperstimulation is best summarized in American Society for Reproductive Medicine (ASRM) guidelines but revolves around fluid and electrolyte management, anticoagulation, and supportive care (Practice Committee of the ASRM 2006).

Table of treatment

Treatment	Comments
Conservative • Lifestyle modification	All patients should receive counseling on diet and exercise.
Medical • OCPs regulate irregular bleeding and decrease hair growth. • Anti-androgens (spironolactone, finasteride, flutamide) can be used with OCPs for hirsutism. • Metformin may decrease the progression of metabolic disease • Letrozole (2.5 mg–7.5 mg PO daily x5 days) or clomiphene citrate (50 mg–150 mg PO daily x5 days) are the first choice for ovulation induction; injectable gonadotropins in the context of ovulation induction or in vitro fertilization are second- or third-line options.	Clinical pearls • Some women may have medical contraindications to OCPs.* • Conflicting evidence for one OCP versus another in management of PCOS • Spironolactone may worsen menstrual irregularity. • Flutamide is of limited clinical utility due to risk of hepatotoxicity. • All anti-androgens must be used with contraception given the risk of fetal toxicity. • Metformin often induces GI side effects and the dose should be escalated slowly (over weeks). • Given potential hepatotoxicity of metformin, many providers will confirm normal liver function tests before prescribing, but no guidelines exist for routine monitoring during treatment.
Surgical • Ovarian diathermy (drilling)	• Surgery is an alternative therapy to assist with ovulation induction in those patients failing oral agents.
Radiological • No radiological treatments	
Psychological • Psychotherapy and pharmacological treatments should be utilized for diagnoses of anxiety and/or depression.	• Patients with symptoms of mood disorder should be screened for anxiety and depression and referred to a mental health provider as appropriate.
Complementary • Inositols • Herbal medication	• More data are needed; however, patients who do not tolerate or have contraindications to hormonal therapy may consider treatment with inositols or herbal medication to help regulate their cycles.**
Other	

* See https://www.cdc.gov/reproductivehealth/unintendedpregnancy/pdf/legal_summary-chart_english_final_tag508.pdf for medical eligibility for OCP use.
** For further information on herbal medication and PCOS: https://dx.doi.org/10.1186%2F1472-6882-14-511

Prevention/management of complications
- The main complications in PCOS relate to side effects from hormonal contraceptives or from the treatment of infertility.
- OCPs slightly increase the risk of venous thromboembolism (VTE). As described previously, patients should be appropriately selected for OCP use and evaluated for any symptoms (limb pain, edema, and/or erythema) of VTE.
- The use of ovulation induction agents and particularly injectable gonadotropins increase the risk of multiple gestation. Patients should receive letrozole therapy as first line to minimize this risk, as it is most associated with monofollicular response. Injectable gonadotropins outside of an in vitro fertilization (IVF) cycle should be used very judiciously, and the cycle cancelled if too many follicles develop (>4 or as per provider judgment).
- In an IVF cycle, PCOS patients are at risk for development of severe ovarian hyperstimulation (OHSS). Protocols should be designed to mitigate this risk, using measures such as low dosing, gonadotropin-releasing hormone antagonist with Lupron trigger, deferment of embryo transfer to subsequent cycle, and cabergoline.

CLINICAL PEARLS
- Evaluate each treatment domain (irregular bleeding, weight, hirsutism, mood, and infertility) at regular intervals to ensure all symptoms are addressed.
- All women with PCOS, regardless of weight, have elevated cardiometabolic risks and should be screened more frequently than women without PCOS.
- Encourage young women considering conception in the near future to work on preconception health optimization, including weight and glycemic control, and management of any associated comorbidities.
- Metformin should not be routinely prescribed based on PCOS diagnosis alone, but rather used primarily to slow the progression to type 2 diabetes mellitus for women who appear at risk for development of metabolic syndrome.

Special populations
Pregnancy
- Early screening (around 12 weeks) for gestational diabetes mellitus
- Nutrition and lifestyle counseling throughout pregnancy to prevent excessive weight gain

Children
- Though diagnosis should be delayed until approximately 8 postmenarcheal years so that a mature menstrual cycle can be observed, adolescent females 2–3 years postmenarcheal who display signs or symptoms of PCOS can be considered "at risk". If PCOS is suspected, the diagnosis should be explained to the patient (and her parents or guardians) to diminish anxiety about future fertility or health and treated with lifestyle modification to make improvements in diet and exercise and prevent early weight gain.

Elderly
- PCOS primarily seems to increase health risks during the pre-menopausal years. After the menopausal transition, health risks appear primarily linked to other comorbidities (Kudesia and Neal-Perry 2014).

Others
- The safety profile and efficacy of hormonal contraception and ovulation induction may be diminished in obese women. These risks and the value of preconception optimization of health status, especially in young women looking to conceive, should be discussed.

Prognosis

> **BOTTOM LINE/CLINICAL PEARLS**
> - When managed proactively, most PCOS symptoms can be brought under control; however, the diagnosis is linked to diminished quality of life and women need thorough counseling and an appropriate care team to ensure best prognosis.
> - Long periods of unopposed estrogen predispose to endometrial pathology; however, proper use of progesterone-induced withdrawal bleeds, and endometrial biopsy when appropriate, can minimize this risk.
> - PCOS alone is highly amenable to fertility treatment, and women should feel reassured that barring any additional fertility diagnoses, they will be able to conceive – albeit with assistance in most cases.
> - Based on the available evidence on PCOS women as they pass through the menopausal transition, it appears that health risks post menopause relate primarily to accumulated comorbidities, particularly obesity, and chronologic age.

Natural history of untreated disease
- If untreated, women with PCOS have a much higher risk of weight gain and metabolic disease, as well as infertility and obstetric complications if they conceive (including abnormal birth weights, gestational diabetes, and hypertensive disorders, as well as preterm delivery). They also remain at risk for mood disorders and diminished quality of life.

Prognosis for treated patients
- Most PCOS symptoms can be controlled or at least improved significantly with treatment.
- Postmenopausal women who have avoided cardiometabolic diagnoses during their premenopausal years have a similar overall health prognosis as non-PCOS women in their age group.

Follow-up tests and monitoring
- Enhanced screening throughout the premenopausal years is indicated, given the elevated risks of comorbidities.
- Postmenopause, it appears that women with PCOS can likely follow the same monitoring and screening guidelines as women without PCOS, taking into account any comorbidities they may have developed.

Reading list

American Academy of Pediatrics Committee on Adolescence; American College of Obstetricians and Gynecologists Committee on Adolescent Health Care, Diaz A, Laufer MR, Breech LL. Menstruation in girls and adolescents: using the menstrual cycle as a vital sign. *Pediatrics* 2006 Nov;118(5):2245-50.

Azziz R, Marin C, Hoq L, et al. Health care-related economic burden of the polycystic ovary syndrome during the reproductive life span. *J Clin Endocrinol Metab* 2005 Aug;90(8):4650-8. Epub 2005 Jun 8.

Committee on Practice Bulletins—Gynecology. Practice bulletin no. 136: management of abnormal uterine bleeding associated with ovulatory dysfunction. *Obstet Gynecol* 2013 Jul;122(1):176-85. doi: 10.1097/01.AOG.0000431815.52679.bb.

Dewailly D, Lujan ME, Carmina E, et al. Definition and significance of polycystic ovarian morphology: a task force report from the Androgen Excess and Polycystic Ovary Syndrome Society. *Hum Reprod Update* 2014 May-Jun;20(3):334-52. http://www.ae-society.org/pdf/guidelines/morphology.pdf.

Dunaif A. Insulin resistance and the polycystic ovary syndrome: mechanism and implications for pathogenesis. *Endocr Rev* 1997 Dec;18(6):774-800. https://doi.org/10.1210/edrv.18.6.0318.

Fauser BCJM, Tarlatzis BC, Rebar RW, et al. Consensus on women's health aspects of polycystic ovary syndrome (PCOS): the Amsterdam ESHRE/ASRM-Sponsored 3rd PCOS Consensus Workshop Group. *Fertil Steril* 2012;97(1):28-38.e25. https://doi.org/10.1016/j.fertnstert.2011.09.024.

Kudesia R, Neal-Perry GS. Menopausal implications of polycystic ovarian syndrome. *Semin Reprod Med* 2014 May;32(3):222-9. doi: 10.1055/s-0034-1371094. Epub 2014 Apr 8.

Kudesia R, Illions EH, Lieman HJ. Elevated prevalence of polycystic ovary syndrome and cardiometabolic disease in South Asian infertility patients. *J Immigr Minor Health* 2017 Dec;19(6):1338-42. doi: 10.1007/s10903-016-0454-7.

Legro RS, Dodson WC, Kris-Etherton PM, et al. Randomized controlled trial of preconception interventions in infertile women with polycystic ovary syndrome. *J Clin Endocrinol Metab* 2015 Nov;100(11):4048-58. doi: 10.1210/jc.2015-2778. Epub 2015 Sep 24.

Moran LJ, Hutchison SK, Norman RJ, et al. Lifestyle changes in women with polycystic ovary syndrome. *Cochrane Database Syst Rev* 2011 Feb 16;(2):CD007506. doi: 10.1002/14651858.CD007506.pub2.

Noncontraceptive uses of hormonal contraceptives: ACOG practice bulletin no. 110. http://www.acog.org/Resources-And-Publications/Practice-Bulletins/Committee-on-Practice-Bulletins-Gynecology/Noncontraceptive-Uses-of-Hormonal-Contraceptives.

Practice Committee of the American Society for Reproductive Medicine. Prevention and treatment of moderate and severe ovarian hyperstimulation syndrome: a guideline. *Fertil Steril* 2016 Dec;106(7):1634-47. doi: 10.1016/j.fertnstert.2016.08.048. Epub 2016 Sep 24.

Rotterdam ESHRE/ASRM-Sponsored PCOS Consensus Workshop Group. Revised 2003 consensus on diagnostic criteria and long-term health risks related to polycystic ovary syndrome (PCOS). *Hum Reprod* 2004;19:41-7.

Teede, HJ, Misso ML, Costello MF, et al. International evidence-based guideline for the assessment and management of polycystic ovary syndrome. *Fertil Steril* 2018;110(3):364-79.

Thessaloniki ESHRE/ASRM-Sponsored PCOS Consensus Workshop Group. Consensus on infertility treatment related to polycystic ovary syndrome. *Hum Reprod* 2008 Mar;23(3):462-77. doi: 10.1093/humrep/dem426.

Wang S, Alvero R. Racial and ethnic differences in physiology and clinical symptoms of polycystic ovary syndrome. *Semin Reprod Med* 2013 Sep;31(5):365-9. doi: 10.1055/s-0033-1348895. Epub 2013 Aug 9.

Zhao Y, Qiao J. Ethnic differences in the phenotypic expression of polycystic ovary syndrome. *Steroids* 2013 Aug;78(8):755-60. doi: 10.1016/j.steroids.2013.04.006. Epub 2013 Apr 25.

Suggested websites

Androgen Excess and Polycystic Ovary Syndrome Society. www.ae-society.org
ASRM Polycystic Ovary Syndrome. http://www.asrm.org/topics/topics-index/polycystic-ovary-syndrome-pcos
Endocrine Society. https://www.endocrine.org/topics/female-reproductive-endocrinology

Guidelines
National society guidelines

Title	Source	Date/URL
Diagnosis & treatment of polycystic ovary syndrome	Endocrine Society	2013 http://www.endocrine.org/~/media/endosociety/Files/Publications/Clinical%20Practice%20Guidelines/120513_PCOS_FinalA_2013.pdf
Guide to the best practices in the evaluation and treatment of polycystic ovary syndrome parts 1 & 2	American Association of Clinical Endocrinologists; American College of Endocrinology; Androgen Excess & Polycystic Ovary Syndrome Society	2015 https://doi.org/10.4158/EP15748.DSC https://doi.org/10.4158/EP15748.DSCPT2
Polycystic ovary syndrome	American College of Obstetricians & Gynecologists	2015 https://doi.org/10.1097/AOG.0b013e3181bd12cb

International society guidelines

Title	Source	Date/URL
International evidence-based guideline for the assessment and management of polycystic ovary syndrome	ASRM, ESHRE, Monash University, and CREPCOS	2018 https://www.monash.edu/medicine/sphpm/mchri/pcos/guideline

Evidence

Type of evidence	Title and comment	Date/URL
Randomized controlled trial (RCT)	Clomiphene, metformin, or both for infertility in the polycystic ovary syndrome Comment: Demonstrated superiority of clomiphene over metformin alone or dual therapy for ovulation induction.	2007 https://doi.org/10.1056/NEJMoa063971
RCT	Letrozole versus clomiphene for infertility in the polycystic ovary syndrome Comment: Demonstrated superiority of letrozole over clomiphene for ovulation induction.	2014 https://doi.org/10.1056/NEJMoa1313517
RCT	Randomized controlled trial of preconception interventions in infertile women with polycystic ovary syndrome Comment: Demonstrated positive impact of preconception health optimization with a lifestyle program as compared to oral contraceptive therapy.	2015 https://doi.org/10.1210/jc.2015-2778
Cohort	Benefit of delayed fertility therapy with preconception weight loss over immediate therapy in obese women with PCOS Comment: Compared data from two separate clinical trials to show improved ovulation and live birth with delayed therapy preceded by lifestyle modification.	2016 https://doi.org/10.1210/jc.2016-1659

Images

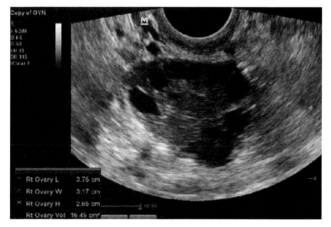

Figure 35.1 A stereotypical image of a polycystic ovary on transvaginal ultrasound, with enlarged ovarian volume and peripheral follicles in a "string of pearls" morphology. Credit: Rashmi Kudesia, MD MSc.

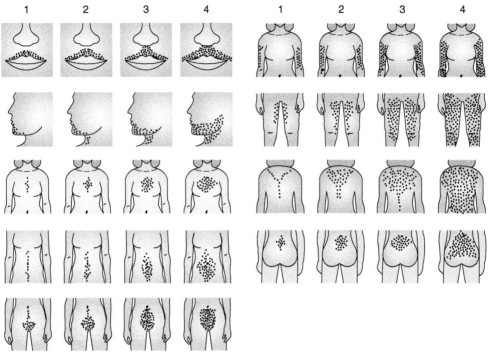

Figure 35.2 Modified Ferriman-Gallwey scoring for hirsutism. Scores from 0–4 are assigned at each of nine body sites. In most ethnicities, a score ≥ 8 is consistent with hirsutism. In East Asian women, lower cutoffs of 3–5 have been used. Credit: Azziz R et al. *Androgen Excess Disorders in Women: Polycystic Ovary Syndrome and Other Disorders.* 2nd ed. Totowa, NJ: Humana Press; 2006.

Additional material for this chapter can be found online at:
www.wiley.com/go/sperling/mountsinai/obstetricsandgynecology

This includes a case study, advice for patients, and ICD codes.

CHAPTER 36

Recurrent Pregnancy Loss

Daniel E. Stein and Alan B. Copperman

Reproductive Medicine Associates of New York; Division of Reproductive Endocrinology and Infertility, Icahn School of Medicine at Mount Sinai, New York, NY

OVERALL BOTTOM LINE
- RPL is commonly defined as two or more clinical miscarriages.
- Etiologies include idiopathic, genetic, anatomic, endocrinological, immunological, thrombotic, and environmental.
- Evaluation requires a history and physical examination, assessment of the uterine cavity, and genetic, hormonal, and immunologic testing.
- Management is focused on treatment of correctable factors and/or selection of euploid embryos by preimplantation genetic testing (PGT).

Background
Definition of disease
- Currently there is no universal consensus on the definition of RPL. The medical literature is replete with definitions ranging from three or more consecutive pregnancy losses before 22 weeks of gestation to simply two or more clinical miscarriages, the definition used by the American Society for Reproductive Medicine (ASRM). In this review, the ASRM definition is used.

Incidence/prevalence
- The prevalence of RPL depends on the definition used. Despite a wide range of prevalence estimates throughout the RPL literature, RPL is generally estimated to occur in approximately 1 to 5% of women trying to conceive.

Etiologies
- Approximately half of cases of RPL can be attributed to identifiable causes. The remaining cases are considered idiopathic.

Idiopathic
Chromosomal/genetic abnormalities
- Sporadic embryo aneuploidy during gametogenesis
  - Meiotic nondisjunction
  - Premature separation of sister chromatids
  - Postmeiotic events
- Inherited aneuploidies
- Transmission to conceptus of a parental structural chromosomal rearrangement (e.g. balanced reciprocal or Robertsonian translocations, or inversions)
- Possible mutations in genes involved with spindle formation, oxidative stress, and mitochondrial function

---

Mount Sinai Expert Guides: Obstetrics and Gynecology, First Edition. Edited by Rhoda Sperling.
© 2020 John Wiley & Sons Ltd. Published 2020 by John Wiley & Sons Ltd.
Companion Website: www.wiley.com/go/sperling/mountsinai/obstetricsandgynecology

Anatomical
- Congenital anomalies (septate, unicornuate, and bicornuate uteri)
- Acquired uterine abnormalities (leiomyomata, polyps, and synechiae)

Immunologic
- Abnormal maternal immune response to the conceptus
- Antiphospholipid antibody syndrome (discussed later)

Endocrine
- Thyroid
  - Frank hypothyroidism
  - Elevated in-range thyroid stimulating hormone (TSH) levels in euthyroid women
  - Elevated antithyroid antibodies in euthyroid women
- Hyperprolactinemia
- Polycystic ovary syndrome (PCOS)
- Obesity
- Insulin resistance
- Diabetes mellitus

Environmental and lifestyle
- Smoking
- Alcohol

Genetic
- Karyotyping studies of abortus tissue have shown that approximately 60% of first-trimester miscarriages are cytogenetically abnormal, a likely underestimate as karyotypes may not detect mosaicism, microdeletions or duplications, and/or single gene mutations. Additional limitations of karyotyping include culture failure and contamination with maternal cell DNA.
- Chromosome abnormalities during gametogenesis result from meiotic nondisjunction, premature separation of sister chromatids, and postmeiotic events. Germline mosaicism and/or structural chromosome abnormalities in one or both parents (e.g. translocations and inversions) may also contribute to recurrent aneuploidy. Abnormal karyotypes have been detected in approximately 7% of couples. RPL has also been linked to sperm aneuploidy and DNA damage.
- Limitations of karyotyping have led to the development of newer technologies including array comparative genomic hybridization (array CGH), quantitative fluorescent polymerase chain reaction (QF-PCR), and next generation sequencing (NGS) to improve the detection of chromosome defects such as mosaicism and segmental aneuploidies. Currently, the percentage of RPL due to chromosome or subchromosome abnormalities is estimated to be 40–50%.
- Parental karyotyping might in some cases help determine the risk of future miscarriages, yet some data suggest that when one partner carries a structural chromosome rearrangement there is a similar chance of live birth compared to noncarrier couples. The ASRM, however, continues to recommend parental karyotyping as part of the standard evaluation of couples with RPL.

Anatomical
- Approximately 10–15% of miscarriages are the result of congenital or acquired anatomic abnormalities. Although it is unclear how uterine anomalies lead to RPL, a mass effect, diminished uterine vascular flow, and/or local inflammation might be involved. Congenital abnormalities in the development of the müllerian duct(s) include unicornuate, bicornuate, didelphic, and septate uteri. An increased rate of spontaneous abortions, preterm labor, and abnormal presentations have been demonstrated in women

with bicornuate uteri and didelphic uteri but normal reproductive outcomes are common. The most common anomaly, uterine septae, are associated with a 45–65% risk of miscarriage, three times the rate of women with normal uteri. Hysteroscopic resection of septae have been shown to lower miscarriage rates from > 60% to 10–15%. There is a lack of prospective, randomized studies, however, some studies have demonstrated the benefits of hysteroscopic resection of uterine septae.

- Acquired uterine anomalies include intrauterine adhesions, leiomyomata, and endometrial polyps. Women with RPL have a higher prevalence of uterine leiomyomata than women without RPL. Submucosal leiomyomata can distort the endometrial cavity resulting in early pregnancy loss. The benefit of myomectomy on miscarriage rates has not been established in well-controlled, randomized trials. Few data exist regarding the role of endometrial polyps and/or uterine synechiae on pregnancy loss, and prospective, well-controlled studies on the effects of correcting these conditions in couples with RPL are lacking.

Immune

- Implantation failure might result from abnormal alloimmune or autoimmune responses to the conceptus. Phospholipids (PL) are involved with cohesion of cytotrophoblasts and syncytiotrophoblasts and invasion of the placenta into the myometrium and spiral arteries. Antiphospholipid antibodies (APA) are linked to an increased incidence of first- and second-trimester miscarriages, intrauterine growth restriction, and placental insufficiency. Repeated miscarriages occur more frequently in women with elevated APAs than in women without these antibodies, and the prevalence of APAs has been found to be higher in women with RPL than those without RPL. Common APAs that have been linked to pregnancy loss include lupus anticoagulants (LA), anticardiolipin antibodies (aCL), and antibodies that target phospholipid binding proteins (e.g. [beta]$_2$-glycoprotein-1 [ß$_2$ GLP-1]). Standardized clinical assays for these three APAs have been well established; it is not recommended to test for other APAs.

- The diagnosis of antiphospholipid antibody syndrome (APS) requires at least one clinical criterion and at least one of each of the following clinical and laboratory criteria:

CLINICAL CRITERIA
- Vascular thrombosis
- Pregnancy morbidity:
  - ≥1 death of a morphologically-normal fetus (by ultrasonography or direct exam of fetus) after 10 weeks gestation
  - ≥1 delivery of a morphologically-normal neonate before 34 weeks gestation due to eclampsia, severe preeclampsia, or placental insufficiency
  - ≥3 unexplained, consecutive spontaneous abortions before 10 weeks gestation (must exclude maternal and paternal chromosome abnormalities and maternal anatomic causes)

LABORATORY CRITERIA
- Lupus anticoagulant (LAC) (antibodies that prolong phospholipid-dependent coagulation assays)
  - Measure in plasma on at least two occasions at least 12 weeks apart
- Anticardiolipin antibody (ACA)
  - Measure IgG or IgM (>40 GPL or MPL, or >99th percentile) on at least two occasions at least 12 weeks apart
- Anti-β2-glycoprotein-1 (antibodies that target phospholipid binding proteins)
  - Measure IgG or IgM in serum or plasma at a titer of >99th percentile for that laboratory (ELISA) on at least two occasions at least 12 weeks apart

---

- Heparin interferes with binding of immune complexes to trophoblast cells. For women with APS-related RPL, low-dose aspirin and subcutaneous heparin twice a day is standard treatment.

Thrombosis

- Pregnancy is a hypercoagulable state. Circulating levels of clotting factors (II, VII, VIII, X, and XII) and fibrinogen are elevated and fibrinolysis is diminished. Although some studies have reported an association between hereditary thrombophilias (e.g. factor V Leiden and factor II genes) and fetal loss, prospective, well-controlled studies have failed to confirm the association and there is little evidence that anticoagulation therapy reduces miscarriage rates in women with inherited thrombophilias. Routine testing for inherited thrombophilias in women with RPL is not currently recommended.

Endocrine factors

- Thyroid: The most common cause of hypothyroidism in pregnancy is Hashimoto's thyroiditis. Hypothyroidism is associated with unexplained RPL although a causative role for low thyroid function and recurrent pregnancy loss has not been established. In euthyroid pregnant women with no antithyroid antibodies, a TSH level > 2.5 mIU/L has been associated with an elevated miscarriage risk. An association between RPL and antithyroid antibodies has also been established. Levothyroxine reduces the miscarriage rate in women with frank hypothyroidism and in euthyroid women with high, in-range, TSH levels.
- Prolactin: Hyperprolactinemia is associated with diminished GnRH and LH secretion and ovulatory dysfunction. Prolactin modulates progesterone secretion by granulosa cells of human corpora lutea. In hyperprolactinemic women with RPL, prospective randomized data revealed a significant improvement in live birth rates in the group treated with dopamine agonists compared to an untreated group.
- Diabetes: Early miscarriage rates may be threefold higher in women with pregestational diabetes as in normoglycemic women. Among women with poorly controlled diabetes, one study reported a 3% increase in miscarriage rate with each one standard deviation increase in glycosylated hemoglobin levels. RPL is not increased in women with well-controlled diabetes. Glycosylated hemoglobin testing is recommended in women with RPL.
- A diagnosis of PCOS requires having at least two of three diagnostic criteria: chronic anovulation, hyperandrogenism (and/or hyperandrogenemia), and polycystic-appearing ovaries on ultrasound. The prevalence of PCOS among women with RPL may be as high as 10%. Some studies have demonstrated a higher rate of pregnancy loss in PCOS women than in normal women. The mechanism(s) for the increased miscarriage rate is unclear. Women with PCOS often present with obesity, hyperinsulinemia, insulin resistance, and/or hyperandrogenism, each of which might affect the risk of pregnancy loss. Obesity is associated with hyperinsulinemia and insulin resistance (IR). Miscarriage rates have been found to be higher in women with a body mass index (BMI) $\geq 25\,kg/m^2$ than in leaner women with the highest rate seen in obese women (BMI $\geq 30\,kg/m^2$). An association between IR and RPL has also been reported. Hyperandrogenemia is associated with an increased incidence of RPL but a reduction in miscarriage risk in women treated with anti-androgen medications has yet to be established.

Infectious factors

- Several bacterial and viral pathogens associated with an increased risk of RPL include *Chlamydia trachomatis*, *Ureaplasma urealyticum*, *Mycoplasma hominis*, *Listeria monocytogenes*, rubella, and herpes virus. There are currently insufficient data to establish any particular pathogen as a cause for RPL. Neither diagnostic testing for infectious pathogens nor antimicrobial therapy is currently recommended.

Environmental factors

- Environmental toxins including organic solvents, radiation, and pesticides have been linked to pregnancy losses but most studies have been uncontrolled and retrospective. There are extensive data demonstrating a significant increase in miscarriage rates in smokers and in women exposed to secondary smoke compared to unexposed women, as well as in women who consumed > 300 mg per day of caffeine compared to noncaffeine users. Moderate alcohol consumption has been shown to increase the miscarriage rate but not significantly. Studies are limited by multiple confounding variables including the level and duration of exposure. Few data exist regarding the role of environmental factors on pregnancy outcomes.

Diagnosis
Diagnostic evaluation
- Serum karyotype analyses on both parents (recommendations regarding the value of parental karyotypes are conflicting)
- Cytogenetic analysis of abortus tissue
- Uterine assessment (saline hysterosonogram [3D] or diagnostic hysteroscopy)
- Antiphospholipid antibodies
- Endocrine studies – Glycosylated hemoglobin, TSH, and free thyroid hormone (free T4) (note: routine testing for antithyroid peroxidase antibodies is controversial and not recommended), prolactin

Treatment
- In couples with RPL and no correctable causes (i.e. genetic factors or idiopathic RPL), there is no consensus on appropriate management. The rationale for assisted reproductive technologies like intrauterine insemination and IVF includes the possible correction of potential endocrine, immunologic and sperm factors. Preimplantation genetic screening of embryos for aneuploidy (PGT-A) allows selection of euploid embryos for transfer. Studies are conflicting on the value of IVF and PGT-SR (preimplantation genetic screening of embryos for structural rearrangements of chromosomes) for reducing RPL in couples in which one partner carries a structural chromosomal rearrangement. Despite some data showing the benefits of PGT-A and/or PGT-SR in the management of RPL, the American Society of Reproductive Medicine does not presently support routine use of PGT-A or PGT-SR in the management of couples with RPL.
- Etiology-specific treatments are discussed later.

Table of treatment

Psychological and emotional support of all couples	
Idiopathic	Continued intercourse
Chromosomal	Continued intercourse
	IVF with PGT-A or PGT (insufficient data)
Anatomical	
Polyps	Hysteroscopic polypectomy (insufficient data)
Leiomyomata	Myomectomy if submucosal (conflicting data)
	No treatment if intramural or subserosal
Septate uterus	Hysteroscopic resection (insufficient data)
Other congenital anomalies	No treatment
Immunological	
APS	Heparin or low-molecular-weight heparin and low-dose aspirin
Endocrine	
Hypothyroidism	Levothyroxine to achieve euthyroid state
Elevated TSH but euthyroid	Levothyroxine to bring TSH to < 2.5 mIU/L
Diabetes	Hypoglycemic agents
Hyperprolactinemia	Dopamine agonists
Obesity	Weight loss
Insulin resistance	Weight loss and metformin (insufficient data)

(Continued)

(Continued)

Psychological and emotional support of all couples	
Environmental	Recommend that patient reduces caffeine to < 300 mg per day and ceases smoking and alcohol consumption
Other	Progesterone supplementation* (insufficient data)

*The role of progesterone supplementation in early pregnancy in patients with RPL is controversial. A Cochrane database systematic review and the well-publicized PROMISE trial each failed to show an association between progesterone supplementation in the first trimester and reduced miscarriage rates.

Reading list

American College of Obstetricians and Gynecologists Women's Health Care Physicians. ACOG practice bulletin no. 138. Inherited thrombophilias in pregnancy. *Obstet Gynecol* 2013;122(3):706-17.

Bosteels J, Kasius J, Weyers S, et al. Hysteroscopy for treating subfertility associated with suspected major uterine cavity abnormalities. *Cochrane Database Syst Rev* 2015 Feb 21;(2):CD009461.

Chan YY, Jayaprakasan K, Tan A, et al. Reproductive outcomes in women with congenital uterine anomalies: a systematic review. *Ultrasound Obstet Gynecol* 2011;38:371-82.

Coomarasamy A, Williams H, Truchanowicz E, et al. PROMISE: first-trimester progesterone therapy in women with a history of unexplained recurrent miscarriages – a randomised, double-blind, placebo-controlled, international multi-centre trial and economic evaluation. *Health Technol Assess* 2016;20(41):1-92.

Evaluation and treatment of recurrent pregnancy loss: a committee opinion. The Practice Committee of the American Society for Reproductive Medicine. *Fertil Steril* 2012;98:1103-11.

Hodes-Wertz B, Grifo J, Ghadir S, et al. Idiopathic recurrent miscarriage is caused mostly by aneuploid embryos. *Fertil Steril* 2012;98(3):675-80.

Iews M, Tan J, Taskin O, et al. Does preimplantation genetic diagnosis improve reproductive outcome in couples with recurrent pregnancy loss owing to structural chromosomal rearrangement? A systematic review. *Reprod Biomed Online* 2018 Jun;36(6):677-85.

Kutteh WH. Antiphospholipid antibody–associated recurrent pregnancy loss: treatment with heparin and low-dose aspirin is superior to low-dose aspirin alone. *Am J Obstet Gynecol* 1996;174:1584-9.

Pluchino N, Drakopoulos P, Wenger JM, et al. Hormonal causes of recurrent pregnancy loss (RPL). *Hormones* 2014;13(3):314-22.

Shahine LK, Lathi RB. Embryo selection with preimplantation chromosomal screening in patients with recurrent pregnancy loss. *Semin Reprod Med* 2014 Mar;32(2):93-9.

Guidelines
National society guidelines

Title	Source	Date/full reference
Evaluation and treatment of recurrent pregnancy loss: a committee opinion	The Practice Committee of the American Society for Reproductive Medicine.	*Fertil Steril* 2012;98:1103-11.

International society guidelines

Title	Source	Date/full reference
European Society of Human Reproduction and Embryology (ESHRE) Guideline for recurrent pregnancy loss	European Society of Human Reproduction and Embryology (ESHRE)	*Human Reproduction Open* 2018.

Additional material for this chapter can be found online at:
www.wiley.com/go/sperling/mountsinai/obstetricsandgynecology

This includes a case study.

CHAPTER 37

Fertility Preservation

Lucky Sekhon[1], Nola S. Herlihy[2], and Alan B. Copperman[1]
[1] Reproductive Medicine Associates of New York; Division of Reproductive Endocrinology and Infertility, Icahn School of Medicine at Mount Sinai, New York, NY
[2] Reproductive Endocrinology and Infertility, IVIRMA, New Jersey, NJ

Indications

- To circumvent age-related fertility decline:
  - Women or couples who wish to delay childbearing
- To preserve fertility in women with genetic conditions associated with:
  - accelerated or premature ovarian failure
  - cancer predisposition, where prophylactic removal of ovaries may have a protective benefit
- To preserve fertility in women before they undergo surgery that may affect their ovarian reserve (removal of benign ovarian cysts such as endometriomas or mature teratomas).
- To preserve fertility in cancer patients before they undergo gonadotoxic chemotherapy, radiation, or surgery:
  - Chemotherapy and radiation may result in infertility and premature ovarian failure. The extent of damage is determined by the patient's age, type, and cumulative dose of chemotherapeutic drug and/or radiation used.
  - Radiation induces direct DNA damage, causing a loss in the number of ovarian follicles, impaired follicle maturation, and cortical and capsular damage. A radiation dose of 2.5–5 Gy causes permanent ovarian failure in 60% of women aged 15–40 years (as compared to a dose of 0.3 to 3 mGy in a standard diagnostic X-ray).
  - Chemotherapy can cause delayed or arrested puberty in young girls and oligomenorrhea/amenorrhea in young, postpubertal women. Alkylating agents such as cyclophosphamide and heavy metals (i.e. carboplatin and cisplatin) are most associated with ovarian dysfunction.
  - Surgical removal of pelvic organs may lead to infertility, not only through removing organs vital for conception but also from resulting adhesions, pelvic pain, and sexual dysfunction.

Procedures

- Controlled ovarian hyperstimulation (COH):
  - The use of injectable, exogenous gonadotropins (follicle stimulating hormone [FSH] and luteinizing hormone [LH]) to induce growth of multiple ovarian follicles while suppressing ovulation using a gonadotropin-releasing hormone (GnRH) agonist or antagonist.
  - Letrozole, an aromatase inhibitor, may be used to decrease endogenous estrogen levels and minimize the risk of stimulating estrogen receptor positive tumors.
  - The response to stimulation is monitored with serial serum estradiol levels and transvaginal ultrasound every 1–3 days to assess the progress and growth of the follicles and adjust the gonadotropin dosing.
  - When the follicles are mature, final maturation and luteinization of follicles is triggered using human chorionic gonadotropin (hCG) with or without a GnRH agonist.

Mount Sinai Expert Guides: Obstetrics and Gynecology, First Edition. Edited by Rhoda Sperling.
© 2020 John Wiley & Sons Ltd. Published 2020 by John Wiley & Sons Ltd.
Companion Website: www.wiley.com/go/sperling/mountsinai/obstetricsandgynecology

- Oocyte retrieval
  - Oocytes are retrieved under light sedation anesthesia via ultrasound-guided transvaginal aspiration.
- In vitro maturation (IVM) of oocytes
  - As follicles are stimulated and approach > 18 mm size, the ovulation trigger administered (hCG and/or GnRH agonist) prior to retrieval stimulates oocytes to resume meiosis after previously arresting at prophase I. Oocytes develop from the immature stage (germinal vesicle [GV] and metaphase I [MI] oocytes) to the mature stage (metaphase II [MII]).
  - After retrieval, oocyte maturity can be assessed by removing the surrounding cumulus cells. Mature (MII) oocytes have extruded the first polar body. Approximately 30% of retrieved oocytes remain immature at the time retrieval.
  - Mature MII oocytes are required in order for successful fertilization and subsequent embryonic development to take place.
  - IVM involves coaxing immature oocytes in culture to mature, in vitro, to the MII stage.
  - As currently existing IVM protocols have had yielded suboptimal implantation and pregnancy rates, IVM is still considered experimental. If effective, reliable protocols are developed, IVM could be clinically useful to preserve fertility in women who are prepubertal and would not respond to COH, those who cannot delay lifesaving, gonadotoxic treatment to undergo COH, those at high risk of ovarian hyperstimulation syndrome, and those with medical contraindications to sustained elevated levels of estradiol.
- Cryopreservation:
  - Methods:
    - Slow freezing – a technique in which programmable freezers allow the cell(s) to cool at a slow enough rate to permit sufficient cellular dehydration. One of the main factors affecting survival is intracellular ice formation, which can disrupt the cell membrane and cause cell lysis. Cryoprotectants are added to minimize intracellular ice formation.
    - Vitrification – a more recently developed method of cryopreservation that utilizes high initial concentrations of cryoprotectant and rapid cooling to transform the cell(s) into a solid, glass-like state. Vitrification involves "flash freezing" to minimize the rate of ice crystal formation and it has been shown to result in higher rates of post-thaw survival of oocytes and embryos.
  - Oocyte cryopreservation
    - Oocytes may be cryopreserved using either slow freezing or vitrification.
    - Both immature and mature oocytes may be cryopreserved; however, the current practice is to perform IVM prior to cryopreservation in order to freeze oocytes at the MII stage.
    - Oocytes that have undergone cryopreservation followed by thawing/warming tend to have a hardened zona pellucida. As such, these warmed/thawed oocytes are often inseminated using intracytoplasmic sperm injection (ICSI) to maximize the odds of successful fertilization.
  - Embryo cryopreservation
    - Oocytes are fertilized on the day of retrieval and allowed to develop in culture. They may be cryopreserved using slow freezing or vitrification at any stage, from zygote to blastocyst.
    - Prior to cryopreservation, embryos that reach the blastocyst stage (day 5 to 7 of development) can undergo biopsy and removal of four to nine trophectoderm cells for the purpose of preimplantation genetic testing (PGT) to screen for aneuploidy and/or single gene disorders. PGT allows patients to bank chromosomally normal, healthy embryos for future use.
    - When patients/couples are ready to conceive, the recipient of the cryopreserved embryo(s) undergoes programmed hormonal preparation of their endometrium using oral/intramuscular/ transdermal estradiol followed by oral/vaginal/intramuscular progesterone starting 5 days prior to embryo transfer. Cryopreserved embryo(s) are thawed/warmed and are transferred into the uterine cavity, under transabdominal ultrasound guidance. A pregnancy test is performed approximately 1.5 weeks later and if pregnancy is achieved, estradiol and progesterone supplementation

is continued for luteal support until the luteal-placental shift takes place at 7–10 weeks gestation.

- Ovarian tissue/whole ovary cryopreservation
  - Cryopreservation of the entire ovary with its vascular supply theoretically could minimize transplantation-related ischemia and maximize the number of primordial follicles preserved. However, a reliable technique to cryopreserve the ovary with its vascular pedicle has yet to be developed and remains an active field of research.
  - Ovarian tissue cryopreservation is another experimental technique that could allow for preservation of thousands of ovarian primordial follicles at a time. This technique has been suggested primarily for pre-pubertal girls (with immature hypothalamic-pituitary-ovarian axes that do not respond to COH), those with cancer diagnoses who cannot undergo COH to harvest oocytes due to critical illness, the need to expedite lifesaving gonadotoxic treatment or the presence of hormonally stimulated tumors.
  - Ovarian cortical tissue (the outer 1 mm) is removed either by laparoscopy or laparotomy and cryopreserved using either slow freezing or vitrification.
  - Cryopreserved tissue can be thawed/warmed and undergo retransplantation that is either orthotopic (i.e. on the remaining ovary or pelvic peritoneum) or heterotopic (i.e. in the abdominal wall, forearm, chest wall). COH can be attempted to stimulated retransplanted tissue in order to harvest oocytes for in vitro fertilization (IVF). In addition, successfully retransplanted ovarian tissue may continue to produce endogenous hormones and allow for natural ovulation and conception.
  - There are multiple reports of naturally conceived and IVF-derived live births after orthotropic transplantation. The first reported ongoing pregnancy from heterotopically transplanted cryopreserved ovarian tissue occurred in 2013. Large clinical trials are required to determine the true success rate of ovarian tissue cryopreservation and transplantation. A difficult challenge in interpreting the current literature, which consists mainly of case reports and small case series, is the need to discern successful treatment outcomes from cases of spontaneous recovery of function of residual ovarian tissue.
  - Immature oocytes can be harvested from strips of removed ovarian cortical tissue and cryopreserved separately. IVM of immature oocytes can be attempted prior to cryopreservation or after thawing/warming.
- Sperm cryopreservation
  - Semen samples are collected by masturbation after 2–3 days of abstinence. In patients with obstructive azoospermia, sperm may be collected by extraction of sperm from the testes or epididydmis.
  - Semen analysis is performed prior to cryopreservation.
  - Semen is combined with cryoprotectants to maximize post-thaw survival and antibiotics to prevent bacterial contamination.
  - Semen is stored in straws or vials kept in liquid nitrogen and can be warmed for intrauterine insemination or conventional insemination/intracytoplasmic sperm injection in IVF.
- Protecting native ovarian function
  - Opting for conservative, nonsurgical management of gynecologic cancers where possible or performing fertility-sparing surgery where deemed safe and appropriate by the patients' oncology team
    - Cervical cancer: in select women with cervical cancer, radical trachelectomy can be performed instead of a radical hysterectomy to preserve the uterus for future childbearing.
    - Endometrial cancer: in cases of low-grade tumor where myometrial invasion and lymph node metastases are ruled out by magnetic resonance imaging, carefully selected patients may be treated medically with high-dose progestins and close interval follow-up.
    - Ovarian cancer: Ovarian cancer is more common in postmenopausal women. Premenopausal women tend to have malignant germ cell and sex cord-stromal tumors that have an overall excellent prognosis – frequently confined to one ovary and almost always presenting at an early stage.

Conservative surgery and staging in which the uterus and the contralateral ovary are maintained can be performed. Chemotherapy is used as indicated. Premenopausal women with epithelial ovarian tumors often have borderline tumors that can also be treated via a conservative surgical approach. Studies have demonstrated that patients with borderline ovarian tumors who are treated conservatively have similar survival rates to those treated with a hysterectomy and bilateral salpingo-oophorectomy. Therefore, surgical staging of these patients is not considered necessary if invasive disease is ruled out on final pathological analysis.

- Prior to radiation:
  - Protective shields may be used to prevent damage to the ovaries from radiation therapy.
  - Oophoropexy may be warranted in female patients with gynecologic cancers involving the cervix, vagina, uterus, and ovary prior to undergoing pelvic radiation.
  - Oophoropexy involves detaching the ovaries from the uterus by transecting the utero-ovarian ligament and transposing the ovaries, along with their respective blood supplies via the infundibulopelvic (IP) ligaments, to the anterior-abdominal wall.
  - There are multiple reports of return of normal ovarian function and successful pregnancy following pelvic radiation preceded by protective oophoropexy.
  - Although there are relatively few risks associated with oophoropexy, it may limit the future accessibility of the ovaries to transvaginal retrieval of oocytes.
- Prior to chemotherapy:
  - Clinicians may offer GnRH agonist treatment in an effort to preserve ovarian function when cryopreservation of oocytes/embryos are not an option (due to limited access to IVF, need to expedite initiating gonadotoxic therapy or medical conditions precluding COH and oocyte retrieval, etc.).
  - GnRH agonists suppress the hypothalamic-pituitary-ovarian axis and theoretically decrease perfusion to the ovary, minimizing ovarian exposure to systemic gonadotoxic medications.
  - This treatment is of unproven benefit for fertility preservation. Limited data from studies with small sample sizes suggest GnRH agonist may improve rate of menses resumption and ovulation after chemotherapy. However, these surrogate markers of clinical outcome have failed to translate into improved live birth rates. Resumption of menses is an unreliable predictor of fertility. Studies that focus on ovarian reserve, measured by anti-Müllerian hormone (AMH) and basal antral follicle count, suggest that GnRH agonist treatment does little to protect patients from diminished ovarian reserve after exposure to gonadotoxic chemotherapy. Patients should be counseled regarding the lack of evidence for efficacy of GnRH agonist therapy as a primary method of fertility preservation.

Management of complications

- Risks of controlled ovarian hyperstimulation:
  - Ovarian hyperstimulation syndrome (OHSS)
    - OHSS is a complex syndrome of increased vascular permeability leading to fluid shifts from the intravascular to the third space.
    - Mild disease may present as abdominal distention and discomfort in the setting of enlarged ovaries, whereas severe disease can result in nausea, vomiting, abdominal ascites, pleural effusion, acute renal failure, cardiac arrhythmia, and disseminated intravascular coagulation.
    - Treatment is supportive and largely targeted at symptom resolution as the physiologic hormonal milieu is restored, with hospitalization reserved for severe cases.
    - The incidence of OHSS has diminished with increased utilization of a dual ovulation trigger (consisting of GnRH agonist combined with low-dose hCG) and the ability to cryopreserve embryos in order to defer embryo transfer to a subsequent cycle.
  - Ovarian torsion
    - As the ovary enlarges during COH it may twist around its ligamentous support, leading to compromised vascular supply and decreased perfusion and necrosis if not recognized in a timely fashion.

- Torsion typically presents as sudden-onset, intermittent, severe abdominal pain with associated nausea and vomiting.
- Diagnosis is made by diagnostic laparoscopy, and treatment involves de-torsion to preserve ovarian function or oophorectomy/salpingo-oophorectomy if the ovary/fallopian tube are found to be completely necrotic at the time of surgery.
- Stimulation of hormonally sensitive tumors
  - COH results in supraphysiologic levels of estrogen, which may stimulate hormonally sensitive cancers.
  - Letrozole, an aromatase inhibitor, has been used as an adjunct to exogenous gonadotropins to minimize estrogen exposure in breast cancer patients undergoing COH for fertility preservation. Studies show no short-term increase in the rate of recurrence of breast cancer with when COH protocols involving aromatase blockade are used.
  - Multiple large-scale studies of healthy patients that have undergone COH have demonstrated no increased risk of developing breast cancer from cumulative exposure to exogenous gonadotropins.
- Risks of orthotopic or heterotopic transplantation of cryopreserved ovarian tissue
  - Ovarian tissue cryopreservation is not an option for patients with ovarian cancer or those with a high likelihood of developing ovarian cancer (i.e. BRCA carriers).
  - In patients with nonovarian cancers (i.e. hematologic malignancies), there is concern regarding potential risk of reseeding malignant cells at the time of tissue thawing/warming and transplant. To minimize the risk, portions of cryopreserved ovarian tissue should undergo a thorough histological evaluation to rule out micrometastases.

Follow-up

- Women who have delayed childbearing for elective reasons and those who have undergone gonadotoxic therapies in the past may return for an assessment of their ovarian reserve once they are ready to conceive. This includes:
  - Transvaginal ultrasound during the early follicular phase of the menstrual cycle to assess the basal antral follicle count (BAFC)
  - Serum measurement of AMH
  - Early follicular basal serum estrogen and FSH
- Men who have undergone gonadotoxic treatments may return for a semen analysis to assess their gonadal function.
  - World Health Organization lower reference limits for semen analysis
    - Volume – 1.5 mL
    - Sperm concentration – 15 million spermatozoa/mL
    - Total sperm number – 39 million spermatozoa per ejaculate
    - Morphology – 4% normal forms
    - Vitality – 58% alive
    - Total motility – 40%
- Surveillance for recurrence of primary cancer, in conjunction with oncologist
- Future use of cryopreserved sperm, oocytes, and/or embryos to conceive
  - ICSI is used to improve fertilization rates and overcome zona pellucida hardening in previously cryopreserved oocytes.
  - Frozen-thawed embryos may be transferred in a natural cycle or one in which the endometrium is artificially prepared with estrogen and progesterone supplementation.
  - Pregnancy success rates from frozen embryo transfer are similar to those achieved with fresh IVF, owing to reduced ice crystal formation with vitrification. An increasing body of literature suggests that frozen embryo transfer may lead to improved implantation and placentation due to the more physiologic hormonal milieu achieved during a frozen embryo transfer.

Algorithm 37.1 Fertility preservation management/treatment algorithm

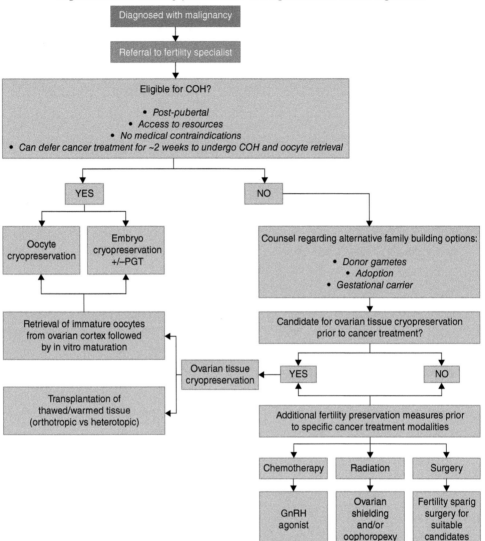

- Future use of cryopreserved ovarian tissue/whole ovaries to conceive:
  - The tissue or ovary may be transplanted back to the original site (orthotopic transplantation) or to another site such as the abdominal wall (heterotopic transplantation).

Reading list

American College of Obstetricians and Gynecologists. Committee opinion no. 607: Gynecologic concerns in children and adolescents with cancer. *Obstet Gynecol* 2014;124:403-8.

Borini A, Setti PE, Anserini P, et al. Multicenter observational study on slow-cooling oocyte cryopreservation: clinical outcome. *Fertil Steril* 2010 Oct 31;94(5):1662-8.

Chen H, Li J, Cui T, et al. Adjuvant gonadotropin-releasing hormone analogues for the prevention of chemotherapy induced premature ovarian failure in premenopausal women. *Cochrane Database Syst Rev* 2011 Nov 9;(11):CD008018.

Chian RC, Huang JY, Tan SL, et al. Obstetric and perinatal outcome in 200 infants conceived from vitrified oocytes. *Reprod Biomed Online* 2008 Dec 31;16(5):608-10.

Cobo A, Rubio C, Gerli S, et al. Use of fluorescence in situ hybridization to assess the chromosomal status of embryos obtained from cryopreserved oocytes. *Fertil Steril* 2001 Feb 28;75(2):354-60.

Fabbri R, Porcu E, Marsella T, et al. Oocyte cryopreservation. *Hum Reprod* 1998 Dec 1;13(Suppl 4):98-108.

Fabbri R, Porcu E, Marsella T, et al. Human oocyte cryopreservation: new perspectives regarding oocyte survival. *Hum Reprod* 2001 Mar 1;16(3):411-6.

Moawad NS, Santamaria E, Rhoton-Vlasak A, et al. Laparoscopic ovarian transposition before pelvic cancer treatment: ovarian function and fertility preservation. *J Minim Invasive Gynecol* 2017 Jan 1;24(1):28-35.

Noyes N, Porcu E, Borini A. Over 900 oocyte cryopreservation babies born with no apparent increase in congenital anomalies. *Reprod Biomed Online* 2009 Dec 31;18(6):769-76.

Practice Committee of the American Society for Reproductive Medicine. Fertility preservation in patients undergoing gonadotoxic therapy or gonadectomy: a committee opinion. *Fertil Steril* 2013 Nov 30;100(5):1214-23.

Practice Committee of the American Society for Reproductive Medicine, Practice Committee of the Society for Assisted Reproductive Technology. Mature oocyte cryopreservation: a guideline. *Fertil Steril* 2013;99(1):37-43.

Smith GD, Serafini PC, Fioravanti J, et al. Prospective randomized comparison of human oocyte cryopreservation with slow-rate freezing or vitrification. *Fertil Steril* 2010 Nov 30;94(6):2088-95.

Ubaldi F, Anniballo R, Romano S, et al. Cumulative ongoing pregnancy rate achieved with oocyte vitrification and cleavage stage transfer without embryo selection in a standard infertility program. *Hum Reprod* 2010 May 1;25(5):1199-205.

Suggested websites

ASRM patient website. http://www.reproductivefacts.org

ASRM video on fertility preservation for cancer patients. https://www.youtube.com/watch?v=li2xFMNlYM8&feature=youtu.be&rel=0

ASRM fact sheets and informational booklets. http://www.asrm.org/FactSheetsandBooklets/

PART 4

Gyn Oncology

CHAPTER 38

Ovarian Cancer

Elena Pereira[1], Jeannette Guziel[2], and Amy Tiersten[3]

[1] Gynecologic Oncology – Department of Obstetrics and Gynecology, Donald and Barbara Zucker School of Medicine at Hofstra/Northwell Health, New York, NY

[2] Hematology/Medical Oncology – Kaiser Permanente, Southern California Permanente Medical Group, Woodland Hills, CA

[3] Department of Medicine, Division of Hematology and Medical Oncology, Icahn School of Medicine at Mount Sinai, New York, NY

OVERALL BOTTOM LINE
- Ovarian cancer is the leading cause of death from gynecologic malignancies in the United States and the fifth most common cause of cancer mortality in females.
- The incidence of ovarian cancer increases with age. The average age at diagnosis of ovarian cancer in the US is 63 years old. The age at diagnosis of ovarian cancer is younger among women with a hereditary ovarian cancer syndrome.
- High-grade epithelial tumors are the most common malignant subtype and the majority are diagnosed at an advanced stage. Less common subtypes include germ cell and stromal cell tumors.

Background
Definition of disease
- Ovarian cancer is a type of cancer that arises from the ovaries.
- Serous carcinomas of the ovary, fallopian tube, and peritoneum are the most common malignant subtype. All originate from the Müllerian epithelium and exhibit similarities in histology and clinical behavior.

Disease classification
- Generally, ovarian neoplasms are grouped into five larger categories based on histologic subtype. The most commonly encountered are epithelial, germ cell, and sex cord-stromal; all three can exist as benign or malignant entities (Table 38.1).
- Epithelial ovarian malignancies are the most common and account for 90–95% of ovarian malignancies. The subtypes are serous, mucinous, endometrioid, and clear cell tumors.
- Epithelial type tumors are classified as either benign, malignant, or tumors of low malignant potential. Tumors of low malignant potential are neither malignant nor benign. They represent a group of tumors that demonstrate a pattern of proliferation greater than those found in benign tumors, but lacking destructive invasion of the stromal components of the ovary. In other words, they do not invade underlying stroma and therefore do not fulfill the definition of malignancy.

Table 38.1 Malignant ovarian histologic subtypes.

Ovarian cancer pathology	Frequency
Epithelial carcinoma	90%
Germ cell	2%
Sex cord-stromal tumors	7%
Miscellaneous	1%

Mount Sinai Expert Guides: Obstetrics and Gynecology, First Edition. Edited by Rhoda Sperling.
© 2020 John Wiley & Sons Ltd. Published 2020 by John Wiley & Sons Ltd.
Companion Website: www.wiley.com/go/sperling/mountsinai/obstetricsandgynecology

Incidence/prevalence
- Worldwide, 295 414 women were diagnosed with ovarian cancer and 184 799 died from this disease (2018).
- In the US, approximately 21 750 cases are expected to be diagnosed in 2020 with an expected 13 940 deaths. This makes ovarian cancer the second most common gynecologic malignancy, the most common cause of gynecologic cancer death, and the fifth leading cause of cancer death in women.
- The lifetime risk of developing ovarian cancer is 1.4%. In other words, 1 in 70 women will develop ovarian cancer.

Etiology
- Although the precise etiology of ovarian cancer is unknown there are several known risk factors that ultimately result in genetic and epigenetic changes causing the defining early events in cancer development, which lead to uncontrolled cell division and growth.
- The majority of ovarian cancer is sporadic and occurs as a result of an accumulation of multiple genetic changes caused by both extrinsic and intrinsic factors.
- About 10% of ovarian cancers arise in women who carry germline mutations in known cancer susceptibility genes such as *BRCA1* and *BRCA2*.

Pathology/pathogenesis
- The various ovarian cancer subtypes are distinct entities and therefore the pathogenesis of each must be thought of as distinct.
- High-grade serous carcinomas of the ovary, fallopian tube, and peritoneum originate from the epithelial cells of the tubal fimbria and are associated with serous tubal in situ carcinomas, which often demonstrate TP53 mutations as a defining early event.
- The pattern of spread among ovarian tumors is unique in that it involves exfoliation of surface ovarian tumor into the peritoneal cavity, resulting in peritoneal surface spread.
- Endometrioid and clear cell ovarian cancers often arise in a background of endometriosis, either on the ovarian surface of the pelvic peritoneum, and more commonly have mutations in the following genes: *ARID1A*, *PIK3CA*, and *PTEN*.

Predictive/risk factors
- Lifetime risk if positive family history:
  - One second-degree relative: 3%
  - One first-degree relative: 5%
  - Two first-degree relatives: 11%
- Genetics: About 20–25% of women diagnosed with ovarian cancer will have a hereditary predisposition to development of the disease, with the most significant being one of the breast cancer genes (*BRCA1* and *BRCA2*). Risk assessment criteria have been defined by the United States Preventive Task Force regarding which patients should be offered genetic testing for BRCA mutations (Tables 38.2A, 38.2B).
  - BRCA1: lifetime risk 40–60%
  - BRCA2: lifetime risk 15–25%
  - Mismatch repair genes (hereditary nonpolyposis colorectal cancer; HNPCC): lifetime risk 6–10%
- Endometriosis increases risk of clear cell and endometrioid ovarian cancers 2–3x.
- Risk increases with age; median age of onset is 63.
- Reproductive history: likely influenced by number of lifetime menstrual cycles
  - Early menarche, late menopause, nulliparity, obesity, and infertility associated with increased risk of ovarian cancer

Table 38.2A   United States Preventive Services Task Force recommendations for *unaffected patients*: who should be offered genetic testing for BRCA mutations?*

For non-Ashkenazi Jewish women:
Two first-degree relatives with breast cancer, one of whom was diagnosed at age 50 or younger
A combination of three or more first- or second-degree relatives with breast cancer regardless of age at diagnosis
A combination of both breast and ovarian cancer among first- and second-degree relatives
A first-degree relative with bilateral breast cancer
A combination of two or more first- or second-degree relatives with ovarian cancer, regardless of age at diagnosis
A first- or second-degree relative with both breast and ovarian cancer at any age
History of breast cancer in a male relative
For women of Ashkenazi Jewish descent:
Any first-degree relative (or two second-degree relatives on the same side of the family) with breast or ovarian cancer

* These recommendations do not apply to women with a family history of breast or ovarian cancer that includes a relative with a known deleterious BRCA mutation.

Table 38.2B   Risk assessment criteria for hereditary breast-ovarian cancer syndrome of *affected patients*: who should be offered genetic testing for BRCA mutations?

Referral should be considered any individual with a personal history of or first-degree relative with:
Breast cancer diagnosed at or before age 50
Triple-negative breast cancer diagnosed at or before age 60
Two or more primary breast cancers in the same person
Ovarian, fallopian tube, or primary peritoneal cancer
Ashkenazi Jewish ancestry and breast or pancreatic cancer at any age
Male breast cancer
Individuals with a family history of three or more cases of breast, ovarian, pancreatic, and/or aggressive prostate cancer (Gleason score ≥ 7)

Prevention

> **BOTTOM LINE/CLINICAL PEARLS**
> - Use of oral contraceptives, multiple pregnancies, breastfeeding, and bilateral tubal ligation are associated with decreased risk of ovarian cancer.
> - Risk reducing salpingo-oophorectomy (RRSO) in patients with known *BRCA1* or *BRCA2* mutation can result in a 70–96% reduction in gynecologic cancer risk (as well as a 47–72% reduction in breast cancer).
> - RRSO should be considered in patients with *BRCA1* mutation between the age of 35–40 and between the age of 40–45 for patients with *BRCA2* mutation, or when childbearing is complete.

Screening
- **There is currently no evidence to support routine screening for prevention of ovarian cancer.**
  - The Prostate, Lung, Colorectal and Ovarian Cancer (PLCO) Screening Trial, which randomized 78 216 women to either undergo annual screening with pelvic ultrasound and CA-125 serum levels or usual medical care, showed no survival advantage with respect to cancer-specific mortality in the

screening group. The number of patients diagnosed at a late stage were also similar between the two groups.
- The United Kingdom Collaborative Trial of Ovarian Cancer Screening (UKCTOCS) randomized 202 638 postmenopausal women to either a multimodality algorithm (risk of ovarian cancer algorithm; ROCA) with annual CA-125 serum levels followed by ultrasound when indicated, annual transvaginal ultrasound (TVUS) alone or no intervention. The multimodality screening algorithm was both sensitive and specific (89.5% and 99.8%) and resulted in a more favorable stage distribution. Preliminary survival data did not show a significant mortality benefit, but continued follow-up is underway.
- For women with identified hereditary ovarian cancer syndromes, the Society of Gynecologic Oncologists (SGO) and the National Comprehensive Cancer Network (NCCN) recommend screening every six months with CA 125 and TVUS beginning between the ages of 30 and 35 years or 5–10 years earlier than the earliest age of first ovarian cancer diagnosis in the family.

Primary prevention
- Avoiding risk factors and increasing protective factors (listed previously) may help prevent cancer, although in many circumstances this is unrealistic.
- Risk-reducing salpingo-oophorectomy (70–96% risk reduction) is recommended for women who have inherited *BRCA1* and *BRCA2* genes or have an inherited ovarian cancer syndrome as soon as childbearing is completed or by age 35–40 for *BRCA1* mutation and age 40–45 for *BRCA2* mutation. RRSO can also decrease breast cancer risk in premenopausal BRCA-positive women (Figure 38.1).

Diagnosis

BOTTOM LINE/CLINICAL PEARLS
- Symptoms associated with ovarian cancer are often nonspecific and include bloating, pelvic pain, changes in bowel or bladder habits, nausea, and weight loss.
- Ovarian masses can be palpated on pelvic exam and are best visualized with pelvic ultrasound (transvaginal and transabdominal).
- If ovarian cancer is suspected, imaging of the chest, abdomen, and pelvis with CT will allow for assessment of the extent of disease.
- Tumor markers (Table 38.3), although helpful, are not diagnostic.

- Definitive diagnosis requires a tissue evaluation that will allow for the distinction between benign and malignant lesions, as well as differentiate between primary ovarian and metastatic tumors.

Differential diagnosis
Differential diagnosis of adnexal masses is provided in Table 38.4. See Algorithm 38.1 for diagnostic workup.

Table 38.3 Tumor markers in ovarian cancers.

Histology	Tumor marker
Epithelial Type	
Serous	CA 125
Mucinous	CEA, CA 19-9
Germ cell tumors	Alpha fetal protein (AFP)
Yolk sac tumor	Lactate dehydrogenase
Choriocarcinoma	β-HCG
Granulosa cell tumor	Inhibin B and A, estradiol

Table 38.4 Differential diagnosis of an ovarian mass.

Ovarian masses	Extraovarian masses
Physiologic cyst	Ectopic pregnancy
Endometrioma	Hydrosalpinx
Theca lutein cysts	Paraovarian cyst
Primary ovarian neoplasm: benign, malignant, or borderline	Peritoneal inclusion cyst
Metastatic carcinoma (breast, colon, uterine)	Pedunculated fibroid
	Diverticular/appendiceal abscess
	Inflammatory or malignant bowel disease

Typical presentation
- Symptoms associated with ovarian cancer are often nonspecific, which results in a typically late stage at presentation.
- Common presentations include an adnexal mass, pelvic or abdominal pain, bloating, dysuria, early satiety, difficulty eating, and abnormal vaginal bleeding.
- Can also be discovered incidentally at the time of surgery performed for another indication.

Clinical diagnosis
History
- Assess for symptoms of abdominal pain, bloating, vaginal bleeding, and difficulty eating.
- Discuss family history of cancer with special attention to a history of gynecologic, breast, and colon malignancies (Figure 38.1).

Physical examination
- Ovarian masses can represent either primary ovarian tumors or metastatic lesions from other cancer sites. In addition, primary ovarian tumors are often metastatic at time of diagnosis and therefore, a complete physical exam is vital to proper diagnosis.
- Chest: assess for evidence of pleural effusions and supraclavicular lymphadenopathy
- Breast: assess for primary breast lesions and axillary lymphadenopathy

Algorithm 38.1 Diagnostic workup

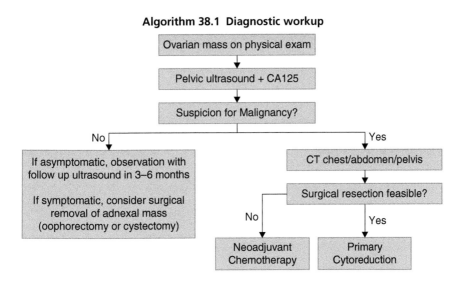

- Abdomen: assess for increasing abdominal girth, ascites, groin lymphadenopathy
- Pelvis: ovarian masses are best assessed on bimanual rectovaginal exam. This allows one to assess if the masses are fixed/mobile or contain nodularity. A thorough exam of the cervix and uterus should also be performed.
- Extremities: assess for edema, which may be an indication that the pelvic mass is impeding venous return from the lower extremities.

Useful clinical decision rules and calculators
- Ovarian cancer is **surgically staged** according to the Joint International Federation of Gynecology and Obstetrics (FIGO)/Tumor, Nodes, Metastasis (TNM) classification system.

FIGO OVARIAN CANCER STAGING 2014:
Stage I: Cancer confined to the ovaries:

IA	Tumor limited to 1 ovary, capsule intact, no tumor on surface, negative washings
IB	Tumor involves both ovaries otherwise like IA.
IC	Tumor limited to 1 or both ovaries
IC1	Surgical spill
IC2	Capsule rupture before surgery or tumor on ovarian surface
IC3	Malignant cells in the ascites or peritoneal washings

Stage II: Tumor involves 1 or both ovaries with pelvic extension (below the pelvic brim) or primary peritoneal cancer

IIA	IIA extension and/or implant on uterus and/or fallopian tubes
IIB	Extension to other pelvic intraperitoneal tissues

Stage III: Tumor involves 1 or both ovaries with cytologically or histologically confirmed spread to the peritoneum outside the pelvis and/or metastasis to the retroperitoneal lymph nodes

IIIA	Positive retroperitoneal lymph nodes and/or microscopic metastasis beyond the pelvis
IIIA1	Positive retroperitoneal lymph nodes only IIIA1(i) Metastasis ≤ 10 mm IIIA1(ii) Metastasis > 10 mm
IIIA2	Microscopic, extrapelvic (above the brim) peritoneal involvement $\pm$ positive retroperitoneal lymph nodes.
IIIB	Macroscopic, extrapelvic, peritoneal metastasis ≤ 2 cm $\pm$ positive retroperitoneal lymph nodes. Includes extension to capsule of liver/spleen.
IIIC	Macroscopic, extrapelvic, peritoneal metastasis > 2 cm $\pm$ positive retroperitoneal lymph nodes. Includes extension to capsule of liver/spleen.

Stage IV: Distant metastasis excluding peritoneal metastasis

IVA	Pleural effusion with positive cytology
IVB	Hepatic and/or splenic parenchymal metastasis, metastasis to extra-abdominal organs (including inguinal lymph nodes and lymph nodes outside of the abdominal cavity)

Table 38.5 Risk of Malignancy Index (RMI), a product that combines three presurgical features: serum CA125 (CA125), menopausal status (M), and ultrasound score (U) [RMI = U x M x CA125].

Ultrasound	1 point for each of the following characteristics: multilocular cysts, solid areas, metastases, ascites, and bilateral lesions. U = 0 (for an ultrasound score of 0) U = 1 (for an ultrasound score of 1) U = 3 (for an ultrasound score of 2-5)
Menopausal Status*	M = 1 (premenopausal) M = 3 (postmenopausal)
CA-125	Serum CA 125 level (U/ml)
RMI	**> 200 = high risk of malignancy**

* Postmenopausal is defined as no menses for more than 1 year.
Jacobs et al. 1990

Disease severity classification
- The goal of surgery is optimal cytoreduction (removal of all visible disease) and volume of residual disease is directly correlated with survival.
- Other prognostic factors include age, stage, histologic grade and type, and performance status.

Laboratory diagnosis
List of diagnostic tests
- The goal of preoperative diagnostic studies is to assess the extent of disease and to determine primary vs metastatic disease as best as possible.
- Tumor markers are not diagnostic but can be useful in guiding management (Table 38.3).
- Colonoscopy: if there is suspicion for nonovarian primary, a colonoscopy should be considered in order to rule out a primary colon cancer metastatic to the ovary.

List of imaging techniques
- Transvaginal and transabdominal ultrasound is the imaging modality of choice for adnexal masses. A composite of ultrasound findings and CA 125, known as the Risk of Malignancy Index, can be used to predict of likelihood of malignancy (Table 38.5).
- CT chest/abdomen/pelvis: if ovarian malignancy is suspected, CT imaging of the chest, abdomen, and pelvis is recommended for assessment of extent of disease and feasibility of surgical resection.
- MRI and/or PET-CT are recommended only as clinically indicated and are not a component of routine evaluation.

Treatment
Treatment rationale
High-grade primary epithelial ovarian carcinomas
Early Stage Disease = Stage I (limited to ovaries) and II (limited to pelvis)
- Stage IA/B:
  - Grade 1: No adjuvant chemotherapy
  - Grade 2: Consider IV carboplatin/paclitaxel x 3–6 cycles
  - Grade 3/Clear Cell: IV carboplatin/paclitaxel x 3–6 cycles
- Stage IC: Adjuvant IV carboplatin/paclitaxel x 3–6 cycles
- Stage II: Adjuvant IV carboplatin/paclitaxel x 6 cycles

Advanced Stage Disease = Stage III (IP or nodal spread) and IV (distant disease)
- *Adjuvant chemotherapy with carboplatin and paclitaxel after maximal attempt at surgical cytoreduction is the standard of care treatment for advanced disease.*

- **Neoadjuvant chemotherapy (NACT)** followed by interval cytoreduction is a management option for patients with bulky, unresectable disease. It is also an option for patients who are felt to be poor candidates for extensive abdominal surgery (Algorithm 38.2).
  - The EORTC-GCG/NCIC-CTG trial (Vergote et al. 2010) demonstrated that NACT followed by interval cytoreductive surgery was not inferior to primary cytoreductive (PCS) surgery followed by chemotherapy.
    - Subset analysis stratified patients by size of largest metastatic lesion. Results favored PCS in patients with stage IIIC disease and ≤ 45 mm metastatic lesions, and favored NACT in patients with stage IV disease > 45 mm metastatic lesions.
  - An expert panel convened by the American Society of Clinical Oncology and the Society of Gynecologic Oncology released a joint statement with recommendations for NACT in patients with newly diagnosed advanced ovarian cancer. The committee compiled data from randomized phase III trials comparing NACT to PCS as well as data regarding risk stratification of patients who are at increased risk for perioperative morbidity and mortality.
    - After a review of four phase III clinical trials the committee concluded that NACT is not inferior to PCS with respect to overall survival (OS) and progression-free survival (PFS). NACT is associated with less peri- and postoperative morbidity and mortality.
    - For women with likelihood of optimal cytoreduction to <1 cm, with acceptable morbidity, PCS is recommended over NACT.
- Combination carboplatin and paclitaxel is standard first-line treatment for ovarian high-grade epithelial carcinomas. Optimal administration of this regimen is an area of continued research.
- **Intravenous (IV) paclitaxel/carboplatin every 3 weeks** became standard adjuvant chemotherapy based on the following studies:
  - Paclitaxel/cisplatin is superior to cyclophosphamide/cisplatin. GOG 111 demonstrated a HR of 0.61 (95%CI 0.47–0.79) for overall survival favoring paclitaxel/cisplatin. This survival benefit was confirmed in EORTC-NCIC OV10 trial.
  - Carboplatin/paclitaxel is at least equivalent in efficacy to cisplatin/paclitaxel with improved toxicity profile (AGO Trial, GOG 158).
- **IV carboplatin given every 3 weeks with weekly IV paclitaxel** was shown to improve overall survival, quality of life, and toxicity when compared to every 3-week paclitaxel/carboplatin in a trial performed in Japan. However, these survival benefits have not been duplicated in subsequent studies. The maximal benefit of this regimen is likely achieved in patients with high tumor burden. Using weekly paclitaxel (vs every 3-week dosing) in combination with carboplatin is also considered standard of care adjuvant therapy.
  - Japanese Trial (Katsumada et al. 2009): Conventional Carbo/Taxol (every 3 weeks, AUC 6) vs dose dense (weekly paclitaxel, AUC6) carboplatin/taxol showed a PFS of 17 vs 28 months ($P = 0.0014$) and a 65% vs 72% 3-year OS ($P = 0.03$) all favoring dose dense therapy. Grade 3/4 anemia more common in DD arm but other toxicities not significant.
  - A confirmatory European trial ASCO 2013 (LBA 5501) comparing weekly carboplatin/taxol vs every 3-week regimen showed no difference in PFS but better quality of life (QOL) and toxicity with weekly paclitaxel.
  - GOG 262 (weekly vs every 3-week paclitaxel/carboplatin, bevacizumab optional) showed a better progression free survival in the weekly paclitaxel group (14 vs 10 months, HR 0.60, 95% CI) in patients that did not receive bevacizumab, but no difference in overall survival.
  - A weekly carboplatin + weekly paclitaxel regimen based on the MITO-7 phase III trial may also be considered in poor performance status patients or patients with multiple comorbidities. Weekly carboplatin/paclitaxel yielded a similar PFS to standard of care with less toxicity and better QOL.
- **Intraperitoneal (IP) chemotherapy with cisplatin and paclitaxel** is considered a standard treatment for small volume residual disease, as issued by the National Cancer Institute (NCI) with the advantage of maximal drug delivery and an overall survival benefit.

- Three large randomized, phase III clinical trials of IP chemotherapy (GOG 104, 114, and 172) demonstrated a superior progression-free and overall survival with IP chemotherapy compared with IV chemotherapy.
- GOG 172 showed a 68-month vs 50-month median OS advantage for IP cisplatin/IP + IV paclitaxel vs IV cisplatin/IV paclitaxel in optimally debulked stage III ovarian cancer.
- IP therapy is associated with greater grade 3/4 toxicities (myelosupression, metabolic abnormalities, catheter complications, bowel complications, abdominal pain), decreased compliance, and decreased QOL. However, at 12-month follow-up, the groups experienced no difference in quality of life, except that paresthesias were more likely to persist in the IP arm.
- IP therapy is therefore recommended only if there is a trained staff to administer it and only after careful patient selection with a discussion of risks/benefits.
- Bevacizumab can be added to adjuvant chemotherapy with an additional progression free survival benefit, but an OS benefit has not been shown (GOG 218 and ICON 7).
- Results from GOG 252, did not demonstrate an advantage to IP chemotherapy over IV. Median PFS was similar among the three arms 24.9 mos (IV carboplatin), 27.3 mos (IP carboplatin), and 26 mos (IP cisplatin). In general, carboplatin was better tolerated than cisplatin. This trial enrolled patients with minimal residual disease ≤ 1 cm with a goal of determining optimal treatment in terms of efficacy and toxicity for advanced ovarian cancer incorporating both dose dense schedules and IP vs IV regimens in the adjuvant setting.
  - Treatment arms:
    - Paclitaxel 80 mg/m2 IV weekly + carboplatin AUC 6 IV + bevacizumab
    - Paclitaxel 80 mg/m2 IV weekly + carboplatin AUC 6 IP + bevacizumab
    - Paclitaxel 135 mg/m2 IV over 3 hours day 1, cisplatin75 mg/m2 IP on day 2, paclitaxel 60 mg/m2 IP on day 8 + bevacizumab
- Maintenance therapy: After front-line therapy, treatment with maintenance therapy has demonstrated benefit in PFS, but not in OS.
  - Paclitaxel: For patients in a complete clinical response, the SWOG S9761/GOG 178 collaborative trial randomized patients to receive either 3 or 12 cycles of monthly paclitaxel (175 mg/m2). Updated data confirmed an 8-month PFS advantage in the 12-cycle arm (22 vs 14 months, $P = 0.006$), but no overall survival advantage (53 vs 48 months, $P = 0.34$).
  - Pazopanib: maintenance with pazopanib, a multikinase inhibitor of the vascular endothelial growth factor (VEGF)-receptor, PDGFR-receptor and c-kit, prolonged PFS (17.9 mos vs 12.3 mos; $P = 0.0021$) compared to placebo in patients with advanced ovarian cancer who had not progressed after first-line chemotherapy. There was no overall survival advantage.

Recurrent high-grade epithelial ovarian carcinoma

- The Risk of Recurrence After 1° Treatment:
  - Early Stage, Low Risk = 10%
  - Early Stage, High Risk = 20% (after adjuvant therapy)
  - Low Volume Residual Disease = 60 to 70%
  - Large Volume Residual Disease = 80 to 85%
- Most recurrences occur within the first 3 years
- Surveillance: a multi-institutional European trial found no advantage to receiving early treatment based on a rising CA-125. The Society of Gynecologic Oncologists consider surveillance with CA-125 as "optional." The NCCN panel suggests that surveillance with CA-125 should be offered to patients after discussion of risks and benefits.
- Each subsequent line of therapy in the recurrent setting is associated with shorter disease-free intervals
- Treatment of recurrent disease is based on response to first-line treatment and the platinum free interval (PFI) and is dichotomized to:

Table 38.6 Combination therapies in recurrent platinum sensitive epithelial ovarian cancer.

Phase III trial	Regimen	Median PFS (months)	Median OS (months)
ICON-4	Carbo vs Carbo/Paclitaxel	9 vs 12	24 vs 29
AGO-AVAR	Carbo vs Carbo/Gemcitabine	5.8 vs 8.6	Not powered for OS
CALYPSO	Carbo/Paclitaxel vs Carbo/PLD	9.4 vs 11.3	Data immature for final analysis
OCEANS	Carbo/Gem vs Carbo/Gemcitabine + Bevacizumab followed by Bevacizumab Maintenance	8 vs 12	33 vs 35

- Platinum-sensitive = PFI > 6 months
- Platinum-resistant = PFI ≤ 6 months
- Platinum Sensitive (PS) Disease: retreat with carboplatin based doublet (RR ≈ 60%, survival is 30 + mos). Treat until progression of disease, unacceptable toxicity, or complete clinical response. Treatment options for platinum sensitive disease are outlined in Table 38.6.
- Poly (ADP-ribose) polymerase (PARP) inhibition maintenance therapy in recurrent, platinum-sensitive disease:
  - Olaparib: there was a PFS advantage with olaparib but no OS difference was seen. (Ledermann et al. 2012).
  - Niraparib: an even more significant PFS advantage (21 mos vs 5 mos in BRCA mutated patients) was demonstrated with niraparib. Overall survival data is not yet available.
- Platinum Resistant Disease: treat with alternative drug therapy (RR ≈ 12–32%, survival 8 + mos). Treat until progression of disease, unacceptable toxicity, or complete clinical response.
  - Single-agent sequential therapies are preferred to combination since this approach may offer a potential balance between efficacy of treatment and an acceptable toxicity profile.
  - An overall response rate (ORR) of 50% has been shown with single-agent paclitaxel. Other active single-agents include pegylated liposomal doxorubicin, topotecan, gemcitabine, etoposide, and bevacizumab.
  - Bevacizumab in platinum-resistant recurrent disease: In the AURELIA trial, bevacizumab was added to either paclitaxel, pegylated liposomal doxorubicin, or topotecan. The addition of bevacizumab to single-agent chemotherapy improved PFS but not OS.
- PARP Inhibition in heavily pretreated patients
  - Olaparib is a PARP inhibitor Food and Drug Administration (FDA)-approved for patients with advanced ovarian cancer who have received treatment with 3 or more lines of chemotherapy and who have a germline BRCA mutation.
  - Single-agent olaparib showed a response rate of 31% and stable disease > 8 weeks rate of 40% for germline BRCA mutated ovarian cancer. (Kaufman et al. 2014).
  - FDA-approved BRACAnalysis CDx (Myriad), a companion diagnostic that will detect the presence of BRCA mutations in blood samples from patients with ovarian cancer.
- Rucaparib: the results from two phase II trials were presented at the 2016 ESMO Congress. Patients with heavily pretreated high-grade ovarian cancer and either germline or somatic BRCA mutations showed a durable response to Rucaparib with a median PFS of 10 months (range: 0–22.1). The ORR by RECIST v1.1 was 53.7% (95% CI, 43.6–63.5). Response was better in platinum-sensitive patients (ORR: 65.5%) than in platinum-resistant (ORR: 25%) and platinum-refractory (0%) disease.

Low-grade epithelial tumors
- Stage IA-IB: considered low risk if no extraovarian spread, negative peritoneal washings, and no ascites. Associated with a 10% risk of recurrence. *No benefit to adjuvant therapy*
- Stage IC-IV: Maximal effort at cytoreduction recommended. Low-grade tumors are classically poorly responsive to chemotherapy and therefore the role of adjuvant treatment is controversial.

Postoperative options include observation, platinum-based therapy, and hormonal therapy such as anastrazole, leuprolide, or tamoxifen.

Malignant germ cell tumors
- Dysgerminoma
  - If fertility is desired, fertility-sparing staging procedure with preservation of the uterus and contralateral ovary may be offered. Otherwise, a complete surgical staging (total hysterectomy, bilateral salpingo-oophorectomy, pelvic and paraaortic lymph node dissection, and omentectomy) is recommended.
  - Stage I: surgical staging followed by observation.
  - Stage II–IV: surgical staging followed by adjuvant chemotherapy with BEP (bleomycin, etoposide, cisplatin) is generally recommended.
- Immature Teratoma
  - If fertility is desired, fertility-sparing staging procedure may be offered. Otherwise, a complete surgical staging (total hysterectomy, bilateral salpingo-oophorectomy, pelvic and paraaortic lymph node dissection and omentectomy) is recommended.
  - Stage I, low grade: surgical staging followed by observation
  - Stage I (grade 2–3) and Stage II–IV: complete surgical staging followed by adjuvant chemotherapy with BEP (bleomycin, etoposide, cisplatin) is generally recommended.
- Embryonal Tumor
  - Stage I–IV: complete surgical staging followed by adjuvant chemotherapy with BEP is generally recommended.

Malignant sex-cord stromal tumors
- Stage I
  - If fertility is desired, fertility-sparing staging procedure may be offered. Otherwise, a complete surgical staging (total hysterectomy, bilateral salpingo-oophorectomy, pelvic and paraaortic lymph node dissection, and omentectomy) is recommended.
  - Low-risk patients: surgical staging followed by observation
  - High-risk patients (defined as ruptured stage IC or poorly differentiated) can be offered either observation or adjuvant chemotherapy with BEP (bleomycin, etoposide, cisplatin) or carboplatin/paclitaxel.
- Stage II–IV
  - Complete surgical staging followed by adjuvant chemotherapy with BEP or carboplatin/paclitaxel is recommended.

When to hospitalize
- Acute conditions can be both related to treatment and the disease process itself.
  - Malignant bowel obstruction: secondary to the peritoneal pattern of spread, bowel obstruction is a common sequela of ovarian cancer. Management of bowel obstruction can be either conservative (nasogastric tube) or surgical (bowel resection, diverting ostomy, percutaneous endoscopic gastrostomy tube).
  - Pleural effusions: can be secondary to ascites or metastatic tumor spread to the lung. Patients present with worsening shortness of breath. Management options include thoracentesis, chest tube placement, and pleurodesis.
  - Febrile neutropenia: defined as an oral temperature >38.5°C or two consecutive readings of >38.0°C for 2 hours associated with an absolute neutrophil count $<0.5 \times 10^9$/l. Patients should be admitted for antibiotics and neutropenia precautions. Consideration for possible sources of infection is vital (ex: indwelling IV catheter, intraabdominal abscess).
  - Dehydration: often the result of decreased oral intake, emesis, and diarrhea (either secondary to side effects of chemotherapy or a result of the disease process).

Algorithm 38.2 Management of primary and recurrent ovarian cancer

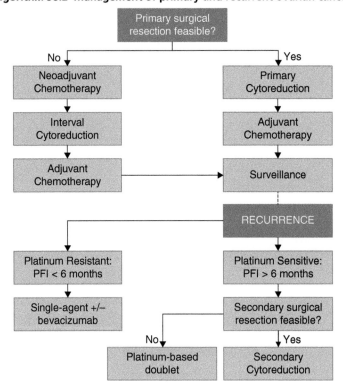

PFI: platinum free interval.

Table of treatment

See Algorithm 38.2 for management/treatment.

Treatment	Comments
Medical **Chemotherapy following surgery:** **Limited stage (I and II):** Low risk: Observation High risk: IV carboplatin/paclitaxel **Advanced stage (III and IV):** IV paclitaxel 175 mg/m2/3 h IV carboplatin AUC 6 Repeat every 3 weeks x 6 cycles *Or* IV paclitaxel (80 mg/m2/1 h) weekly IV carboplatin AUC 6 every 3 weeks 21-day cycle x 6 cycles **Recurrent or persistent disease:** **Platinum sensitive disease**: Carboplatin AUC 5 + paclitaxel 175 mg/m2 every 3 weeks or carboplatin AUC 5 + doxorubicin 30 mg/m2 every 4 weeks Carboplatin AUC 4 day 1 + gemcitabine 1000 mg/m2 day 1 and 8 every 3 weeks +/- Bevacizumab 10–15 mg/kg	Clinical pearls **Can consider:** Addition of bevacizumab IP therapy in small volume disease

(Continued)

Treatment	Comments
Platinum resistant disease: Single-agent sequential therapy **BRCA1/BRCA1 mutation with chemorefractory disease:** Olaparib	
Surgical **Staging vs cytoreduction** Staging procedures are performed to assess the extent of microscopic disease. In patients with bulky tumor a cytoreductive surgery is indicated. **Staging**: includes total hysterectomy, BSO, pelvic washings, pelvic and paraaortic lymph node dissection and omentectomy. Can be performed via laparotomy or laparoscopically. **Primary cytoreduction**: laparotomy, TAH, BSO, omentectomy, tumor debulking with the goal of optimal cytoreduction (no visible disease). **Secondary cytoreduction:** can be considered for recurrence in patients with platinum sensitive disease in whom optimal cytoreduction is deemed possible. No evidence to support second look surgery. Palliative Surgery: Individualized	Neoadjuvant chemotherapy, followed by interval cytoreduction, may be offered to patients who are considered poor surgical candidates, or in whom primary optimal cytoreduction is deemed impossible.

TAH, total abdominal hysterectomy; BSO, bilateral salpingo-oophorectomy

Prevention/management of complications
- Treatment of ovarian cancer with chemotherapeutic agents can be associated with acute drug reaction, which can be largely prevented with appropriate pre-medications.
  - Taxanes: tend to be infusion-related drug reactions (hot flushing, rash), often attributed to a solvent in the formulation (Cremophor®). These reactions are notable because they tend to occur within the *first* cycle of treatment. Pretreatment with steroids indicated for prevention.
  - Platinum agents: produce a true hypersensitivity allergic reaction (shortness of breath, hives/itching, changes in blood pressure). These reactions tend to occur following reexposure to the drug. Mild reactions can be managed with an antihistamine. More severe reactions should be managed with an antihistamine, epinephrine, and corticosteroids.
  - Doxorubicin: is a vesicant and extravasation can cause damage to the tissues surrounding the venous access. Must be managed swiftly with neutralizing agents: dexrazoxane. For this reason, administration through a central line is recommended.

> **CLINICAL PEARLS**
> - Optimal cytoreduction with no visible gross residual disease is the goal of primary cytoreductive surgery and is the standard of care.
> - IV carboplatin/paclitaxel (given every 3 weeks or weekly) is standard adjuvant therapy for high-risk limited stage disease and for advanced disease after primary cytoreduction.
> - Intraperitoneal (IP) chemotherapy is standard of care for small volume residual disease as issued by the NCI but requires expertise in administration and is associated with greater toxicity.
> - In the recurrent setting, treatment choice and response to therapy is determined by the PFI.
> - All patients with ovarian cancer should be tested for germline *BRCA1* and *BRCA2* mutations.

Special populations
Elderly
- Patients with advanced disease who are elderly, have poor performance status, and have comorbidities may not tolerate standard IP or IV combinations of chemotherapy. Single-agent platinum agents may be appropriate for these patients.

- The risks and benefits of cytoreductive surgery must be considered in elderly patients. For patients who may not tolerate upfront surgery, neoadjuvant therapy followed by interval debulking is an option.

Prognosis

> **BOTTOM LINE/CLINICAL PEARLS**
> - Survival from ovarian cancer is related to the stage at diagnosis; 5-year survival is over 90% for the minority of women with stage I disease. This number drops to about 75 to 80% for regional disease and 25% for those with distant metastases.
> - Patients with BRCA mutations may have a better prognosis due to increased sensitivity to platinum-based chemotherapy and the efficacy of PARP inhibitors.
> - The majority of high-grade epithelial ovarian cancers are chemosensitive diseases; however, with subsequent recurrences disease-free interval and chemosensitivity largely decrease ultimately making this a very challenging disease.

Reading list

Aghajanian C, Blank SV, Goff BA et al. OCEANS: a randomized, double-blinded, placebo-controlled phase III trial of chemotherapy with or without bevacizumab (BEV) in patients with platinum-sensitive recurrent epithelial ovarian (EOC), primary peritoneal (PPC), or fallopian tube cancer (FTC). *J Clin Oncol* 2012;30:2039.

Jacobs I, Oram D, Fairbanks J, et al. A risk of malignancy index incorporating CA125, ultrasound and menopausal status for accurate preoperative diagnosis of ovarian cancer. *Br J Obstet Gynaecol* 1990;97:922-29.

Katsumata N, Yasuda M, Takahashi F, et al. Dose-dense paclitaxel once a week in combination with carboplatin every 3 weeks for advanced ovarian cancer: a phase 3, open-label, randomised controlled trial. *Lancet* 2009;374(9698):1331-38.

Kaufman B, Shapira-Frommer R, Schmutzler RK, et al. Olaparib monotherapy in patients with advanced cancer and a germline BRCA1/2 mutation. *J Clin Oncol* 2015;33:244-50.

Ledermann J, Harter P, Gourley C, et al. Olaparib maintenance therapy in platinum-sensitive relapsed ovarian cancer. *N Engl J Med* 2012;366:1382.

Markman M, Liu PY, Moon J, et al. Impact on survival of 12 versus 3 monthly cycles of paclitaxel (175 mg/m2) administered to patients with advanced ovarian cancer who attained a complete response to primary platinum-paclitaxel: follow-up of a Southwest Oncology Group and Gynecologic Oncology Group phase 3 trial. *Gynecol Oncol* 2009;14(2):195-98.

Parmer MK, Ledermann JA, Colombo N, et al. Paclitaxel plus platinum-based chemotherapy versus conventional platinum-based chemotherapy in women with relapsed ovarian cancer: the ICON4/AGO-OVAR-2.2 trial. *Lancet* 361(9375):2099-106.

Pfisterer J, Plante M, Vergote I, et al. Gemcitabine plus carboplatin compared with carboplatin in patients with platinum-sensitive recurrent ovarian cancer: an intergroup trial of the AGO-OVAR, the NCIC CTG, and the EORTC GCG. *J Clin Oncol* 2006 Oct 10;24(29):4699-707.

Pujade-Lauraine E, Mahner S, Kaern J, et al. A randomized, phase III study of carboplatin and pegylated liposomal doxorubicin versus carboplatin and paclitaxel in relapsed platinum-sensitive ovarian cancer (OC). CALYPSO study of the Gynecologic Cancer Intergroup (GCIG). *J Clin Oncol* 2009;27.

Pujade-Lauraine E, Hilpert F, Weber B, et al. AURELIA: A randomized phase III trial evaluating bevacizumab (BEV) plus chemotherapy (CT) for platinum (PT)-resistant recurrent ovarian cancer (OC). *J Clin Oncol* 2012;30.

Toss A, Tomasello C, Razzaboni E, et al. Hereditary ovarian cancer: not only BRCA1 and 2 genes. *BioMed Res Intl* 2015:1-11.

Vergote I, Trope CG, Amant F, et al. Neoadjuvant chemotherapy or primary surgery in stage IIIC or IV ovarian cancer. *N Engl J Med* 2010;363:943-53.

Suggested websites

American Society of Clinical Oncology (ASCO). www.asco.org/
National Comprehensive Cancer Network (NCCN). http://www.nccn.org/professionals/physician_gls/

Guidelines
National society guidelines

Title	Source	Date/URL
NCCN guidelines for ovarian cancer	National Comprehensive Cancer Network (NCCN)	2019 http://www.nccn.org/professionals/physician_gls/pdf/ovarian.pdf
Clinical practice guidelines	Society of Gynecologic Oncology (SGO)	www.sgo.org/clinical-practice/guidelines

International society guidelines

Title	Source	URL
	International Federation of Gynecologists and Obstetricians (FIGO)	www.figo.org

Images

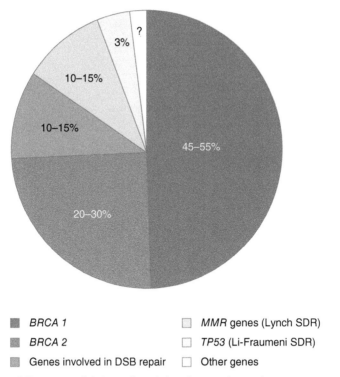

Figure 38.1 Susceptibility genes and their prevalence in hereditary ovarian syndromes. From Toss et al. 2015.

CHAPTER 39

Cervical Cancer

Navya Nair[1], Ann Marie Beddoe[2], and Peter Dottino[2]

[1] Division of Gynecologic Oncology – Department of Obstetrics and Gynecology, Louisiana State University School of Medicine, New Orleans, LA
[2] Division of Gynecologic Oncology – Department of Obstetrics, Gynecology and Reproductive Science, Icahn School of Medicine at Mount Sinai, New York, NY

OVERALL BOTTOM LINE
- Cervical cancer is a major source of morbidity and mortality worldwide, with most cases occurring in developing nations.
- With screening and treatment of preinvasive disease, cervical cancer can be prevented.
- Most cervical cancers are the end result of a long process that begins with human papillomavirus (HPV) infection.
- Vaccines against HPV can prevent preinvasive disease that leads to cervical cancer.
- Treatment of cervical cancer is dependent on stage and can include surgery, radiation therapy, and chemotherapy.

Background
Definition of disease
- Cancer arising from the cervix (lower segment of the uterus)
- Due to abnormal growth of cells that have the potential to invade neighboring tissue and spread

Disease classification
- Majority of cervical cancers are squamous cell type (75–80%)
- Most of the remainder are adenocarcinomas

Incidence/prevalence
- In the United States, it is estimated that there will be 13 170 new cases of cervical cancer and 4250 cervical cancer deaths (Siegel et al. 2019).
- Worldwide, cervical cancer is the fourth most common cancer in women with an estimated 569 800 new cases and 311 400 deaths in 2018 (American Cancer Society 2018) (Figure 39.1).

Economic impact
- In high-income countries, the incidence of cervical cancer has declined through the combined strategy of early detection and treatment of precancerous lesions and vaccination programs.
- The implementation of organized screening has not been effective in low-resource settings – where 85% of the global cervical cancer burden resides – due to the lack of health delivery infrastructure and limited financial resources.
- In low-resource settings a 10-year rollout of the HPV vaccination could avert up to 4.8 million cervical cancer cases and 3.3 million cervical cancer deaths (Campos et al. 2016).
- In low-resource settings, rollout of a one-time cervical cancer screening program could avert as many as 1.4 million cervical cases and 968 000 cervical cancer deaths (Campos et al. 2016).

Mount Sinai Expert Guides: Obstetrics and Gynecology, First Edition. Edited by Rhoda Sperling.
© 2020 John Wiley & Sons Ltd. Published 2020 by John Wiley & Sons Ltd.
Companion Website: www.wiley.com/go/sperling/mountsinai/obstetricsandgynecology

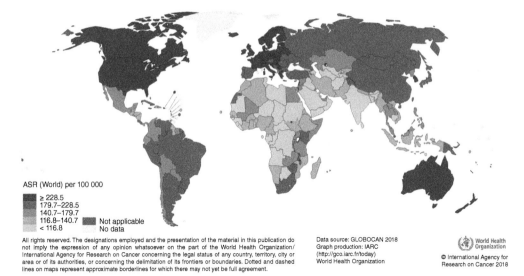

ASR (World) per 100 000

- ≥ 228.5
- 179.7–228.5
- 140.7–179.7
- 116.8–140.7   Not applicable
- < 116.8   No data

Data source: GLOBOCAN 2018
Graph production: IARC
(http://gco.iarc.fr/today)
World Health Organization

World Health Organization

© International Agency for Research on Cancer 2018

Figure 39.1 Global distribution of cervical cancer cases in 2018. Available from: http://globocan.iarc.fr (accessed 28 June 2019).

Etiology

- Cervical cancer is typically the end result of a process that begins with infection with HPV.
- Chronic HPV infection leads to cervical dysplasia (preinvasive disease) and subsequently cervical cancer (Figure 39.2).
- HPV strains 16 and 18 account for over 70% of cervical cancer cases.

Pathology/pathogenesis

- Presenting symptoms including abnormal vaginal bleeding (including postcoital bleeding) and/or abnormal vaginal discharge.
- Symptoms of advanced disease include hematuria, rectal bleeding, referred leg or flank pain, and lymphedema.

Predictive/risk factors

Risk factor	Odds ratio
HPV infection	81.3 (95% confidence interval [CI]: 42.0, 157.1) (Castellsagué et al. 2006)
HIV	12.2 (95% CI: 9.4, 15.6) (Patel et al. 2008)*
Cigarette smoking	1.5 (95% CI: 1.0, 2.2) (Gram et al. 1992)

* Standard Rate Ratio: observed cases in HIV population to general population

Prevention

> **BOTTOM LINE/CLINICAL PEARLS**
> - Papanicolaou smear/HVP screening, treatment of preinvasive disease, and HPV vaccination can prevent development of cervical cancer.

Screening
- Papanicolaou smear screening in adult women
- Papanicolaou smear screening with HPV co-testing in adult women 30 years and older
- Cobas HPV screening in adult women

Primary prevention
- Cervical cancer screening has been shown to decrease the incidence of cervical cancers.
- Treatment of high-grade cervical dysplasia decreases rate of progression to cervical cancer.
- HPV vaccination decreases rates of cervical dysplasia.

Diagnosis

> **BOTTOM LINE/CLINICAL PEARLS**
> - History of no prior cervical cancer screening or untreated prior cervical dysplasia.
> - Exam findings can be variable: visible exophytic polypoid friable mass, barrel-shaped cervix on palpation, visible ulcerative lesion.
> - Biopsy must be done to confirm diagnosis. Staging includes thorough clinical evaluation that includes physical examination and additional evaluation as needed (cystoscopy, proctoscopy, chest X-ray, intravenous pyelogram).

Differential diagnosis
See Algorithm 39.1.

Differential diagnosis	Features
Cervical polyp or nabothian cyst	On exam, a benign polyp or cyst is uniform with smooth edges; however, pathology will confirm diagnosis.
Ulcerative lesion	Infections such as herpes in the cervix will typically presents with multiple vesicles and tender ulcers.
Other malignancies	Bladder cancer, endometrial cancer, rectal cancer can infiltrate the cervix.

Typical presentation
- The most common presentations include abnormal vaginal bleeding and vaginal discharge. Women can also be asymptomatic and diagnosis is made on biopsy following examination or Papanicolaou smear screening (Figure 39.3).
- As the tumor enlarges, it can cause symptoms of pelvic pain. If the tumor starts to invade toward the bladder or rectum, symptoms with urination and/or defecation can develop. In advanced cases, back pain, lower extremity swelling, and back pain can be present.

Clinical diagnosis
History
- Key factors that must be elicited from the history are prior abnormal Papanicolaou smears, chronic HPV infection, and history of cervical dysplasia.
- History of immunosuppression including HIV (cervical cancer is an AIDS-defining illness in HIV patients), history of organ transplant, chronic use of steroids or other immunomodulators place patients at higher risk of developing cervical cancer.

Algorithm 39.1 Diagnostic algorithm for cervical cancer

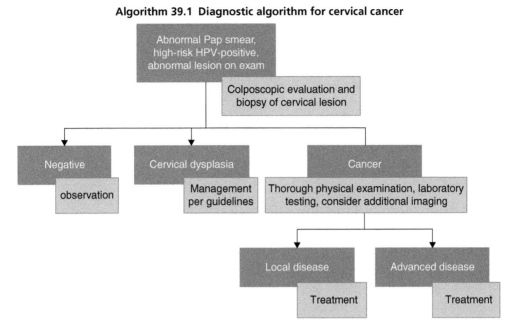

- Additional risk factors that must be ascertained include smoking history, history of oral contraceptive use, multiple sexual partners, early age of first intercourse.

Physical examination
- A clinician skilled in evaluating patients for cervical cancer must perform the physical examination. Examination includes a speculum exam to visualize the mass and its extent as well as a rectovaginal examination to evaluate for spread of disease to the parametria and/or pelvic side walls. Other areas that must be examined include regional and distant lymph nodes, specifically the superficial inguinal, femoral, and supraclavicular lymph nodes.

Laboratory diagnosis
List of diagnostic tests
- Biopsy of the abnormal lesion – this is done to confirm the diagnosis.
- Complete blood count – to evaluate for anemia. Thrombocytosis may also be present in a fraction of patients.
- Serum chemistry – specifically creatinine level to evaluate the kidney function. Abnormal kidney function may be a sign of advanced stage disease. Assessment of kidney function is also important in patients who will need platinum chemotherapy.
- Urinalysis – can be considered for patients with urinary symptoms.

List of imaging techniques
- International Federation of Gynecology and Obstetrics (FIGO) system for staging historically included only clinical evaluation. In 2018, FIGO updated staging to include use of imaging and pathology modalities when available (Bhatla et al. 2018).
- Computed tomography (CT), positron emission tomography (PET), and magnetic resonance imaging (MRI) can be performed when available to assess extent of disease.

Potential pitfalls/common errors made regarding diagnosis of disease
- Inexperienced examiner not skilled in recognizing the disease
- Lesion missed on exam/biopsy
- Delay in seeking care

Treatment
Treatment rationale
- Early stage disease is treated with surgery or radiation. Bulky disease and advanced stage disease are mainly treated with concurrent chemoradiation.
- Stage 1A1 disease is treated by cervical conization or simple hysterectomy.
- Stage 1A2 disease can be treated by modified radical hysterectomy or trachelectomy +/- pelvic and paraaortic lymph node dissection.
- Early stage (1B-2A), nonbulky disease is treated by radical hysterectomy or trachelectomy with pelvic and paraaortic lymph node dissection or external beam radiotherapy. In those undergoing radical hysterectomy, laparotomy is the preferred over minimally invasive techniques (Ramirez et al. 2018).
- Bulky early stage disease and advanced stage disease are treated with external beam radiotherapy and intracavitary brachytherapy with concurrent cisplatin chemotherapy.
- For patients with metastatic disease at diagnosis, systemic chemotherapy (carboplatin, paclitaxel, bevacizumab) is recommended.

When to hospitalize
- Patients must be hospitalized following radical surgery (hysterectomy, trachelectomy) for postoperative care.
- Patients who have active heavy bleeding from their tumor or are severely anemic must be hospitalized.
- Patients with treatment-related complications must be hospitalized.

Managing the hospitalized patient
- Close observation for postoperative complications
- Transfusion of blood products for anemic patients
- Emergency radiation therapy for patients actively bleeding, requiring urgent hemostasis
- Antibiotic therapy for infections

Table of treatment
See Algorithm 39.2.

Treatment	Comments
Conservative	Cervical conization can be considered for treatment of 1A disease in patients who desire to preserve fertility.
Medical	Chemotherapy (cisplatin) given concurrently with radiation therapy is standard treatment for those with advanced stage or bulky early stage disease. Chemotherapy (carboplatin, paclitaxel, +/- bevacizumab) is primary treatment for metastatic disease.
Surgical	Stage 1A: cervical conization or simple hysterectomy Stage 1B or 2A (nonbulky): radical hysterectomy or trachelectomy with pelvic and paraaortic lymph node dissection
Radiological	External beam radiation therapy with intracavitary brachytherapy has been shown to be most effective in treating advanced stage and bulky early stage disease. Cisplatin is given concurrently to sensitize the cancer cells to radiation treatment.

Algorithm 39.2 Treatment algorithm for cervical cancer, based on stage of disease

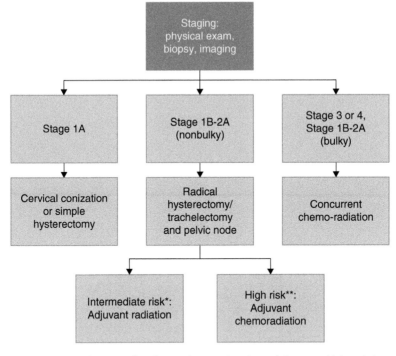

* Intermediate risk based on Sedlis criteria (lymphovascular space invasion and deep one-third cervical stromal invasion and tumor of any size, lymphovascular space invasion and middle one-third stromal invasion and tumor size $\geq$ 2 cm, lymphovascular space invasion and superficial one-third stromal invasion and tumor size $\geq$ 5 cm, no lymphovascular space invasion with deep or middle one-third stromal invasion and tumor size $\geq$ 4 cm)
** High risk based on Peters' criteria (positive surgical margins, pathologically confirmed involvement of pelvic lymph nodes, microscopic involvement of parametrium)

Prevention/management of complications
- Complications of surgery include infection, blood loss, damage to nearby structures. Complications of radical surgery include postoperative vesico- or uretero-vaginal fistula formation, ureteral strictures, bladder dysfunction, lymphedema, lymphocyst formation.
  - Infection: surgical infection can be prevented with preoperative antibiotics, adherence to sterile technique.
  - Blood loss and damage to nearby structures: risk is lower in experienced surgeons.
  - Vesicovaginal fistulas can be managed conservatively with continuous drainage of urine from bladder and treatment of existing urinary tract infection. Ureterovaginal fistulas can be managed with ureteral stent placement or percutaneous nephrostomy tube placement to drain the urinary system.
  - Ureteral stricture can be managed by placement of ureteral stents and/or nephrostomy tube placement.
  - Bladder dysfunction can be managed with bladder training, intermittent self-catheterization, prolonged catheter placement, medical therapy.
  - Lymphedema is treated with supportive care.
  - Lymphocysts can be managed with observation or drainage.
- Complications of chemotherapy can include nephrotoxicity, peripheral neuropathy, and bone marrow suppression. Nephrotoxicity can be prevented with adequate hydration with chemotherapy. Neuropathy can be managed by dose reduction and/or drug therapy for more severe neuropathy. Colony stimulating factors can be used to treat bone marrow suppression. Bone marrow suppression can place patients at risk for neutropenic sepsis, which is managed by intravenous antibiotics.

- Complications of radiation therapy include radiation proctitis, radiation cystitis, and vaginal stricture. Radiation proctitis and cystitis can be prevented with minimizing exposure of nearby structures to radiation field. Dilators are used for treatment of vaginal stricture.

> **CLINICAL PEARLS**
> - Accurate clinical staging is essential to treatment in cervical cancer.
> - Treatment of cervical cancer is dependent on stage of disease.
> - Early stage disease is treated with surgery.
> - Advanced stage disease is treated with concurrent chemo-radiation.

Special populations
Pregnancy
- The majority of cervical cancer diagnosed in pregnancy is stage 1 disease. Patients 20 weeks gestation can opt to delay treatment until fetal lung maturity is documented and then undergo cesarean delivery with radical surgery.

Elderly
- In patients who are frail or have numerous comorbid conditions, treatment with concurrent chemo-radiation is preferable to radical surgery.

Others
- HIV patients: treatment of HIV is important in maintaining the immune system to decrease rates of recurrence of cancer and/or dysplasia.

Prognosis

> **BOTTOM LINE/CLINICAL PEARLS**
> - Cervical cancer spreads through direct extension and through lymphatic channels.
> - Untreated disease can lead to invasion of surrounding structures and subsequently patients can develop life-threatening complications such as renal failure and rectal obstruction.
> - Prognostic factors include stage, tumor size, tumor volume, margin status, nodal status, lymphovascular space invasion.

Natural history of untreated disease
- Untreated disease will spread locally and through lymphatic channels.
- Disease can spread to neighboring organs such as the bladder and/or rectum.
- Disease can spread through lymphatic channels to the pelvic and para-aortic lymph nodes.

Prognosis for treated patients
- Early stage disease: 5-year survival 58–93%
- Advanced disease: 5-year survival 15–35% (American Cancer Society 2018)

Follow-up tests and monitoring
- Following treatment of cervical cancer, patient should undergo surveillance every 3–6 months based on stage of disease.
- Surveillance should include a review of symptoms, physical examination, and Papanicolaou testing.

Reading list
American Cancer Society. Cervical cancer. Revised 2015. Available from: https://www.cancer.org/cancer/cervical-cancer. html

American Cancer Society. *Global cancer facts & figures*. 4th ed. Atlanta: American Cancer Society; 2018. Available from: https://www.cancer.org/content/dam/cancer-org/research/cancer-facts-and-statistics/global-cancer-facts-and-figures/global-cancer-facts-and-figures-4th-edition.pdf

Bhatla N, Aoki D, Sharma DN, et al. FIGO cancer report 2018. Cancer of the cervix uteri. *Intl J Gynecol Obstet* 2018;143(Suppl):22-36.

Campos NG, Sharma M, Clark A. *Comprehensive global cervical cancer prevention costs and benefits of scaling up within a decade*. Boston, MA: Center for Health Decision Science, Harvard School of Public Health; 2016. Available from: https://www.cancer.org/content/dam/cancer-org/cancer-control/en/reports/the-cost-of-cervical-cancer-prevention.pdf

Castellsagué X, Díaz M, de Sanjosé S, et al. Worldwide human papillomavirus etiology of cervical adenocarcinoma and its cofactors: implications for screening and prevention. *J Natl Cancer Inst* 2006;Mar 1;98(5):303-15.

Chemoradiotherapy for Cervical Cancer Meta-Analysis Collaboration. Reducing uncertainties about the effects of chemoradiotherapy for cervical cancer: a systematic review and meta-analysis of individual patient data from 18 randomized trials. *J Clin Oncol* 2008;Dec 10;26(35):5802-12. doi: 10.1200/JCO.2008.16.4368. Epub 2008 Nov 10.

Gram IT, Austin H, Stalsberg H. Cigarette smoking and the incidence of cervical intraepithelial neoplasia, grade III, and cancer of the cervix uteri. *Am J Epidemiol* 1992;Feb 15;135(4):341-6.

Koh WJ, Greer BE, Abu-Rustum NR, et al. Cervical cancer, Version 2.2015. *J Natl Compr Canc Netw* 2015;Apr;13(4):395-404.

Lowy DR, Schiller JT. Prophylactic human papillomavirus vaccines. *J Clin Invest* 2006;May;116(5):1167-73.

Massad LS, Einstein MH, Huh WK, et al. 2012 updated consensus guidelines for the management of abnormal cervical cancer screening tests and cancer precursors. *J Low Genit Tract Dis* 2013;Apr;17(5 Suppl 1):S1-27.

Patel P, Hanson DL, Sullivan PS, et al. Incidence of types of cancer among HIV-infected persons compared with the general population in the United States, 1992–2003. *Ann Intern Med* 2008;May 20;148(10):728-36.

Ramirez PT, Frumovitz M, Pareja R, et al. Minimally invasive versus abdominal radical hysterectomy for cervical cancer. *N Engl J Med* 2018;Nov 15;379(20):1895-04.

Randall ME, Fracasso PM, Toita I, et al. Chapter 21: Cervix. In: Barakat RR, Berchuck A, Markman M, et al. eds. *Principles and practice of gynecologic oncology*. 6th ed. Philadelphia: Wolters Kluwer Health/Lippincott Williams & Wilkins; 2013:598-660.

Saslow D, Solomon D, Lawson HW, et al. American Cancer Society, American Society for Colposcopy and Cervical Pathology, and American Society for Clinical Pathology screening guidelines for the prevention and early detection of cervical cancer. *J Low Genit Tract Dis* 2012;Jul;16(3):175-204.

Schiffman MH, Bauer HM, Hoover RN, et al. Epidemiologic evidence showing that human papillomavirus infection causes most cervical intraepithelial neoplasia. *J Natl Cancer Inst* 1993;85(12):958-64.

Siegel RL, Miller KD, Jemal A. Cancer statistics 2019. *CA Can J Clin* 2019;69(1):7-34.

Suggested websites

American Society for Colposcopy and Cervical Pathology. www.asccp.org

American Cancer Society. http://www.cancer.org/cancer/cervical-cancer/

Centers for Disease Control and Prevention. http://www.cdc.gov/cancer/cervical/

Guidelines
National society guidelines

Title	Source	Date/full reference
Cervical cancer screening	American Society for Colposcopy and Cervical Pathology	Saslow D, Solomon D, Lawson HW, et al. American Cancer Society, American Society for Colposcopy and Cervical Pathology, and American Society for Clinical Pathology screening guidelines for the prevention and early detection of cervical cancer. *J Low Genit Tract Dis* 2012;Jul;16(3):175-204.
Management of abnormal cervical cancer screening results	American Society for Colposcopy and Cervical Pathology	Massad LS, Einstein MH, Huh WK, et al. 2012 updated consensus guidelines for the management of abnormal cervical cancer screening tests and cancer precursors. *J Low Genit Tract Dis* 2013;Apr;17(5 Suppl 1):S1-27.

(Continued)

(*Continued*)

Title	Source	Date/full reference
Treatment of cervical cancer	National Comprehensive Cancer Network	Koh WJ, Greer BE, Abu-Rustum NR, et al. Cervical cancer, Version 3. 2019 NCCN Clinical Practice Guidelines in Oncology. *J Natl Compr Canc Netw* 2019;Jan;17(1):64-84.
Diagnosis and treatment of cervical cancer	International Federation of Gynecology and Obstetrics	Bhatla N, Aoki D, Sharma DN, et al. FIGO Cancer Report 2018. Cancer of the cervix uteri. *Intl J Gynecol Obstet* 2018;143(Suppl):22-36.
Surveillance	Society of Gynecologic Oncology	Salani R, Khanna N, Frimer M, et al. An update on post-treatment surveillance and diagnosis of recurrence in women with gynecologic malignancies: Society of Gynecologic Oncology (SGO) recommendations. *Gynecol Oncol* 2017 Jul;146(1):3-10.

Evidence

Type of evidence	Title and comment	Date/full reference
Randomized controlled trial	Gynecologic Oncology Group trial 92 established the role of adjuvant postoperative pelvic radiation in intermediate risk patients at reducing recurrence of disease.	Sedlis A, Bundy BN, Rotman MZ, et al. A randomized trial of pelvic radiation therapy versus no further therapy in selected patients with stage IB carcinoma of the cervix after radical hysterectomy and pelvic lymphadenectomy: A Gynecologic Oncology Group Study. *Gynecol Oncol* 1999;May;73(2):177-83.
Prospective surgical/ pathological study	Gynecologic Oncology Group trial 49 found that pelvic nodal metastasis, tumor size, lymphovascular space invasion, and depth of cervical stromal invasion were significant predictive factors in cervical cancer recurrence.	Delgado G, Bundy BN, Fowler WC Jr, et al. A prospective surgical pathological study of stage I squamous carcinoma of the cervix: a Gynecologic Oncology Group Study. *Gynecol Oncol* 1989;Dec;35(3):314-20.
Randomized controlled trial	Gynecologic Oncology Group trial 109 showed that concurrent chemotherapy with radiation therapy improves progression-free and overall survival in patients with high-risk, early-stage disease who have been treated surgically for cervical cancer.	Peters WA, Liu PY, Barrett RJ 2nd, et al. Concurrent chemotherapy and pelvic radiation therapy compared with pelvic radiation therapy alone as adjuvant therapy after radical surgery in high-risk early-stage cancer of the cervix. *J Clin Oncol* 2000;Apr;18(8):1606-13.
Randomized controlled trial	The OUTBACK trial is ongoing and its objective is to evaluate if adjuvant chemotherapy in addition to chemoradiation improves overall survival.	Mileshkin LR, Narayan K, Moore KN, et al. A phase III trial of adjuvant chemotherapy following chemoradiation as primary treatment for locally advanced cervical cancer compared to chemoradiation alone: The OUTBACK TRIAL. *J Clin Oncol* 2012;30(15 Suppl; abstr TPS5116).
Randomized controlled trial	The LACC trial found that minimally invasive radical hysterectomy was associated with lower rates of disease-free survival and overall survival than open abdominal radical hysterectomy among women with early-stage cervical cancer.	Ramirez PT, Frumovitz M, Pareja R, et al. Minimally invasive versus abdominal radical hysterectomy for cervical cancer. *N Engl J Med* 2018;Nov 15;379(20):1895-904.

Images

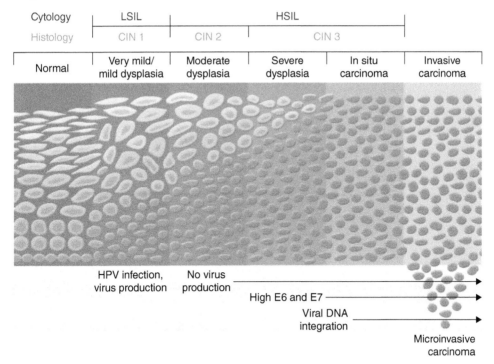

Figure 39.2 Progression from benign cervical lesion to invasive carcinoma. Courtesy of National Cancer Institute. Infection by oncogenic HPV types, especially HPV16, may directly cause a benign condylomatous lesion, low-grade dysplasia, or sometimes even an early high-grade lesion. Carcinoma in situ rarely occurs until several years after infection. It results from the combined effects of HPV genes, particularly those encoding E6 and E7, which are the two viral oncoproteins that are preferentially retained and expressed in cervical cancers; integration of the viral DNA into the host DNA; and a series of genetic and epigenetic changes in cellular genes. HSIL, high-grade squamous intraepithelial lesion; LSIL, low-grade squamous intraepithelial lesion (Lowy and Schiller 2006).

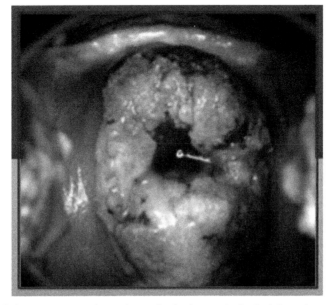

Figure 39.3 Cervical cancer seen on colposcopic examination (personal collection). See color version on website.

Additional material for this chapter can be found online at:
www.wiley.com/go/sperling/mountsinai/obstetricsandgynecology

This includes a case study, multiple choice questions, advice for patients,
and ICD codes. The following image is available in color: Figure 39.3.

CHAPTER 40

Endometrial Cancer

Jamal Rahaman and Carmel J. Cohen

Division of Gynecologic Oncology – Department of Obstetrics, Gynecology and Reproductive Science, Icahn School of Medicine at Mount Sinai, New York, NY

OVERALL BOTTOM LINE

- Endometrial carcinoma is the most frequent gynecologic cancer in the US with over 50 000 new cases diagnosed each year.
- Over 80% have the classic estrogen-dependent endometrioid histology with a favorable prognosis (type I cancers).
- Type II cancers have a different molecular profile associated with more virulent disease and diminished survival and include uterine papillary serous carcinomas (UPSC) and clear cell carcinomas.
- Surgery, where possible, constitutes the definitive primary treatment.
- Primary radiation therapy and primary hormonal therapy are alternatives for inoperable patients.
- Paclitaxel (T), carboplatin (C), cisplatin (P), and doxorubicin (A) are the most active single agents, with TC and TAP being the most effective combination chemotherapy regimens.

Background
Definition of disease

- Endometrioid adenocarcinoma is the most common of the endometrial cancer histologies characterized by the disappearance of stroma between abnormal glands that have enfolding of their linings into the lumens, disordered nuclear chromatin distribution, nuclear enlargement, and a variable degree of mitosis, necrosis, and hemorrhage. It accounts for 80–95% of the adenocarcinomas.
- Other less common histologies include UPSC, clear cell carcinoma, endometrial papillary adenocarcinoma, and adenosquamous carcinoma.

Disease classification

- Type I cancers represent over 80% of endometrial cancers and have the classic estrogen-dependent endometrioid histology with a favorable prognosis.
- Type II endometrial cancers have a distinct phenotype and now are recognized to also have a different molecular profile associated with more virulent disease and diminished survival and includes UPSC and clear cell carcinomas.

Incidence/prevalence

- In 2015, 54 870 new cases of uterine corpus cancer were diagnosed in the US and 10 170 women died from this cancer. Endometrial carcinoma occurs most often in the sixth and seventh decades of life, with an average age at onset of 60 years, and a lifetime risk of 2.6%.
- Compared with white women, black women have a lower incidence of endometrial carcinoma but with less favorable histologies, more advanced stages of disease, more poorly differentiated tumors, and higher mortality.

Mount Sinai Expert Guides: Obstetrics and Gynecology, First Edition. Edited by Rhoda Sperling.
© 2020 John Wiley & Sons Ltd. Published 2020 by John Wiley & Sons Ltd.
Companion Website: www.wiley.com/go/sperling/mountsinai/obstetricsandgynecology

Etiology

- Endogenous or exogenous exposure to estrogen is believed to be an important risk factor for the development of endometrial hyperplasia and type I endometrial cancers. Estrogens not opposed by progestins lead to increased mitotic activity of endometrial cells, resulting in more frequent errors in DNA replication and somatic mutations.
- Type II tumors are estrogen independent and include high-grade endometrioid and serous histologies and are characterized by a high mutational rate of TP53, have high copy numbers, and are microsatellite stable tumors.

Pathology/pathogenesis

- Tumor growth may be confined to the endometrium, invade the underlying myometrium, penetrate to the uterine serosal surface or adjacent bladder or rectum, or extend into the cervical canal and invade cervical glands or stroma.
- Lymphatic spread occurs primarily to pelvic and paraaortic lymph nodes and occasionally involves inguinal nodes.
- Peritoneal disease spreads via transmigration from the fallopian tubes or through serosal penetration.
- Hematogenous spread is not uncommon but usually occurs late.

Predictive/risk factors

Risk factor	Relative risk
Increasing age	Women 50–70 years have a 1.4% risk; the overall lifetime risk is 2.6%
Obesity	2–10
Unopposed estrogen therapy	2–10
Lynch syndrome – genetic mutations *MLH1, MSH2, MSH6, PMS2*	20–70% lifetime risk
Race	White 1.6 times Asian
Tamoxifen therapy	2.5–7.5
Nulliparity	2
Late menopause (after age 55)	2
Polycystic ovary syndrome	3
Cowden syndrome (*PTEN* mutation)	13–19% lifetime risk
Estrogen secreting tumor	NA
Diabetes mellitus	2
Early menarche	NA

Prevention

BOTTOM LINE/CLINICAL PEARLS
- Factors that reduce circulating estrogen levels (weight loss/exercise, cigarette smoking) appear to be protective.
- Progestins antagonize the effects of estrogen on the endometrium and prevent the development of hyperplasia and cancer and can reverse precancerous complex atypical endometrial hyperplasia.
- Prior use of oral contraceptives also appears to be protective.

Screening

- The relatively low prevalence of endometrial carcinoma in the population (5 per 1000 women > 45 years) makes standardized screening inefficient.
- The American College of Obstetrics and Gynecology (ACOG) and the Society of Gynecologic Oncology (SGO) do not recommend routine screening of patients for uterine cancer.
- The American Cancer Society (ACS) does recommend annual endometrial biopsies starting at age 35 for women known to have or be at risk for hereditary nonpolyposis colorectal cancer (HNPCC) and/or Lynch syndrome.

Primary prevention

- The increased risk of endometrial carcinoma associated with unopposed estrogens means that women with an intact uterus should rarely, if ever, be prescribed estrogen-only replacement therapy.
- The use of the estrogen–progesterone oral contraceptive pill decreases the risk by 50% and the protective effect persists for more than 10–20 years after cessation.
- Progestin-only contraception and therapy including depot-medroxyprogesterone acetate, progestin implants, and progestin-releasing intrauterine devices provide protection against development of endometrial cancer.

Diagnosis (Algorithm 40.1)

> **BOTTOM LINE/CLINICAL PEARLS**
> - Over 75% of patients with endometrial carcinoma present with the classic symptom of postmenopausal bleeding or abnormal uterine bleeding. Additionally, patients with endometrial carcinoma present with vaginal discharge or have a thickened endometrium incidentally noted on ultrasound, computed tomography (CT) scan, or magnetic resonance imaging (MRI) performed for another reason.
> - Some patients present with abnormal cervical cytology findings including endometrial cells in women aged over 40, atypical glandular cells, or adenocarcinoma.
> - Pathologic evaluation of the endometrium provides histologic diagnosis and can identify other etiologies of bleeding such as chronic endometritis, atrophy, polyps, cervical cancer, or unusual histologic variants. This can be achieved by an office endometrial biopsy or a dilatation and curettage (D&C) under anesthesia.
> - Hysteroscopy has been advocated as an adjunct to D&C to improve detection of pathology in the evaluation of postmenopausal bleeding.

Algorithm 40.1 Surgical management of endometrial carcinoma

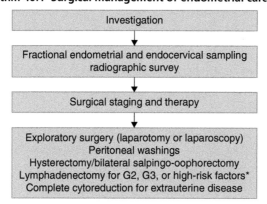

* < 50% myoinvasion, clear cell or papillary serous histology, adnexal metastasis, lymph-vascular space invasion, and/or cervical invasion, > 50% uterine cavity involved, suspicious nodes.

Differential diagnosis

Differential diagnosis	Features
Benign endometrial polyps	Abnormal bleeding and a thickened endometrial stripe on sonography – carcinoma can be excluded only by complete polypectomy at hysteroscopy.
Endometrial hyperplasia	Abnormal bleeding and a thickened endometrial stripe on sonography – carcinoma can be excluded only by thorough global curettage – 25–40% of complex atypical endometrial hyperplasia will have an associated endometrial cancer.
Uterine fibroids	Fibroids (especially submucous) can develop with heavy vaginal bleeding (menorrhagia). Prior to hysterectomy, all women with abnormal uterine bleeding should have endometrial sampling to exclude an endometrial cancer.
Endocervical carcinoma	Can produce identical symptoms including menorrhagia, postmenopausal bleeding, and abnormal cytology on a Pap smear. A fractional curettage to assess the endocervical mucosa should be included in the preoperative evaluation and cervical biopsies and cone biopsy considered in select cases. The appropriate management is surgery with a radical hysterectomy for early stages I and IIA and chemo-radiation for advanced stages of endocervical cancer.
Uterine sarcoma	Uterine sarcomas (especially leiomyosarcomas and endometrial stromal sarcomas) can develop with abnormal bleeding and an enlarging uterus and have negative findings on D&C. The diagnosis is sometimes established only by a hysterectomy.

Typical presentation
- Patients with endometrial carcinoma typically present with abnormal uterine bleeding. It is most commonly found in women who are postmenopausal and with increasing age in premenopausal women.
- Incidental finding on imaging – a thickened endometrial lining is sometimes found incidentally on ultrasound, CT, or MRI performed for another indication.
- Some patients present with abnormal cervical cytology findings including endometrial cells in women aged over 40, atypical glandular cells, or adenocarcinoma.
- Incidental finding at hysterectomy – endometrial carcinoma or hyperplasia is sometimes discovered incidentally when hysterectomy is performed for benign disease. Prior to hysterectomy, all women with abnormal uterine bleeding should have endometrial sampling.

Clinical diagnosis
History
Because patients with endometrial carcinoma typically present with abnormal uterine bleeding the following bleeding patterns should prompt endometrial evaluation.
- **Postmenopausal women:** any bleeding, including spotting or staining. Three to 20% of women with postmenopausal bleeding are found to have endometrial carcinoma and another 5–15% have endometrial hyperplasia.
- **Age 45 to menopause:** any abnormal uterine bleeding, including intermenstrual bleeding in women who are ovulatory, frequent (interval between the onset of bleeding episodes is less than 21 days), heavy (total volume of > 80 mL), or prolonged (longer than 7 days). In addition, endometrial neoplasia should be suspected in women with prolonged periods of amenorrhea (6 months or more) in women with anovulation.
- **Younger than 45 years:** abnormal uterine bleeding that is persistent, occurs in the setting of a history of unopposed estrogen exposure (obesity, chronic anovulation) or failed medical management of the bleeding, or in women at high risk of endometrial cancer (e.g. Lynch and Cowden syndromes).

Physical examination
- Prior to treatment, a complete pelvic and general physical examination should be performed, with particular attention to the size and mobility of the uterus and the presence of extrauterine masses or ascites; potential sites of nodal metastases should also be examined (e.g. supraclavicular nodes). Because surgical staging is the preferred definitive management, a thorough physical examination for preoperative clearance for major surgery is required.

Useful clinical decision rules and calculators
- Endometrial carcinoma is a histologic diagnosis based upon the results of evaluation of an endometrial biopsy, curettage sample, or hysterectomy specimen.
- **Negative endometrial sampling:** the sensitivity for endometrial sampling is 90% or higher. Risk factors for false-negative endometrial sampling include a personal history of colorectal cancer, endometrial polyps, and morbid obesity.
- Women with an endometrial biopsy result that has insufficient endometrial cells should have sampling repeated with a D&C as well as a hysteroscopy to ensure thorough evaluation.
- **Persistent or recurrent bleeding:** if bleeding persists or recurs after endometrial sampling with benign findings, further evaluation is required with a hysteroscopy or, if necessary, a hysterectomy.

Disease severity classification
- Endometrial carcinoma is surgically staged according to the joint 2010 International Federation of Gynecology and Obstetrics/Tumor-Node-Metastasis (FIGO/TNM) classification system (Table 40.1).

Laboratory diagnosis
List of diagnostic tests
- Women of reproductive age with suspected endometrial hyperplasia or carcinoma should have urine or serum human chorionic gonadotropin testing to exclude pregnancy as an etiology of abnormal uterine bleeding and to ensure that endometrial sampling will not disrupt a pregnancy.
- Preoperative blood testing should include a complete blood count (CBC), type and screen, and metabolic profile.
- Measurement of the serum tumor marker CA 125 is a clinically useful test for predicting extrauterine spread of endometrial carcinoma.

List of imaging techniques
- For women with suspected endometrial carcinoma or hyperplasia, pelvic sonography is often the first-line imaging study to evaluate for other etiologies of abnormal uterine bleeding.
- In the infrequent situation in which a patient is staged clinically, contrast-enhanced MRI appears to be the best radiographic modality for detecting myometrial invasion or cervical involvement when compared with nonenhanced MRI, ultrasound, or CT.
- MRI is also the best imaging modality, compared with CT or positron emission tomography (PET) with or without CT, for detecting lymph node metastases.
- A chest radiograph should be performed as part of the initial assessment.
- For patients with advanced or recurrent disease, a metastatic investigation should include a CT scan or MRI of the chest, abdomen, and pelvis.
- PET scans have utility in detecting occult lesions.

Potential pitfalls/common errors made regarding diagnosis of disease
- Prior to hysterectomy, all women with abnormal uterine bleeding should have endometrial sampling to exclude an associated endometrial carcinoma.

Table 40.1 Staging of endometrial carcinoma.

TNM categories	FIGO[a] stages	Definition
Primary tumor (T)		
TX		Primary tumor cannot be assessed
T0		No evidence of primary tumor
Tis[b]		Carcinoma in situ (preinvasive carcinoma)
T1	I	Tumor confined to the corpus uteri
T1a	IA	Tumor limited to the endometrium or invades less than half of the myometrium
T1b	IB	Tumor invades half or more of the myometrium
T2	II	Tumor invades stromal connective tissue of the cervix but does not extend beyond the uterus[c]
T3	IIIA	Tumor involves serosa and/or adnexa (direct extension or metastasis)[d]
T3b	IIIB	Vaginal involvement (direct extension or metastasis) or parametrial involvement[d]
	IIIC	Metastasis to pelvic and/or paraaortic lymph nodes[d]
T4	IVA	Tumor invades bladder mucosa and/or bowel (bullous edema is not sufficient to classify a tumor as T4)
Regional lymph nodes (N)		
NX		Regional lymph nodes cannot be assessed
N0		No regional lymph node metastasis
N1	IIIC1	Regional lymph node metastasis to pelvic lymph nodes (positive pelvic nodes)
N2	IIIC2	Regional lymph node metastasis to paraaortic lymph nodes, with or without positive pelvic lymph nodes
Distant metastasis (M)		
M0		No distant metastasis
M1	IVB	Distant metastasis (includes metastasis to inguinal lymph nodes, intraperitoneal disease, or lung, liver, or bone. It excludes metastasis to paraaortic lymph nodes, vagina, pelvic serosa, or adnexa)

[a] Either G1, G2, or G3.
[b] FIGO no longer includes stage 0 (Tis).
[c] Endocervical glandular involvement should be considered only as stage I and no longer as stage II.
[d] Positive cytology has to be reported separately without changing the stage.

- All patients having a hysterectomy for complex endometrial hyperplasia should have a frozen section taken to exclude an associated endometrial cancer (25–40% risk). If cancer is discovered, a staging procedure can be performed immediately, with a bilateral salpingo-oophorectomy (BSO), pelvic and paraaortic lymphadenectomy and omentectomy (for serous and clear cell cancers).

Treatment (Algorithm 40.2)
Treatment rationale
All women with endometrial cancer should undergo surgical staging, especially if the disease is not suspected to be metastatic. Surgical staging defines the extent of disease and largely defines the risk of recurrence. Adjuvant therapy for stage I disease is determined by age, depth of myometrial invasion, lymph–vascular space invasion, and tumor grade.

Algorithm 40.2 Postoperative management of endometrial carcinoma

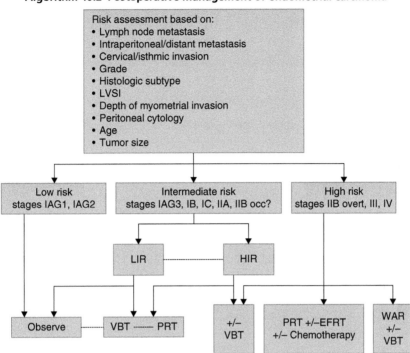

EFRT, extended field radiotherapy; HIR, high intermediate risk based on GOG-99; LIR, low intermediate risk; LVSI, lymph–vascular space invasion; PRT, pelvic radiotherapy; VBT, vaginal brachytherapy; WAR, whole abdominopelvic radiotherapy. Age: < 50, three factors; 50–70, two factors; > 70, one factor. High-risk factors were LVSI, outer one-third invasion, and Grade 2–3.

Surgery, where possible, constitutes the definitive primary treatment for most patients with endometrial carcinoma (Figures 40.1 and 40.2). Primary radiation therapy and primary hormonal therapy are alternatives for inoperable patients.
- Women with low-grade (grade 1 or 2) endometrioid cancers confined to the endometrium (a subset of stage IA disease) are classified as having low-risk endometrial cancer. Because their prognosis following surgery is excellent, no adjuvant treatment is required.
- Women with endometrial cancer that invades the myometrium (stage IA or IB) or demonstrates occult cervical stromal invasion (stage II) have intermediate-risk disease. These patients are candidates for adjuvant radiation therapy. Although there is no clear role for chemotherapy as part of an adjuvant treatment strategy, some clinicians recommend chemotherapy to women with high intermediate-risk disease.
- Women who have any of the following features have high-risk endometrial cancer: stage III disease, regardless of histology or grade; and/or uterine serous carcinoma or clear cell carcinoma of any stage. Women with high-risk disease often receive chemotherapy with or without radiation therapy given their high risk of both distant and locoregional relapse.

Table of treatment

Treatment	Comments
Conservative/hormonal	Women with apparent stage IA grade 1 endometrial carcinoma who wish to preserve fertility can opt to avoid hysterectomy/BSO and undergo progestin therapy. These women should undergo hysterectomy/BSO after completion of childbearing, even in cases with demonstrated tumor regression.

(Continued)

(Continued)

Treatment	Comments
Medical	For patients with early high-risk, advanced, and recurrent disease chemotherapy is recommended. Paclitaxel (T), carboplatin (C), cisplatin (P), and doxorubicin (A) are the most active single agents with TC and TAP being the most effective combination chemotherapy regimens.
Surgical	A total extrafascial hysterectomy with BSO with pelvic and paraaortic lymph node dissection is the standard staging procedure for endometrial carcinoma. Abdominal, vaginal, laparoscopic, or robot-assisted approaches are possible. An omentectomy is frequently carried out for patients with serous or clear cell histology. Cytoreduction is performed when metastases are evident.
Radiation	Radiation therapy can be administered as primary definitive management for inoperable patients. Adjuvant vaginal cuff brachytherapy with or without whole pelvic radiotherapy is recommended for patients with intermediate- or high-risk stage I and II cancer. For advanced stages and recurrent cancer whole pelvic and extended field (to include paraaortic nodes) is appropriate. Targeted radiation to painful bony metastasis is a useful option.

CLINICAL PEARLS
- Surgery constitutes the definitive primary treatment for most patients with endometrial carcinoma.
- Primary radiation therapy and primary hormonal therapy are alternatives for inoperable patients.
- For women with low-risk endometrial cancer no additional treatment is needed after surgery because their prognosis is excellent.
- Women with intermediate-risk disease are candidates for adjuvant radiation therapy.
- Women with high-risk disease may require chemotherapy with or without radiation therapy.

Special populations
Elderly
- Older age has been associated with higher rates of clinical failure and survival in several studies. The association between age and prognosis can be illustrated by data from the Gynecologic Oncology Group (GOG) protocol 33, in which 5-year relative survival rates for women with clinical stage I and II endometrial cancer stratified by age were as follows:
  - ≤ 40 years – 96%.
  - 41–50 years – 94%
  - 51–60 years – 87%
  - 61–70 years – 78%
  - 71–80 years – 71%
  - ≥ 80 years – 54%

Prognosis

BOTTOM LINE/CLINICAL PEARLS
- The prognosis of endometrial carcinoma is determined primarily by disease stage and histology (including both grade and histologic subtype). Fortunately, most women with endometrial carcinoma have a favorable prognosis, because the majority of patients have endometrioid (usually good prognosis) and present with early stage disease because of abnormal uterine bleeding.

- Other histologic types of endometrial carcinoma (e.g. serous, clear cell) as well as other types of uterine cancer are associated with a poorer prognosis. In general, the rate of 5-year survival for stage I disease is approximately 80–90%, for stage II it is 70–80%, and for stages III and IV it is 20–60% (Table 40.2).

Prognosis for treated patients

- This is included in the survival data from both the FIGO report and the Surveillance, Epidemiology, and End Results (SEER) data.

Follow-up tests and monitoring

- Posttreatment surveillance is aimed at the early detection of recurrent disease. For women with endometrial carcinoma, surveillance consists mainly of monitoring for symptoms and physical examination.
- There is no high-quality evidence that any specific posttreatment surveillance strategy is associated with improved outcomes. In the absence of data, we agree with the consensus-based guidelines from the US National Comprehensive Cancer Network (NCCN) and the SGO, which include the following.
  - Review of symptoms and physical examination including speculum and bimanual pelvic examination every 3–6 months for 2 years, then every 6 months or annually. The frequency of examinations depends upon the risk of persistent or recurrent disease. Although surveillance using vaginal cytology is recommended by the NCCN, the SGO does not support this.
- When planning the posttreatment surveillance strategy, care should be taken to limit the number of CT scans, given concerns about radiation exposure and the risk for secondary malignancies.
- CT and MRI should be performed for patients who are symptomatic or have abnormal findings on physical examination.

Table 40.2 Uterine carcinoma: FIGO surgical stage and overall survival (%).

FIGO stage	2 years[a]	5 years[a]	5 years[b]
IA	97	91	90
IB	97	91	78
IC	94	85	–
II	–	–	74
IIA	93	83	–
IIB	85	74	–
IIIA	80	66	56
IIIB	62	50	36
IIIC	75	57	–
IIIC1	–	–	57
IIIC2	–	–	49
IVA	47	26	22
IVB	37	20	21

[a] Data from FIGO for patients treated in 1999–2001, using the original 1988 FIGO surgical staging classification (from Creasman et al. 2006).
[b] Data from SEER database for patients treated in 1988–2006, staged according to the 2010 FIGO staging system (from Lewin et al. 2010).

- PET as a modality for the evaluation of a suspected recurrence has a sensitivity and specificity of 95% and 93%, respectively.

Reading list

Bokhman JV. Two pathogenetic types of endometrial carcinoma. *Gynecol Oncol* 1983;15:10-17.
Boruta DM 2nd, Gehrig PA, Fader AN, et al. Management of women with uterine papillary serous cancer: a Society of Gynecologic Oncology (SGO) review. *Gynecol Oncol* 2009;115:142-53.
Cancer Genome Atlas Research Network, Kandoth C, Schultz N, Cherniack AD, et al. Integrated genomic characterization of endometrial carcinoma. *Nature* 2013;497:67-73.
Cohen CJ, Rahaman J. Endometrial cancer: management of high risk and recurrence including the tamoxifen controversy. *Cancer* 1995;76:2044-52.
Creasman WT, Odicino F, Maisonneuve P, et al. Carcinoma of the corpus uteri. FIGO 26th Annual Report on the Results of Treatment in Gynecological Cancer. *Int J Gynaecol Obstet* 2006;95(Suppl 1):S105.
Gusberg SB. Precursors of corpus carcinoma, estrogen and adenomatous hyperplasia. *Am J Obstet Gynecol* 1947;54:905-27.
Lewin SN, Herzog TJ, Barrena Medel NI, et al. Comparative performance of the 2009 international Federation of Gynecology and Obstetrics staging system for uterine corpus cancer. *Obstet Gynecol* 2010 Nov;116(5):1141-9.
Olawaiye AB, Boruta DM 2nd. Management of women with clear cell endometrial cancer: a Society of Gynecologic Oncology (SGO) review. *Gynecol Oncol* 2009;113:277-83.
Rahaman J, Lu K, Cohen CJ. Chapter 103: endometrial cancer. In: Bast R, Croce CM, Hait WN, et al., eds. *Holland-Frei cancer medicine*. 9th ed. Hoboken, NJ: Wiley; 2017.
Ramirez PT, Frumovitz M, Bodurka DC, et al. Hormonal therapy for the management of grade 1 endometrial adenocarcinoma: a literature review. *Gynecol Oncol* 2004;95:133-8.

Suggested website

National Comprehensive Cancer Network. http://www.nccn.org/professionals/physician_gls

Guidelines
National society guidelines

Title	Source	Date/URL
NCCN clinical practice guidelines in oncology	NCCN	2019 http://www.nccn.org/professionals/physician_gls/
Post-treatment surveillance and diagnosis of recurrence in women with gynecologic malignancies: Society of Gynecologic Oncologists recommendations	Society of Gynecologic Oncologists	2011 https://www.ncbi.nlm.nih.gov/pubmed/21752752

Evidence

Type of evidence	Title and comment	Date/URL
Randomized controlled trial (RCT)	A phase III trial of surgery with or without adjunctive external pelvic radiation therapy in intermediate risk endometrial adenocarcinoma: a Gynecologic Oncology Group study Comment: The GOG 99 is the only randomized trial to evaluate the value of RT in well-staged patients with intermediate risk	2004 https://www.ncbi.nlm.nih.gov/pubmed/14984936
RCT	Surgery and postoperative radiotherapy versus surgery alone for patients with stage-1 endometrial carcinoma: multicentre randomised trial. PORTEC Study Group. Post Operative Radiation Therapy in Endometrial Carcinoma	2000 https://www.ncbi.nlm.nih.gov/pubmed/10791524

(*Continued*)

Type of evidence	Title and comment	Date/URL
RCT	Vaginal brachytherapy versus pelvic external beam radiotherapy for patients with endometrial cancer of high-intermediate risk (PORTEC-2): an open-label, non-inferiority, randomised trial	2010 https://www.ncbi.nlm.nih.gov/ pubmed/20206777
RCT	Randomized phase III noninferiority trial of first line chemotherapy for metastatic or recurrent endometrial carcinoma: a Gynecologic Oncology Group Study Comment: Comment: This GOG 209 study established taxol/carboplatin combination chemotherapy as a better tolerated and equivalent therapeutic option to taxol/doxorubicin/cisplatin	2012 https://www.gynecologi concology-online.net/article/ S0090-8258(12)00228-4/fulltext doi:10.1016/j.ygyno.2012.03.034
RCT	Phase III trial of doxorubicin plus cisplatin with or without paclitaxel plus filgrastim in advanced endometrial carcinoma: a Gynecologic Oncology Group Study. Comment: Demonstrated that TAP was superior PFS to AP but associated with more toxicity	2004 https://www.ncbi.nlm.nih.gov/ pubmed/15169803
RCT	Randomized phase III trial of pelvic radiotherapy versus cisplatin-based combined chemotherapy in patients with intermediate- and high risk endometrial cancer: a Japanese Gynecologic Oncology Group study	2008 https://www.ncbi.nlm.nih.gov/ pubmed/17996926
RCT	Randomized phase III trial of whole-abdominal irradiation versus doxorubicin and cisplatin chemotherapy in advanced endometrial carcinoma: a Gynecologic Oncology Group Study	2006 https://www.ncbi.nlm.nih.gov/ pubmed/16330675
RCT	Phase III trial of doxorubicin with or without cisplatin in advanced endometrial carcinoma: a Gynecologic Oncology Group Study	2004 https://www.ncbi.nlm.nih.gov/ pubmed/15459211
Prospective cohort study	Surgical pathologic spread patterns of endometrial cancer. A Gynecologic Oncology Group Study	1987 https://www.ncbi.nlm.nih.gov/ pubmed/3652025
Prospective cohort study	Relationship between surgical-pathological risk factors and outcome in clinical stage I and II carcinoma of the endometrium: a Gynecologic Oncology Group Study	1991 https://www.ncbi.nlm.nih.gov/ pubmed/1989916

Images

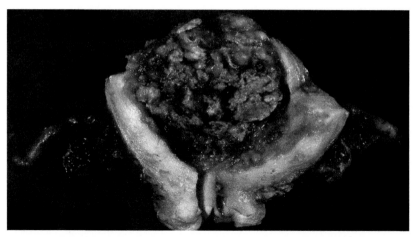

Figure 40.1 Endometrial cancer. Courtesy of Dr. Tamara Kalir, Department of Pathology, Icahn School of Medicine at Mount Sinai. See color version on website.

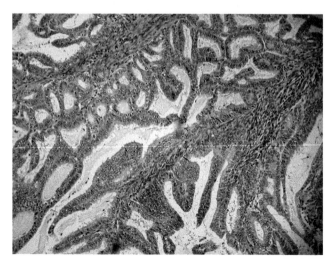

Figure 40.2 Photomicrograph of a well-differentiated endometrioid endometrial adenocarcinoma. Courtesy of Dr. Tamara Kalir, Department of Pathology, Icahn School of Medicine at Mount Sinai. See color version on website.

Additional material for this chapter can be found online at:
www.wiley.com/go/sperling/mountsinai/obstetricsandgynecology

The following images are available in color: Figure 40.1 and Figure 40.2.

CHAPTER 41

Gestational Trophoblastic Disease

Melissa Schwartz[1] and Stephanie V. Blank[2]

[1] Division of Gynecologic Oncology – Department of Obstetrics, Gynecology and Women's Health, Saint Louis University School of Medicine, St. Louis, MO
[2] Division of Gynecologic Oncology – Department of Obstetrics, Gynecology and Reproductive Science, Icahn School of Medicine at Mount Sinai, New York, NY

OVERALL BOTTOM LINE
- Gestational trophoblastic disease (GTD) is a spectrum of premalignant and malignant conditions that arise from the placenta.
- After a molar pregnancy, serial monitoring of serum human chorionic gonadotropin (hCG) is important for early identification of malignant sequelae.
- Treatment of malignant GTD, or gestational trophoblastic neoplasia (GTN), is dependent on stage and prognostic score.

Background
Definition of disease
- Gestational trophoblastic disease (GTD) comprises a spectrum of premalignant to malignant conditions that originate from the placenta. Collectively all malignant forms of disease are known as gestational trophoblastic neoplasia (GTN).

Disease classification
- Histologically distinct diseases within the spectrum of GTD include complete and partial hydatidiform moles (premalignant) to invasive moles, gestational choriocarcinoma, placental site trophoblastic tumor (PSTT), and epithelioid trophoblastic tumor (ETT).

Incidence/prevalence
- Incidence of hydatidiform moles (HMs) is 1-3:1000 pregnancies.
- Approximately 20% of patients with a HM will develop malignant sequelae.
- After a molar pregnancy, risk of recurrence increases to ~1%.

Etiology
- Complete moles are diploid and androgenic in origin. Approximately 80% result from the duplication of the haploid genome of a single sperm, whereas ~20% arise from dispermic fertilization of an ovum.
- Partial moles are almost always triploid and result from the fertilization of a normal ovum by two sperms or occasionally a diploid sperm.

Pathology/pathogenesis
- Complete moles show characteristic villous architecture, associated with abnormal trophoblastic hyperplasia, stromal hypercellularity, stromal karyorrhectic debris, and collapsed villous blood vessels.

Mount Sinai Expert Guides: Obstetrics and Gynecology, First Edition. Edited by Rhoda Sperling.
© 2020 John Wiley & Sons Ltd. Published 2020 by John Wiley & Sons Ltd.
Companion Website: www.wiley.com/go/sperling/mountsinai/obstetricsandgynecology

- Partial moles show patchy villous hydropic change with scattered abnormally shaped irregular villi with trophoblastic pseudoinclusions and patchy trophoblastic hyperplasia.
- An invasive mole develops after molar pregnancy and is characterized by edematous chorionic villi with trophoblastic proliferation that invades into the myometrium.
- Choriocarcinoma is malignant and includes both neoplastic syncytiotrophoblast and cytotrophoblastic elements without chorionic villi.
- Placental site trophoblastic tumors are rare and characterized by absence of villi with proliferation of intermediate trophoblast cells.

Predictive/risk factors
- Age: for moles, young or old age is a risk factor
- History of prior molar pregnancy
- Asian or African descent
- History of spontaneous abortion
- Infertility
- Family history of GTD

Prevention

BOTTOM LINE/CLINICAL PEARLS
- Effective birth control can prevent this disease.

Primary prevention
- Contraception

Diagnosis

BOTTOM LINE/CLINICAL PEARLS
- The most common symptom is abnormal vaginal bleeding.
- Transvaginal ultrasonography is used to establish the diagnosis of molar pregnancy in combination with abnormally high level of hCG (>100 000 mIU/mL).
- Serial monitoring of hCG is used for identification of postmolar gestational trophoblastic neoplasia.

Differential diagnosis

Differential diagnosis	Features
Early normal intrauterine pregnancy (IUP)	• IUP may or may not be noted on transvaginal ultrasound (TVUS), dependent on gestational age
Threatened abortion	• IUP noted on TVUS • Vaginal bleeding • Cervical os closed
Incomplete abortion	• Cervical os open
Complete abortion	• TVUS could show thickened endometrial echo • Cervical os closed

Typical presentation
- Reproductive age woman who presents with abnormal vaginal bleeding and an abnormally elevated β-hCG level (>100 000 mIU/mL). Other signs and symptoms include uterine size greater than expected for gestational age, absence of fetal heart tones, bilateral ovarian enlargement (theca lutein cysts), and hyperemesis gravidarum. Less commonly, patients may present with thyroid storm or preeclampsia. Transvaginal ultrasound shows diffuse mixed echogenic pattern replacing the placenta.

Clinical diagnosis
History
- Date of last menstrual period should be obtained. A complete obstetrical history should be taken, including dates, duration, and outcomes of all prior pregnancies. Medical, gynecologic, and surgical histories should be taken. Review of systems should include common symptoms associated with molar pregnancy, such as painless vaginal bleeding and emesis.

Physical examination
- A pelvic exam, including speculum exam, should be performed. On bimanual exam, uterine size might be larger than expected for gestational age. Bilateral adnexal masses may be present if ovarian theca lutein cysts are present. On speculum exam, the vagina should be examined for metastases. Focused physical exam should be done to exclude metastases to common sites, such as the lungs, vagina, liver, and central nervous system.

Useful clinical decision rules and calculators
- After molar evacuation, it is important to monitor serial serum quantitative hCG in order to promptly diagnose and treat malignant sequelae. Serum hCG should be obtained within 24 hours after evacuation, then weekly while elevated, and then monthly for 6 additional months.
- The following criteria are used for identification of postmolar gestational trophoblastic disease: (a) hCG level plateau of 4 values (+/- 10%) over 3 weeks, (b) hCG level increase of > 10% of 3 values recorded over 2 weeks, (c) persistence of detectable hCG level for > 6 months after molar evacuation.

Disease severity classification
- Staging for GTN

Stage I	Confined to uterus
Stage II	Tumor outside the uterus, but localized to pelvis and/or vagina
Stage III	Pulmonary metastases on chest X-ray
Stage IV	Metastatic disease outside of the lungs/pelvis/vagina

- 2000 International Federation of Gynecology and Obstetrics (FIGO) modification of the World Health Organization (WHO) prognostic index score for risk assessment for GTN – more clinically important than staging

FIGO score	0	1	2	4
Age (y)	≤39	>39	-	-
Antecedent pregnancy	Hydatidiform mole	Abortion	Term pregnancy	-
Interval from index pregnancy (mo)	<4	4-6	7–12	>12

(Continued)

(Continued)

FIGO score	0	1	2	4
Pretreatment hCG level (mIU/mL)	<1000	1000–10 000	>10 000–100 000	>100 000
Largest tumor size including uterus (cm)	3–4	5	-	-
Site of metastases	Lung, vagina	Spleen, kidney	Gastrointestinal tract	Brain, liver
Number of metastases identified	0	1–4	4–8	>8
Previous failed chemotherapy	-	-	Single drug	2 or more drugs

Total score 0–6 = low-risk; ≥7 = high-risk. Treatment is based on score. Low-risk patients can be treated with single-agent chemotherapy, whereas high-risk patients require multiagent chemotherapy.

Laboratory diagnosis

List of diagnostic tests
- Complete blood count
- Clotting function studies
- Renal, liver, thyroid function studies
- Blood type
- hCG level

List of imaging techniques
- Transvaginal ultrasound
- Chest X-ray
- If there is evidence of metastatic disease on initial evaluation, should include CT of the abdomen and pelvis and magnetic resonance imaging of the brain

Potential pitfalls/common errors made regarding diagnosis of disease
- Patient noncompliance with serial assessments of hCG levels.
- New pregnancy. Pregnancy obscures hCG monitoring during interval after molar evacuation.
- "Phantom hCG." False-positive hCG values due to nonspecific heterophilic antibodies. Should be suspected if hCG values plateau at low levels and do not respond to therapeutic measures.

Treatment

Treatment rationale
- Patients with nonmetastatic GTN (Stage I) or low-risk metastatic GTN (Stage II or III) can be treated with single-agent chemotherapy. In patients with nonmetastatic disease GTN, early hysterectomy may decrease the number of cycles of chemotherapy needed to induce remission. Patients with FIGO high-risk GTN require treatment with multiagent chemotherapy. For patients with cerebral metastases, radiation therapy to the brain in combination with systemic chemotherapy should be considered in order to limit acute hemorrhagic complications. Serum hCG should be serially monitored prior to administration of chemotherapy and be continued until values are normal. An additional two doses of consolidation chemotherapy should then be given after hCG levels normalize. If hCG plateaus or increases during therapy, the patient should be switched to an alternative regimen.

When to hospitalize
- If patient is hemodynamically unstable.
- If patient has high-risk GTN and needs multiagent chemotherapy.
- Neurologic symptoms.

Table of treatment

Treatment	Comments
Medical Methotrexate: 30–50 mg/m2 IM weekly vs 0.4 mg/kg/day IV or IM for 5 days (considered better) until serum hCG undetectable Actinomycin D: 1.25 mg/m2 IV every 2 weeks EMA/CO Etoposide: 100 mg/m2 IV over 30 min (D1, D2) Methotrexate 300 mg/m2 IV over 12 hrs (D1) Actinomycin D: 0.5 mg IV (D1, D2) Cyclophosphamide: 600 mg/m2 IV over 30 min (D8) Vincristine: 1 mg/m2 IV bolus, max 2 mg (D8)	Single-agent regimen for low risk vs multiagent for high-risk GTN
Surgical Suction D&C Hysterectomy	Uterine curettage is controversial, but can be considered as initial treatment in low-risk, nonmetastatic GTN. Hysterectomy can be considered in patients with nonmetastatic GTN and may shorten duration and amount of chemotherapy needed to effect remission.

Prevention/management of complications
• Folinic acid (leucovorin) rescue has been widely adopted in order to prevent high-dose methotrexate toxicity, which can lead to renal dysfunction and delayed methotrexate elimination.

Management/treatment algorithm
• Once patients are risk stratified into nonmetastatic or metastatic and low- or high-risk GTN, treatment is either single agent or multiagent, respectively. Chemotherapy is continued until hCG levels are undetectable, followed by at least two additional consolidation doses.

> **CLINICAL PEARLS**
> • A WHO prognostic score ≥ 7 indicates a high risk of resistance to single agent treatment.
> • Nonmetastatic and metastatic low-risk GTN should be treated with a single-agent regimen.
> • High-risk GTN should be treated with aggressive multiagent chemotherapy and be referred to specialists with experience treating this disease.

Prognosis

> **BOTTOM LINE/CLINICAL PEARLS**
> • Essentially all patients with low-risk GTN can be cured.
> • Survival rates for high-risk GTN are around 80–90%.
> • Recurrence rates are < 5% and up to 13% for low- and high-risk GTN, respectively.

Prognosis for treated patients
• Single-agent treatment for low-risk GTN is 50–90% effective at inducing remission. Patients initially failing first-line therapy, can easily be salvaged with second- or third-line chemotherapy with an overall survival of ~100%. Recurrence rate <5% among low-risk patients successfully treated versus up to 13% for patients with high-risk disease. Risk of recurrence after 1 year of remission is <1%. 1–2% risk of second mole in subsequent pregnancy.

Follow-up tests and monitoring

- Following completion of chemotherapy and after hCG remission has been achieved, hCG levels are monitored every 2 weeks for the first 3 months and then at 1-month intervals until monitoring has shown normal hCG levels for 1 year.

Reading list

American College of Obstetricians and Gynecologists. *ACOG practice bulletin no. 53: Diagnosis and treatment of gestational trophoblastic disease.* June 2004.

Berkowitz RS, Goldstein DP. Molar pregnancy. Clinical Practice. *N Engl J Med* 2009;360:1639-45.

Deng L, Zhang J, Wu T, et al. Combination chemotherapy for primary treatment of high-risk gestational trophoblastic tumour. *Cochrane Database Syst Rev* 2013;31(1):CD005196.

Lawrie TA, Alazzam M, Tidy J, et al. First-line chemotherapy in low-risk gestational trophoblastic neoplasia. *Cochrane Database Syst Rev* 2016;9(6):CD007102.

Lurain JR, Singh DK, Schink JC. Primary treatment of metastatic high-risk gestational trophoblastic neoplasia with EMA-CO chemotherapy. *J Reprod Med* 2006;51(10):767.

McNeish IA, Strickland S, Holden L, et al. Low-risk persistent gestational trophoblastic disease: outcome after initial treatment with low-dose methotrexate and folinic acid from 1992 to 2000. *J Clin Oncol* 2002;20(7):1838.

Seckl MJ, Sebire NJ, Fisher RA, et al. Gestational trophoblastic disease: ESMO Clinical Practice Guidelines for diagnosis, treatment and follow-up. *Ann Onc* 2013;24(Suppl 6):vi39-50.

Yarandi F, Mousavi A, Abbaslu F, et al. Five-day intravascular methotrexate versus biweekly actinomycin-D in the treatment of low-risk gestational trophoblastic neoplasia: a clinical randomized trial. *Int J Gynecol Cancer* 2016;26(5):971-6.

Guidelines
National society guidelines

Title	Source	Date/URL
Diagnosis and treatment of gestational trophoblastic disease	American College of Obstetricians and Gynecologists	2004 https://www.ncbi.nlm.nih.gov/pubmed/15172880

Evidence

Type of evidence	Title and comment	Date/URL
Meta-analysis	First-line chemotherapy in low-risk gestational trophoblastic neoplasia Comment: Cochrane review of efficacy and safety of first-line chemotherapy in the treatment of low-risk GTN	2016 https://www.ncbi.nlm.nih.gov/pubmed/27281496
Meta-analysis	Combination chemotherapy for primary treatment of high-risk gestational trophoblastic tumour Comment: Cochrane review of efficacy and safety of combination chemotherapy in treating high-risk GTN	2013 https://www.ncbi.nlm.nih.gov/pubmed/23440800

Additional material for this chapter can be found online at:
www.wiley.com/go/sperling/mountsinai/obstetricsandgynecology

This includes ICD codes.

CHAPTER 42

Vulvar Cancer

Melissa Schwartz[1] and Stephanie V. Blank[2]

[1] Division of Gynecologic Oncology – Department of Obstetrics, Gynecology and Women's Health, Saint Louis University School of Medicine, St. Louis, MO

[2] Division of Gynecologic Oncology – Department of Obstetrics, Gynecology and Reproductive Science, Icahn School of Medicine at Mount Sinai, New York, NY

OVERALL BOTTOM LINE
- Vulvar cancer is a rare disease that mainly affects elderly women.
- The most common symptom of vulvar cancer is vulvar itching, which is also common to other vulvar disorders.
- Biopsy of any suspicious vulvar lesions is important for diagnosis.
- Treatment is primarily surgical and dependent on stage of disease.

Background
Definition of disease
- Vulvar cancer refers to cancer originating from the female external genitalia, which includes the labia, mons pubis, clitoris, and perineum. Most vulvar cancers (70%) involve the labia.

Disease classification
- Over 90% of vulvar cancers are squamous cell carcinomas (SCC). Other histologic subtypes include verrucous carcinomas, melanomas, basal cell carcinomas, sarcomas, and extramammary Paget disease.

Incidence/prevalence
- Vulvar cancer is a rare disease.
- It is the fourth most common gynecologic cancer, accounting for approximately 5% of all gynecologic cancers.
- In the United States, there are around 6000 new cases of vulvar cancer and 1100 deaths annually.
- Median age of diagnosis is 65 years.

Etiology
- Currently, it is believed that vulvar carcinogenesis occurs via one of two independent pathways. The first pathway is thought to be mediated by human papillomavirus (HPV) and the second is related to chronic vulvar inflammation and vulvar dystrophies. Vulvar cancer is usually preceded by vulvar intraepithelial neoplasia (VIN).

Pathology/pathogenesis
- Classic or warty type vulvar SCC is associated with persistent HPV infection, specifically HPV 16, 18, and 31. Differentiated or keratinizing vulvar SCC usually occurs in older women and is associated with vulvar dystrophies, such as lichen sclerosis.

Mount Sinai Expert Guides: Obstetrics and Gynecology, First Edition. Edited by Rhoda Sperling.
© 2020 John Wiley & Sons Ltd. Published 2020 by John Wiley & Sons Ltd.
Companion Website: www.wiley.com/go/sperling/mountsinai/obstetricsandgynecology

- Verrucous carcinoma is a slow-growing variant of SCC with a cauliflower-like appearance that rarely metastasizes to the lymph nodes.
- Melanoma is the second most common type of vulvar cancer and lesions typically develop within a preexisting nevus.
- Basal cell carcinoma accounts for 2% of vulvar cancers and is characterized by rolled edges with central ulceration.
- Extramammary Paget disease accounts for less than 1% of vulvar malignancies and has an eczematoid appearance.

Predictive/risk factors

- Age
- Cigarette smoking
- Lichen sclerosis
- Human papillomavirus infection
- Immunodeficiency (i.e. HIV infection)
- Vulvar or cervical intraepithelial neoplasia
- History of cervical cancer

Prevention

> **BOTTOM LINE/CLINICAL PEARLS**
> - Early detection and treatment of vulvar precancers may help to prevent progression to vulvar cancer.

Primary prevention

- Early detection and treatment of vulvar intraepithelial neoplasia

Diagnosis

> **BOTTOM LINE/CLINICAL PEARLS**
> - Vulvar cancer is a histologic diagnosis
> - Most women present with a unifocal lesion on the labia.
> - The most common symptom is vulvar pruritis.

Differential diagnosis

Differential diagnosis	Features
Lichen sclerosis	• Characterized by marked inflammation and epithelial thinning. Benign, chronic, progressive condition. Can cause pruritus and pain.
Condyloma acuminata	• Commonly known as warts. Can be single or multiple, flat or cauliflower shaped, and variable in color. Typically asymptomatic, but can cause pruritus.
Seborrheic keratosis	• Benign, common epidermal tumor. Caused by benign proliferation of immature keratinocytes.
Lentigo	• Benign pigmented lesion. Occurs as a result of increased activity of epidermal melanocytes.
Epidermal inclusion cyst	• Most common cutaneous cyst. Typically skin-colored nodule.
Disorders of the Bartholin gland	• Located in the lower medial labia majora. Can range from cyst to abscess.
Acrochordons	• Commonly known as skin tags. Outgrowth of normal skin.

Typical presentation
- The clinical presentation of vulvar cancer of all histologic subtypes is similar. Most patients present with a unifocal vulvar lesion or skin changes on the labia, which can be raised, ulcerated, and of variable coloration (red, pink, white, brown). Vulvar itching that does not go away is the hallmark complaint of patients. Other common symptoms include pain, vulvar bleeding or discharge, and dysuria.

Clinical diagnosis
History
- A complete gynecologic history should be taken, including history of abnormal pap smears. The patient should be asked about all potential risk factors, including but not limited to cigarette smoking. Complete medical and surgical histories should be taken. Review of systems should include vulvar pruritus, vulvar bleeding or discharge, and urinary complaints.

Physical examination
- A pelvic exam, including rectal and speculum exam should be performed. Attention should be taken with regards to examination of the vulva. Size, location, and distance from the midline of any suspicious lesions should be recorded. Careful palpation of the any vulvar lesions and inguinofemoral lymphadenopathy should be done. Bimanual exam should be performed to assess for local extension of any invasive disease. On speculum exam, the vagina and cervix should be assessed for any concurrent lesions. A focused physical exam should be done to exclude metastases, including palpation of supraclavicular lymph nodes. A thorough dermatologic examination should be performed to rule out systemic processes.

Disease severity classification
- Vulvar cancer is staged surgically
- 2014 International Federation of Gynecology and Obstetrics (FIGO) staging

Stage I	Tumor confined to the vulva or perineum with no nodal metastasis
IA	Lesions ≤ 2 cm in size and with stromal invasion ≤ 1.0 mm, confined to the vulva or perineum
IB	Lesions > 2 cm in size or with stromal invasion > 1.0 mm, confined to the vulva or perineum
Stage II	Tumor of any size with extension to adjacent perineal structures (1/3 lower urethra, 1/3 lower vagina, anus) with negative nodes
Stage III	Tumor of any size with or without extension to adjacent perineal structures (1/3 lower urethra, 1/3 lower vagina, anus) with positive inguinofemoral lymph nodes
IIIA	(i) With 1 lymph node metastasis (≥ 5 mm), or (ii) 1–2 lymph node metastasis(es) (< 5 mm)
IIIB	(i) With 2 or more lymph node metastases (≥ 5 mm), or (ii) 3 or more lymph node metastases (< 5 mm)
IIIC	With positive nodes with extracapsular spread
Stage IV	Tumor invades other regional (2/3 upper urethra, 2/3 upper vagina) or distant structures and/or fixed or ulcerated inguinofemoral lymph nodes
IVA	Tumor invades any of the following: (i) Upper urethral and/or vaginal mucosa, bladder mucosa, rectal mucosa, or fixed to pelvic bone, or (ii) Fixed or ulcerated inguinofemoral lymph nodes
IVB	Any distant metastasis including pelvic lymph nodes

FIGO Committee on Gynecologic Oncology 2014

Laboratory diagnosis

List of diagnostic tests
- Vulvar colposcopy
- Direct vulvar punch biopsies
- Histology from clinically suspicious nodes

List of imaging techniques
- Diagnostic imaging should be dependent on physical exam findings.
- Choice of imaging modality to evaluate locoregional and/or distant spread is not standardized.
- Magnetic resonance imaging (MRI) of the pelvis: Can be used to help define local extent of disease for surgical planning.
- Positron emission tomography/computed tomography (PET/CT): Can be used to asses for locoregional and distant metastases.
- Chest X-ray: Can be obtained if there is clinical suspicion of lung metastases and if no other chest imaging has been done.

Potential pitfalls/common errors made regarding diagnosis of disease
- Because signs and symptoms of early vulvar cancer are common to many different benign vulvar conditions, women often present late to medical care.
- Often patients are prescribed topical remedies for symptomatic relief without biopsy. Tissue diagnosis should be obtained when evaluating symptomatic vulvar lesions.

Treatment

Treatment rationale
- Vulvar cancer treatment is dependent on stage of disease. Vulvar cancer spreads by (a) direct extension to adjacent structures, (b) lymphatic spread to regional nodes, or (c) hematogenous spread (which typically occurs late in the course of disease). Treatment is primarily surgical. Extent of excision is dependent on tumor size and depth and can range from wide local excision to radical vulvectomy. Resection includes removing diseased tissue with adequate margins.
- Evaluation of inguinofemoral lymph nodes, via sentinel lymph node biopsy (SLNB) if possible, is done when a patient has greater than stage IA disease. Unilateral lymphadenectomy is preferred over bilateral whenever possible to avoid postoperative morbidity and can be performed if the primary lesion is <1 cm from the vulvar midline. SLNB is preferred over full inguinofemoral lymphadenectomy when the primary lesion is <4 cm in the absence of clinically suspicious nodes. Women with palpable groin nodes are typically managed with debulking of affected nodes.
- Certain women are unable to be managed surgically – patients with tumor fixed to vital structures, patients who are medically unable to tolerate surgery, or patients with distant metastases. In these cases, chemoradiation, radiation, or chemotherapy is offered, respectively.
- For patients with inconveniently located disease or initially inoperable disease, neoadjuvant chemoradiation can help reduce tumor size and improve chances of surgical excision.
- Adjuvant radiation is usually given to patients with positive inguinofemoral nodes.
- In cases of recurrent disease in previously irradiated areas, there is a lack of effective treatment.

When to hospitalize
- If patient is hemodynamically unstable

Table of treatment

Treatment	Comments
Surgery 1. Wide local excision 2. Radical partial vulvectomy 3. Pelvic exenteration +/- SLNB or inguinofemoral lymphadenectomy or debulking of groin lymph nodes	Cornerstone of treatment. Radicality of surgery is dependent of tumor size and depth of invasion.
Radiation – Irradiation of ipsilateral or bilateral groin and hemipelvis. – Target tissues treated once daily, 5 days per week. Total dose ranges from 60–70 Gy.	Used in advanced vulvar cancers. May be done in adjuvant setting or in place of surgery for select patients. Can be combined with chemotherapy in cases of unresectable disease or in neoadjuvant setting.

Chemotherapy
1. Alone:
  – Cisplatin
  – Carboplatin
  – Cisplatin + paclitaxel
  – Cisplatin + vinorelbine
  – Paclitaxel
  – Erlotinib – biologic
2. Combined with radiation therapy:
  – Cisplatin
  – Cisplatin + 5-FU
  – 5-FU + mitomycin-C
	Used in neoadjuvant setting to reduce size of tumor in cases of initially inoperable disease.
	Can be considered for patients who present with stage IVB or recurrent disease. Can also be combined with radiation therapy as a radiosensitizer.

Prevention/management of complications

- For patients with stage I or II disease and no palpable groin nodes, SLNB can be used in place of inguinofemoral lymphadenectomy. SLNB has been shown to be effective in detecting inguinofemoral lymph nodes metastases. SLNB also helps patients avoid acute and late morbidities associated with full inguinofemoral lymph node dissection, such as lymphedema, lymphocyst formation, infection, and wound dehiscence.

CLINICAL PEARLS
- The cornerstone for treatment of vulvar cancer is surgery.
- Evaluation of inguinofemoral nodal status is important for prognosis and tailored adjuvant treatments.
- SLNB should be considered over full groin lymphadenectomy for patients with stage I or II disease and no enlarged lymph nodes to avoid morbidity from full lymph node dissection.
- Radiation +/- chemotherapy can be considered in the adjuvant setting or for patients who are ineligible for primary surgical resection of disease.

Prognosis

BOTTOM LINE/CLINICAL PEARLS
- Lymph node involvement is the most important prognostic factor.
- Prognosis is also affected by stage, age, and capillary lymphatic space invasion.

Natural history of untreated disease
- Progression of disease and death

Prognosis for treated patients
- Inguinofemoral lymph node involvement is the most significant prognostic factor for women with vulvar cancer. 5-year survival ranges from 70–93% for women with negative nodes, and 25–41% for women with positive nodes.

Follow-up tests and monitoring
- The majority of vulvar cancer recurrence occur in the first two years; however, up to 10% of women will recur ≥ 5 years after primary treatment. Therefore, long-term follow-up is required. Given the rarity of vulvar cancer, evidence is lacking regarding appropriate surveillance strategies. Most gynecologic oncologists monitor patients with serial physical exams every 3–6 months for the first 2 years after initial treatment, and then at increasing intervals. Patients with concerning symptoms of physical exam findings should have additional imaging performed.

Reading list

FIGO Committee on Gynecologic Oncology. FIGO staging for carcinoma of the vulva, cervix, and corpus uteri. *Int J Gynaecol Obstet* 2014;125(2):97-8. [PUBMED Abstract]

Fuh KC, Berek JS. Current management of vulvar cancer. *Hematol Oncol Clin North Am* 2012 Feb;26(1):45-62.

Hacker NF, Nieberg RK, Berek JS, et al. Superficially invasive vulvar cancer with nodal metastases. *Gynecol Oncol* 1983;15(1):65.

Homesley HD, Bundy BN, Sedis A, et al. Radiation therapy versus pelvic node resection for carcinoma of the vulva with positive groin nodes. *Obstet Gynecol* 1986;68:733-40.

Homesley HD, Bundy BN, Sedlis A, et al. Prognostic factors for groin node metastasis in squamous cell carcinoma of the vulva (a Gynecologic Oncology Group study). *Gynecol Oncol* 1993;49:279-83.

Kunos C, Simpkins F, Gibbons T, et al. Radiation therapy compared with pelvic node resection for node-positive vulvar cancer: a randomized controlled trial. *Obstet Gynecol* 2009;114:537-46.

Salani R, Khanna N, Frimer M, et al. An update on post-treatment surveillance and diagnosis of recurrence in women with gynecologic malignancies: Society of Gynecologic Oncology (SGO) recommendations. *Gynecol Oncol* 2017 Mar 31. pii: S0090-8258(17)30238-X. doi: 10.1016/j.ygyno.2017.03.022. [Epub ahead of print]

Tan J, Chetty N, Kondalsamy-Chennakesavan S, et al. Validation of the FIGO 2009 staging system for carcinoma of the vulva. *Int J Gynecol Cancer* 2012 Mar;22(3):498-502.

Van der Zee AG, Oonk MH, De Hullu JA, et al. Sentinel node dissection is safe in the treatment of early-stage vulvar cancer. *J Clin Oncol* 2008;26(6):884.

Suggested website
Vulvar Cancer Treatment (PDQ®). https://www.cancer.gov/types/vulvar/patient/vulvar-treatment-pdq

Guidelines
National society guidelines

Title	Source	Date/URL
Vulvar Cancer Version 1.2017	National Comprehensive Cancer Network	2017 http://www.jnccn.org/content/15/1/92.full.pdf+html

Evidence

Type of evidence	Title and comment	Date/URL
Meta-analysis	Sentinel lymph node biopsy in vulvar cancer: Systematic review, meta-analysis and guideline recommendations. Comment: Fewer complications with SLNB than full groin lymphadenectomy, but higher rate of recurrence.	2015 https://www.ncbi.nlm.nih.gov/pubmed/25703673
Meta-analysis	Surgical interventions for early squamous cell carcinoma of the vulva. Comment: Comparison of radical local excision with radical vulvectomy.	2000 https://www.ncbi.nlm.nih.gov/pubmed/10796849

Additional material for this chapter can be found online at:
www.wiley.com/go/sperling/mountsinai/obstetricsandgynecology

This includes ICD codes.

PART 5

Family Planning

CHAPTER 43

Unintended Pregnancy

Gillian Dean[1] and Rachel Masch[2]

[1] Planned Parenthood Federation of America; Division of Family Planning – Department of Obstetrics, Gynecology and Reproductive Science, Icahn School of Medicine at Mount Sinai, New York, NY

[2] Division of Family Planning – Department of Obstetrics, Gynecology and Reproductive Science, Icahn School of Medicine at Mount Sinai, New York, NY

OVERALL BOTTOM LINE
- Nearly half of the approximately 6 million pregnancies each year in the United States are unintended; 42% result in abortion.
- Abortion is one of the most common medical procedures performed in the United States and can be safely provided for most patients in the outpatient as well as the hospital setting.
- Most abortions are performed in the first trimester.
- Medical and surgical approaches are safe and effective; eligible patients may choose between the two approaches.
- Complications of abortion are rare.

Background
Definition of disease
- The category unintended pregnancy includes both mistimed pregnancies (wanted but unplanned) and pregnancies that are unwanted.

Incidence/prevalence
- Approximately half of all US pregnancies are unintended; rates are highest among low-income, minority, and young people.
- In 2014, 19% of all pregnancies, excluding miscarriages, were managed with abortion, resulting in approximately 926 200 US abortions that year.
- The abortion rate has declined in recent years to the lowest rate ever in the US (14.6 abortions per 1000 women ages 15–44); the decline is related to the decrease in unintended pregnancies due to increased use of highly effective contraception.

Economic impact
- Unplanned pregnancies result in a higher proportion of births covered by public insurance programs compared with planned pregnancies; nationwide, unintended pregnancies are estimated to cost approximately $21 billion annually.
- Although most abortion patients have medical insurance, many private and most public insurers do not cover abortion services and some patients avoid using insurance because of privacy concerns; thus over half of abortion patients pay out of pocket.

Authors contributed equally to this chapter.

Mount Sinai Expert Guides: Obstetrics and Gynecology, First Edition. Edited by Rhoda Sperling.
Companion Website: www.wiley.com/go/sperling/mountsinai/obstetricsandgynecology

- No federal funding is used to cover abortion services even for patients insured by Medicaid; only 15 states use state funds to pay for some or all eligible abortions.

Etiology

- 54% of unintended pregnancy is due to nonuse of contraception; 41% is due to inconsistent or incorrect use, and < 5% is a result of contraceptive method failure.
- Approximately half of abortion patients use a contraceptive method in the month they become pregnant; the most commonly reported methods are condoms and short-acting hormonal methods such as pill and patch.
- Patients report many reasons for seeking abortion; the most common are related to family and children: (a) concern or responsibility for others; (b) not being able to afford a(nother) child; and (c) belief that a(nother) child would interfere with work, school, or current dependent care.

Pathology/pathogenesis

- 89% of abortions occur at ≤12 weeks, 6.2% at 13–15 weeks, 3.8% at 16–20 weeks, and 1.3% at ≥ 21 weeks.

Predictive/risk factors

Risk factor	Incidence (in year 2014)
Young age	More than half of all abortion patients are in their 20s; 12% are adolescents.
Low income	75% of abortion patients are poor or low income.
Minority race	Abortion patients are 28% black, 25% Hispanic, 39% white, 9% other.
Being a parent	59% of abortion patients have had one or more births.

Prevention

> **BOTTOM LINE/CLINICAL PEARLS**
> - Contraception and abstinence. See "Pregnancy Prevention" (Chapter 44).
> - The CHOICE project, from St. Louis, showed a marked decrease in unintended pregnancies and abortion when people were counseled about highly effective birth control methods and given a choice of contraception at no cost. Abortion rates of the CHOICE project cohort were less than half the regional and national rates.

Screening

- Urine or serum pregnancy tests are both accurate tests to screen for the pregnancy hormone, β-human chorionic gonadotropin (β-hCG).

Primary prevention

- Contraception and abstinence. See "Pregnancy Prevention" (Chapter 44).

Secondary prevention

- Contraception and abstinence. See "Pregnancy Prevention" (Chapter 44).

Algorithm 43.1 Diagnostic algorithm for unintended pregnancy

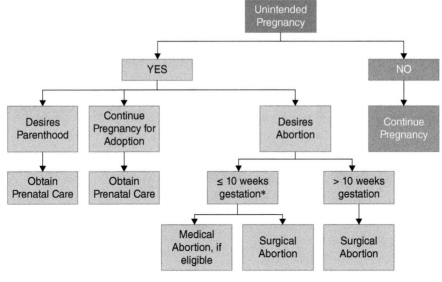

*Some protocols allow medical abortion to ≤ 11 weeks.

Diagnosis

> **BOTTOM LINE/CLINICAL PEARLS**
> - Secondary amenorrhea (missed menses)
> - Positive pregnancy test, either urine or serum
> - Ultrasound findings consistent with pregnancy

Differential diagnosis
See Algorithm 43.1.

Differential diagnosis	Features
Ectopic Pregnancy	History of pelvic inflammatory disease, previous ectopic, or intrauterine device (IUD) in situ; irregular spotting; unilateral pain; ultrasound findings consistent with ectopic pregnancy
Molar Pregnancy	Pregnancy symptoms that are more severe than typical; vaginal spotting; high levels of quantitative hCG; cystic structures in the uterine cavity by ultrasound
Early Pregnancy Loss (EPL)	All or some of a pregnancy noted in the uterus by ultrasound with no fetal heartbeat or fetus markedly lagging in growth; can be totally asymptomatic or present with vaginal spotting, with or without pain

Typical presentation
- Most women (89%) with unintended pregnancies present at ≤12 weeks gestation. They are typically in their 20s–30s, lower socioeconomic status, less educated, have had at least one previous birth, identify as straight or heterosexual, report some religious affiliation, and were using some method of contraception when they became pregnant. All races and ethnicities seek abortions; minority patients are disproportionately represented.

Clinical diagnosis
History
To diagnose an unintended pregnancy the following questions should be asked:
- Date of last menstrual period (LMP). Are menses regular? How often do they usually occur?
- Are you having unprotected sex? Are you using any contraception?
- How do you feel about being pregnant?
  - If unsure, ask if the patient knows how they would like to manage the pregnancy.
  - If undecided, ask:
    - Do you want to be a parent at this time? Do you want to continue this pregnancy and put the child up for adoption? Do you want to have an abortion?

Physical examination
- In an asymptomatic patient with an unintended pregnancy, no physical exam is required.
- Pregnancy location and dating should be confirmed with the LMP, a lab test (either urine or blood), and/or an ultrasound. The patient should then be counseled about her options.

Disease severity classification
- Pregnancies can be dated using the LMP, if known, and/or ultrasonography.

Laboratory diagnosis
List of diagnostic tests
- Lab tests:
  - Urine pregnancy tests (UPTs): hCG can be detected in the urine as early as approximately 6–7 days after implantation, or 2–3 days before a missed menses. Depending on the brand, UPTs have hCG detection thresholds between 10 mIU/ml–100 mIU/ml.
  - Serum pregnancy tests:
    - Qualitative hCG: Is a binary test that indicates the presence or absence of hCG in the serum and is reported as "POSITIVE" or "NEGATIVE"
    - Quantitative hCG: Quantifies the amount of hCG in the blood; most labs can detect serum hCG levels greater than 1 mIU/ml
  - Complete blood count (CBC) and type and screen
    - First trimester:
      - CBC not required, however most providers obtain one.
      - Type and screen: The likelihood of Rh sensitization at gestations ≤10 weeks is unknown; however, most U.S. abortion providers obtain Rh typing and administer Rh immune globulin (RhIg) to Rh negative patients.
    - Second trimester:
      - CBC and type and screen are routine and indicated.

Lists of imaging techniques
- Ultrasonography:
  - In early pregnancy, a transvaginal ultrasound (TVUS) has the greatest sensitivity in diagnosing a pregnancy
    - By 4–5 weeks, a gestational sac (GS) can be seen and grows by 1 mm/day.
    - By 4–5 weeks gestation, the yolk sac can be seen and persists until approximately 10 weeks gestation. It has the appearance of a small circle within the GS with a hypoechoic center.
    - By 5.5–6 weeks gestation, a double-decidual sac sign can be seen, which is the GS surrounded by the thickened decidua (the "double ring" sign). Early GS can sometimes be confused with blood/fluid or a pseudo-sac of an ectopic pregnancy.
  - Depending on a patient's body habitus, a transabdominal ultrasound can be used to discern a pregnancy as early as 7 weeks.

Potential pitfalls/common errors made regarding diagnosis of disease
- Prior to proceeding with a uterine evacuation or medical abortion for an unintended pregnancy, early pregnancy losses, ectopic pregnancies, and molar pregnancies should be ruled out.

Treatment
Treatment rationale
- Pregnancy termination may be accomplished with either medications or surgery.
- For patients seeking abortion, first determine gestational age to determine eligibility for medical as well as surgical abortion. There is no lower gestational age limit for either surgical or medical abortion.
- Determine medical eligibility for method and setting of abortion. See table of treatment for contraindications to medical abortion. For contraindications to office-based surgical abortion, see "when to hospitalize."
- Present options for type and setting of abortion to the patient. For healthy patients presenting at ≤10 weeks, choice of medical versus surgical abortion may be left to patient discretion. Risks of serious adverse events are low with both. 45% of all eligible abortions are medical in the US.
- If patient is Rh NEGATIVE, give RhIg per practice protocol. Some practices forego Rh testing and RhIg provision at < 8 weeks gestation, while others test and administer RhIg to all Rh negative patients regardless of gestational age.

When to hospitalize
- Most surgical abortions may be provided safely in an outpatient (office or health center) setting and many of these offer anesthesia. In 2014, 96% of all US abortions were performed in an outpatient setting.
- First trimester abortion is one of the safest and most common medical procedures in the US. The risk of a complication requiring hospital care or transfer is ≤0.05%.
- Contraindications to outpatient surgical abortion include any conditions requiring hospital care, such as poorly controlled hypertension, significant cardiac disease, suspected placenta accreta, other conditions requiring advanced airway or other specialized anesthesia management, availability of blood products, or the need for an operating room due to an elevated risk of operative complications.

Table of treatment
See Algorithm 43.2.

Algorithm 43.2 Management/treatment algorithm for unintended pregnancy

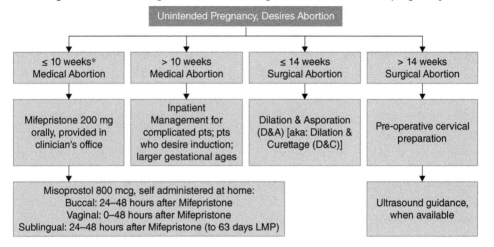

*Some protocols allow medical abortion to ≤ 11 weeks.

Treatment	Comments
Medical abortion • Mifepristone plus misoprostol (preferred) • Misoprostol alone • Methotrexate plus misoprostol	• May be preferred by patients seeking to avoid surgery and to accomplish abortion at home. • Mifepristone in combination with misoprostol is the most effective and safest regimen for first trimester medical abortion with failure rates ≤4%. The regimen is approved by the Food and Drug Administration (FDA) through 10 0/7 weeks LMP; in some practices, it is used to 11 0/7 weeks LMP. Other regimens may be used in geographical regions with no or limited availability of mifepristone. • Contraindications: gestation > 10.0 weeks LMP (or 11.0 days LMP depending on practice guidelines), allergy to mifepristone or misoprostol, IUD in situ, ectopic pregnancy, chronic adrenal failure, long-term systemic corticosteroid therapy, anticoagulant use, hemorrhagic disorders, uncontrolled medical disorders (e.g. seizures, hypertension), porphyria. • Mifepristone 200 mg is administered and taken orally in the office or at home. Misoprostol 800 mcg (buccal or vaginal) is provided for home use within 0–48 hours (depending on route of administration). Bleeding and passage of pregnancy should occur after misoprostol use. • Follow-up (in person with ultrasound or remotely with serum or urine pregnancy test) is required to confirm completion. • Mifepristone and misoprostol may be used inpatient for medical termination > 11 weeks.
Surgical • First trimester: Dilation and Aspiration (D&A), also called Dilation and Curettage (D&C) • Second trimester: Dilation and Evacuation (D&E)	• May be preferred by patients wishing to avoid the heavy bleeding and cramping associated with medical abortion. • Legally permissible in New York State through 24 weeks of pregnancy, defined as 26 weeks LMP. • May be performed in outpatient (office or health center) or hospital (operating room) setting. • D&A is performed using mechanical cervical dilators followed by vacuum aspiration. • D&E requires cervical preparation with osmotic cervical dilators and/or medications (mifepristone and/or misoprostol); uterine evacuation is accomplished using grasping forceps and vacuum aspiration, or manual maneuvers under transabdominal ultrasound guidance, when available. • Completion is confirmed by an empty uterus on ultrasound and/or visualization of complete products of conception (villi plus sac, or fetal parts plus placenta). • Routine follow-up is not required.
Psychological	• Some patients elect to speak with mental health providers before or after making a decision to terminate a pregnancy. • Mental health experts have determined that abortion does not cause depression or other mental health disorders any more than carrying a pregnancy to term.

Prevention/management of complications
• Excessive bleeding/hemorrhage
  • Incidence < 1%
  • Risk factors: Previous cesarean sections, larger gestational ages, multifetal pregnancies

- Defined as > 500 cc
- If excessive bleeding is anticipated, can pretreat with vasopressin (2–4 units) in a paracervical block
- Treated with:
  - Fundal massage
  - Medications (ergot, prostaglandins, oxytocin, vasopressin)
  - Reaspiration
  - Intrauterine foley balloon
  - Interventional radiology (IR) angiographic embolization
  - Additional surgeries (cervical or uterine artery ligation, B-Lynch sutures, hysterectomy)
- Lacerations (cervical, vaginal)
  - Incidence: Up to 3% of second trimester abortions can have cervical lacerations.
  - Risk factors: Previous cesarean sections, young age, nulliparity
  - If excessive bleeding occurs, thorough examination must be performed to rule out lacerations.
  - Repair with hemostatic agents (Monsell's, silver nitrate) or suture.
- Infection
  - Incidence: <1% of abortions
  - Risk factors: Presence of chlamydia and/or gonorrhea
  - Prophylaxis with antibiotics reduces risk up to 40%.
    - Many regimens acceptable
  - Suspect if fever > 100.3°F (38°C), tachycardia, foul-smelling vaginal discharge or amniotic fluid
  - Treatment includes confirmation of empty uterus; initiate outpatient antibiotics unless patient is unstable; arrange follow-up by phone or visit to confirm response to therapy.
- Uterine atony
  - Risk factors: Previous cesarean section, older maternal age, greater gestational age
  - Relaxation of the uterus causing excessive blood loss
  - Treat with manual uterine massage, uterotonic agents, intrauterine tamponade; consider additional surgery to treat hemorrhage
- Abnormal placentation
  - Incidence: Accreta affects ~0.2% of deliveries
  - Risk factors: previous uterine surgery involving entry from the myometrium into the uterine cavity
  - Placental location should always be ascertained prior to second trimester abortion procedure.
  - Patients most at risk: those with a history of uterine surgery that traverses the myometrium and enters the endometrial cavity (cesarean sections, myomectomies, etc.)
  - Preoperative preparation includes communication with anesthesia, IR (if available) and OR teams; readily available blood/blood products, uterotonics, intrauterine balloon
- Uterine perforation
  - Incidence: <1% of abortions
  - Risk factors: Higher gestational ages, abortions taking place in training centers, inadequate cervical dilation, prior cesarean sections, anatomically abnormal uterus.
  - Suspect when: instruments pass farther than expected, there is excessive bleeding, suction not able to be maintained, patient becomes acutely hypotensive, intra-abdominal contents are observed in the cannula or cervix.
  - Small perforations without suspicion of other organ injury can be observed.
  - Larger perforations, or suspicion of entry into other viscera, require surgical intervention.
- Retained products of conception
  - Risk factors: Abnormal uterine anatomy, severe uterine flexion, inexperienced provider
  - All products of conception must be examined and completion confirmed. Fetal parts are visible grossly by approximately 9 weeks.

- Retained products of conception can result in excessive bleeding, lower abdominal pain and/or infection.
  - Products of conception ≤ 10 weeks can typically pass spontaneously.
  - If retained products are suspected greater than 10 weeks, or if the patient is symptomatic, reaspiration must be performed.
- Post-abortal hematometra
  - Incidence: 0.2%
  - Risk factors: Severe uterine anteflexion or retroflexion
  - Accumulation of blood in the uterus following a pregnancy evacuation
  - Treated with reaspiration, typically followed by uterotonics
- Anesthesia complications
  - Lidocaine injection intravascularly – adverse effects most commonly minor and transient. If advances, prepare for seizures and pulmonary/cardiac arrest.
  - Regional or general anesthetic complications to be managed by anesthesiologist
  - Reversal agents may be administered as needed.
- Allergy (to cervical dilators, medications, etc.)
  - Most frequently manifests dermatologically, but can also have acute bronchospasm, profound hypotension, shock, and/or pulmonary edema
  - Withdraw offending agent; administer medications (Benadryl, steroids, epinephrine), ensure airway access, initiate ventilation and cardiac support; maintain fluids.

CLINICAL PEARLS
- Cervical preparation before surgical abortion:
  - May be accomplished with medications (mifepristone or misoprostol) or osmotic dilators (laminaria or synthetic).
  - First trimester: Routine cervical preparation is not recommended; the decision to use should be individualized and based on patient and provider factors.
  - Second trimester: Routine cervical preparation is recommended. May be same day (through 18 weeks) or 1 to 2 days before D&E.
- Pain management:
  - Medical abortion: Anticipatory counseling is important to successful patient management of the cramping associated with medical abortion. Nonsteroidal anti-inflammatory drugs (NSAIDs) are usually sufficient; some people also use Tylenol with codeine or similar medication.
  - Surgical: Anesthesia options include local anesthesia only, moderate or deep sedation, and general or regional anesthesia. Second trimester abortion may be performed with any anesthetic approach but is usually performed with deep sedation or general anesthesia.
- Post-abortion contraception:
  - Medical abortion: All methods except the IUD may be provided at the first medical abortion visit and may be initiated immediately, including the implant and depot-medroxyprogesterone acetate (DMPA).
  - Surgical abortion: All methods may be provided at the time of abortion; IUDs and implants may be placed immediately following the abortion procedure.

Special populations
Children

- New York State does not require parental or judicial consent for minors seeking abortion; in NYS, pregnant minors are emancipated and may make decisions regarding pregnancy, including termination, without parental or judicial consent.

Others

- Advanced gestational age: The skill required to complete abortion and the risk of anesthetic and surgical complications increases with increasing gestational age.
- Obesity: There are no weight restrictions for medical abortion. Recent publications demonstrate that obesity does not appear to increase the risk of surgical complications with surgical abortion; however, anesthetic options may be limited in obese patients.
- History of cesarean section: First trimester medical abortion is not restricted in patients with past cesarean sections. Additional cervical priming steps may be required in patients with multiple past cesarean sections especially at advanced gestations.
- Abnormal placentation: Patients at risk for accreta (increta, percreta) require careful surgical planning. Abortion may be attempted by D&E with preparation for hysterectomy or uterine artery embolization in case of hemorrhage, or abortion may be accomplished by hysterotomy or hysterectomy.
- Serious medical conditions: Careful anesthetic and surgical planning is required for patients with serious medical conditions. Because the risk of complications with abortion increases with gestational age, surgeons often cannot wait for medical conditions to be optimized, especially when the patient presents at an advanced gestation.
- No visible gestational sac: Medical abortion may be performed in the absence of a gestational sac as long as the risk of ectopic pregnancy is low (e.g. at < 35 days LMP in an asymptomatic patient) and completion is confirmed promptly with serial serum hCG levels. Surgical abortion may be performed in the absence of a gestational sac; if no products of conception (sac and villi) are visualized after aspiration, serum hCG levels must be followed until they are negative to confirm complete evacuation and to rule out ectopic pregnancy.
- Uterine anomalies: Most uterine anomalies (except pregnancy in a blind horn) are not a contraindication to early medical abortion. Both congenital (including bicornuate, didelphys, and septate uteri) and acquired (fibroids and synechiae) may increase the difficulty of uterine evacuation during surgical abortion.
- Multiple gestations: First trimester medical abortion is not restricted in multiple pregnancies. With surgical abortion, the surgeon must prepare for a uterus larger than the gestational weeks and confirm removal of all fetal parts.

Prognosis

> **BOTTOM LINE/CLINICAL PEARLS**
> - Medical abortions ≤ 10 wks are 96% effective.
> - Surgical abortions are > 99% effective.
> - Complications for all abortions are rare.
> - Contraception should always be discussed whenever a patient seeks care for an unintended pregnancy.

Follow-up tests and monitoring

- Medical abortion: Follow-up is required to confirm completion. Follow-up can be in person with ultrasound or remotely with serum or urine pregnancy tests.
- Surgical: Routine follow-up is not required.

Reading list

Low N, Mueller M, Van Vliet HA, et al. Perioperative antibiotics to prevent infection after first-trimester abortion. *Cochrane Database Syst Rev* 2012 Mar 14;(3):CD005217.

Okusanya BO, Oduwole O, Effa EE. Immediate postabortal insertion of intrauterine devices. *Cochrane Database Syst Rev* 2014 Jul 28;(7):CD001777.

Paul, M. *Management of unintended and abnormal pregnancy*. Chichester, West Sussex: Wiley-Blackwell; 2009.

Suggested websites

American College of Obstetricians and Gynecologists (ACOG). www.acog.org
CHOICE Project. www.choiceproject.wustl.edu
Guttmacher Institute. www.guttmacher.org
Mifeprex®. www.earlyoptionpill.com
National Abortion Federation. www.prochoice.org
Planned Parenthood Federation of America. www.plannedparenthood.org
Society of Family Planning. www.societyfp.org

Guidelines
National society guidelines

Title	Source	Date/full reference
Medical management of first-trimester abortion	American College of Obstetrics & Gynecology (ACOG)	Practice Bulletin No. 143, March 2014 *Reaffirmed 2016. Replaces Practice Bulletin No. 67, October 2005*
Second-trimester abortion	American College of Obstetrics & Gynecology (ACOG)	Practice Bulletin No. 135, June 2013 *Reaffirmed 2015*
Providing quality family planning services: recommendations of CDC and the U.S. Office of Population Affairs	Centers for Disease Control and Prevention	*MMWR Recomm Rep* 2014 Apr 25;63(RR-04):1-54.
Cervical dilation before first-trimester surgical abortion (<14 weeks' gestation). Guideline no. 2015-1	Society of Family Planning (SFP) Comment: This document revises and replaces the previous version, originally published in #2007-1.	Allen RH, Goldberg AB. *Contraception* 2016 Apr;93(4):277-91.
Medical management of first-trimester abortion. Guideline no. 2014-1	SFP	Committee on Practice Bulletins — Gynecology and the Society of Family Planning, Creinin MD, Grossman DA. *Contraception* 2014 Mar;89(3):148-61.
Cervical preparation for second-trimester surgical abortion prior to 20 weeks' gestation. Guideline no. 2013-4	SFP Comment: This document revises and replaces the previous version, originally published in #2007-2.	Fox MC, Krajewski CM. *Contraception* 2014 Feb;89(2):75-84.
Surgical abortion prior to 7 weeks of gestation. Guideline no. 2013-2	SFP	Lichtenberg ES, Paul M. *Contraception* 2013 Jul;88(1):7-17.
Management of postabortion hemorrhage. Guideline no. 2013-1	SFP	Kerns J, Steinauer J. *Contraception* 2013;87(3):331-42.
First-trimester abortion in women with medical conditions. Guideline no. 2012-2	SFP	Guiahi M, Davis A; S *Contraception* 2012;86(6):622-30.
Labor induction abortion in the second trimester. Guideline no. 2011-1	SFP	Borgatta L, Kapp N. *Contraception* 2011;84(1):4-18.
Prevention of infection after induced abortion. Guideline no. 2010-2	SFP	Achilles SL, Reeves MF. *Contraception* 2011;83(4):295-309.
Cervical preparation for surgical abortion from 20 to 24 weeks' gestation. Guideline no. 2007-3	SFP	Newmann S, Dalve-Endres A, Drey EA. *Contraception* 2008;77(4):308-14.

Evidence

Type of evidence	Title and comment	Date/full reference)
Randomized controlled trial	The CHOICE Project: preventing unintended pregnancies by providing no-cost contraception See ACOG guidelines in the Guidelines section. See SFP guidelines in the Guidelines section.	*Obstet Gynecol* 2012 Dec;120(6):1291-7.

Additional material for this chapter can be found online at:
www.wiley.com/go/sperling/mountsinai/obstetricsandgynecology

This includes a case study, multiple choice questions, advice for patients, and ICD codes.

CHAPTER 44

Pregnancy Prevention

Laura MacIsaac, Geetha N. Fink, and Neha R. Bhardwaj

Division of Family Planning – Department of Obstetrics, Gynecology and Reproductive Science, Icahn School of Medicine at Mount Sinai, New York, NY

OVERALL BOTTOM LINE

- All reproductive age women should be screened for reproductive intentions and started on contraception as appropriate.
- Promote shared decision-making with reproductive intention discussions and contraceptive planning.
- Before starting contraception, pregnancy should be reasonably ruled out; however, when this is not possible, many methods may be initiated using the quick-start approach.
- Most contraceptive methods have significant noncontraceptive indications and benefits, not covered in this chapter.

Background

Definition of disease

- Unintended pregnancies are defined as pregnancies that are reported as mistimed and/or unwanted.

Disease classification

- Increasing the proportion of pregnancies that are planned and desired is a healthcare priority of the US Department of Health and Human Services as well as the World Health Organization.

Incidence/prevalence

- 45% of pregnancies in the United States each year are unintended (Finer and Zolna 2016).
- Approximately half of the unintended pregnancies worldwide result in induced abortion, with more than half of these abortions considered unsafe and causing one in seven maternal deaths (Singh et al. 2010).

Economic impact

- Unintended childbearing, a potential result of unintended pregnancy, is associated with delayed or inadequate prenatal care and premature birth.
- Unintended pregnancies resulted in $21 billion in direct medical costs in the United States in 2015.

Etiology/pathology

- Unintended or mistimed pregnancy is typically the result of incorrect or inconsistent use of contraception or nonuse of contraception.

Predictive/risk factors

- Age
  - Sexually active women aged 15–19 years have the highest unintended pregnancy rate.
  - In addition to young age, the postpartum and perimenopausal periods are also high risk for unintended pregnancy.

Mount Sinai Expert Guides: Obstetrics and Gynecology, First Edition. Edited by Rhoda Sperling.
© 2020 John Wiley & Sons Ltd. Published 2020 by John Wiley & Sons Ltd.
Companion Website: www.wiley.com/go/sperling/mountsinai/obstetricsandgynecology

- Income
  - The rate of unintended pregnancy among women with incomes below the federal poverty level is more than five times the rate of women with incomes at least 200% of the federal poverty level.
- Education
  - Among all educational levels, women without a high school degree have the highest unintended pregnancy rate.
- Race
  - Unintended pregnancy rates among black women are more than double the rates for non-Hispanic white women.
- Healthcare system inequities confound many of these contributing demographic risk factors.

Prevention

> **BOTTOM LINE/CLINICAL PEARLS**
> - Clinical encounters with reproductive age women should include pregnancy intention/protection.
> - Use of contraception, especially highly effective long-acting reversible contraception (LARC), such as intrauterine devices (IUDs) and contraceptive implants, lowers the unintended pregnancy and abortion rates and improves maternal and child health outcomes.
> - Addressing unintended pregnancy requires increasing access to contraception and removing barriers for patients.

Screening
- All reproductive aged women should be screened for pregnancy intention.
- The United States Medical Eligibility Criteria for Contraceptive Use includes guidelines from the US Centers for Disease Control and Prevention (CDC) for the use of contraceptive methods by women who have various medical conditions (CDC 2016).
- Women with complex medical problems can be referred to family planning specialists.

Primary prevention
- Education and counseling around fertility control and contraceptive options
- Increasing access to long and short acting contraception
- Education and access to emergency contraception
- Expand use of highly effective long-acting methods, while avoiding contraceptive coercion

Secondary prevention
- Removing financial and institutional barriers to all contraceptive methods
- Ensuring access to safe abortion services

Diagnosis
- Obtain history about missed menses and sexually activity and urine or serum pregnancy hormone β-human chorionic gonadotropin (β-hCG) when indicated.
- Pregnancy location and gestational age are confirmed by ultrasound when necessary.
- Offer options counseling for patients who are ambivalent about their pregnancy.

Clinical diagnosis
History
- Is the patient sexually active? What is her reproductive life plan? Is contraception indicated? Is there a benefit to starting on a contraceptive method currently, regardless of risk of unintended pregnancy?
- Past gynecologic history, including menstrual, obstetric, family, and sexual history

- Past medical history and current medications
- Prior methods of contraception used and reasons for successes or early discontinuation

Physical examination
- Urine pregnancy test to rule out current pregnancy
- Vital signs, review of medical history and medications
- A gynecologic or pelvic exam and/or testing for sexually transmitted infections (STI) are not necessary to start contraception.
- A pelvic exam is part of the procedure for IUD placement. STI testing is recommended prior to or at the time of IUD placement if it has not been done recently.
- Before starting contraception, pregnancy should be reasonably ruled out. However, when not possible this should not delay quick-starting contraceptive methods. Except for the intrauterine device (IUD); contraceptive hormones do not harm an established pregnancy.

Useful clinical decision rules and calculators
- Most contraceptive methods also have extensive noncontraceptive benefits that may be helpful for women with complex medical problems or menstrual irregularities.
- Continuous use of common hormonal methods to reduce or eliminate the scheduled monthly menses, referred to as "continuous cycling," as well as the use of emergency contraception for any gaps in use, should be explained.

Laboratory diagnosis
- Urine pregnancy test should be completed prior to the start contraception. A negative urine pregnancy test excludes pregnancies that are over 2 weeks from conception, around the time of a missed period.
- Most sensitive urine pregnancy tests will be positive as early as 8 days after conception, when implantation has just started.
- A positive urine pregnancy test reliably diagnoses pregnancy, although not the location or the gestation; a negative urine pregnancy test indicates the patient is not pregnant, or there is a very early pregnancy starting. In the latter case, a repeat urine pregnancy test within a week, or a blood β-hCG test is indicated.
- When starting contraception in the immediate postpartum or post-abortal period a pregnancy test is not indicated; it will be positive from the prior pregnancy event for 1–8 weeks (depending on the duration of the prior pregnancy event).

List of imaging techniques
- No imaging techniques are routinely recommended.
- For women with a suspected uterine anomaly desiring an IUD, an ultrasound and possibly an MRI of the uterus should be completed prior to consideration of placing an IUD.

Diagnostic algorithm to exclude pregnancy
- Centers for Disease Control and Prevention algorithm to be reasonably certain someone is not pregnant: If she has no symptoms or signs of pregnancy and meets any **one** of the following criteria:
  - Is ≤ 7 days after the start of normal menses
  - Has not had sexual intercourse since the start of last normal menses
  - Has been correctly and consistently using a reliable method of contraception
  - Is ≤ 7 days after spontaneous or induced abortion
  - Is within 4 weeks postpartum
  - Is fully or nearly fully breastfeeding (exclusively breastfeeding or the vast majority [≥85%] of feeds are breastfeeds), is amenorrheic, and < 6 months postpartum

Potential pitfalls/common errors made regarding diagnosis of disease
- Providers should ask women about their sexual health history, number and gender of partners, and reproductive health goals.
- Every woman with a newly diagnosed pregnancy should be asked about pregnancy intention.
- A pelvic exam is not needed for uncomplicated women wanting to start contraception.
- Routine screening for STIs and cervical cancer is not required before initiation of contraception; the two should be uncoupled in order to avoid delay of initiation of contraception.

Treatment
Treatment rationale
- Patients should be counseled on all available contraceptive options with an emphasis placed on typical use effectiveness, side effects, and noncontraceptive benefits.
- Although LARC methods are the most effective reversible methods they may not be acceptable to all women given the inability to stop and start the method on one's own, that a procedure is required to initiate, and there are changes to bleeding patterns in most women.

When to hospitalize
- Hospitalization due to contraception is a very rare occurrence. However, the following exceptions should be noted.
  - IUD perforation into the abdomen requiring surgical removal. This is rarely an emergency and can be managed as outpatient surgery with a laparoscopic approach. If there is evidence of perforation into a visceral organ, prompt surgical exploration and general surgery assistance may be required.
  - Difficult contraceptive implant removals may require referral to specialized imaging and providers for the removal procedure.
  - Presence of a deep vein thrombosis concurrent with a combined hormonal contraception (CHC) use. If a deep vein thrombosis is diagnosed CHC should be discontinued immediately and anticoagulation should be initiated. Contraception that avoids an estrogen component is still recommended as pregnancy carries a higher risk for thromboembolism than any contraceptive method. In addition, many anticoagulation medications are teratogenic.

Table of treatment

Permanent Sterilization: lifelong pregnancy prevention
- Advantages: high efficacy, high acceptability, safety, quick recovery, lack of significant long-term side effects, cost effectiveness, and convenience
- Disadvantages: Permanence, surgical and anesthetic risk, expense and time of procedure, need for surgeon, support staff, operating room and specialized equipment, higher probability of ectopic pregnancy in case of method failure
- Tubal Ligation or Occlusion
  - Transabdominal: Tubal ligation is performed at the time of cesarean section, in the immediate postpartum period, or as an interval procedure. Multiple surgical methods exist, including partial salpingectomy, total salpingectomy, occlusion with rings or clips, or electrocoagulation.
  - The added advantage of ovarian cancer protection with salpingectomy provides additional noncontraceptive benefit to women choosing this method of permanent contraception (ACOG committee opinion no. 774 2019).
- Male sterilization can be performed as an outpatient vasectomy. Vasectomy is comparable in effectiveness and is simpler, safer, and less expensive than female sterilization.

Long-Acting Reversible Contraceptive Methods
Contraceptive Implant: Nexplanon®
- Implant placed in the arm under local anesthesia as an outpatient procedure.
- Food and Drug Administration (FDA) approved for 3 years; can be used for up to 5 years.
- Releases a continuous dose of progestin (etonogestrel). Can cause menstrual irregularity. Typically induces a decrease in menstrual bleeding with some women experiencing amenorrhea.

(Continued)

(Continued)

Progestin (Levenorgestrel) Intrauterine Device
- Inert plastic device that is placed in the uterus as an outpatient procedure.
- Releases a low continuous dose of levenorgestrel. Can cause menstrual irregularity. Typically induces a decrease in menstrual bleeding with some women experiencing amenorrhea. Mirena® is FDA approved for treatment of menorrhagia and dysmenorrhea.
- Multiple devices (Mirena, Liletta, Skyla, Kyleena) available in the US with differing sizes, doses of hormone, and duration of use. Food and Drug Administration (FDA) approved for 3–6 years, data supports 3–7 years.

Copper Intrauterine Device: Paragard
- Inert plastic device wrapped in copper placed in the uterus as an outpatient procedure.
- Does not contain hormones. Optimal option for patients that may want or need to avoid hormones.
- Typically, no effect on overall menstrual cycle. However, periods may be heavier and more painful, particularly in the first 3 cycles.
- FDA approved for 10 years; can be used for up to 12 years.
- Can be used as emergency contraception for up to 5 days after unprotected intercourse.

Depot-Medroxyprogesterone Acetate (DMPA) or Depo-Provera®
- Intramuscular injection administered every 12 weeks, requiring a clinic visit.
- Typically causes menstrual irregularity with most women experiencing a decrease in bleeding or amenorrhea, especially with prolonged use.
- Can cause weight gain in some women.
- Noted to cause a decrease in bone density with prolonged use due to unopposed progestin effect. However, this is not of clinical consequence. Recommend normal dietary calcium and vitamin D intake, and encourage weight bearing exercise to increase peak bone density in young women.
- Caution use in patients with depression; there are mixed data on effects on mood of DMPA.
- May delay return to fertility for up to 1 year after discontinuation.

Self-Administered Hormonal Methods
Combined Hormonal Contraception
- Self-administered medication that contains both estrogen and a progestin. Method failure is highly dependent on adherence and more important continuation rates. Gaps in protection from self-discontinuation contribute to the higher failure rates.
- Requires a prescription from healthcare provider, although the American College of Obstetricians and Gynecologists (ACOG) supports over the counter provision of hormonal contraception. The few contraindications to estrogen must be ruled out (refer to Medical Eligibility Criteria guidelines) before initiating an estrogen-containing method. This is done by history and blood pressure check.
- Typically, cause menstrual cycle to be more regular and less painful. Effective in many settings to regulate irregular, heavy, or painful menstrual cycles.
- Can improve acne and premenstrual syndrome symptoms. Many brands of CHC pills are FDA approved for acne and some for treatment of premenstrual dysphoric disorder (PMDD).
- Can "quick-start" on any day of cycle and will take 7 days to be effective, except when started on day 1 of cycle or post-abortal (immediately effective).
- Combined Oral Contraceptive Pills (COCs)
  - Variations in type of progestin, dose of each component, monophasic versus multiphasic, and type of cycling. Typical cycling is 21 days of COCs followed by 7 days of placebo.
- Hormonal Patch: Zulane®: Patch applied to skin weekly for 3 weeks followed by a patch-free week.
- Hormonal Ring: Nuva Ring®: Vaginally inserted ring that is left in place for 3 weeks followed by ring-free placebo week.
- All CHC methods can be used off-label with extended administration, thus avoiding monthly menses, and some are designed to have fewer than once/month menses. Careful education is required to help patient keep on track of when to stop and re-start new pack of the method.

Progestin-only Pills
- Traditional progestin-only pills require very strict adherence because of the narrow window (within 3 hours) of administration each day; an active pill is taken daily without a placebo break for menses.
- A new progestin-only pill, Slynd, with drospirenone, has a 4 day placebo break for a monthly withdrawal menses, similar to a combined hormonal pill, aiming to improve adherence and bleeding patterns compared to traditional progestin-only pills.
- Can be used for women with contraindications to estrogen or immediately postpartum.
- Uptake and continuation rates on this method are low due to strict adherence requires and abnormal bleeding patterns common to progestin-only methods.

(Continued)

Emergency Contraceptive (EC) Pills
- Used postcoitally for unprotected sex up to 5 days after unprotected sex.
- Works best if used as soon as possible after unprotected sex; but any time within 5 days helps.
- Rarely causes any symptoms; can cause menstrual irregularity, nausea, and vomiting.
- Can be combined with other hormonal contraceptive methods for added protection related to unprotected intercourse that could occur after the emergency contraceptive dose. Common regimen: one dose of EC as soon as possible after unprotected intercourse and immediate start of a pack of CHC pills the day after the EC dose and every day until a placebo week in the pill pack. A urine pregnancy test should be done at the completion of that pill pack to ensure no pregnancy resulted from the unprotected intercourse. If pregnancy did occur, and continuation of pregnancy is desired, the contraceptive hormones in EC and in a pack of CHC pills will not harm developing embryo.
- Levenorgestrel: Plan B©
  - Contains 1.5 mg of levenorgestrel
  - Can be obtained over the counter (OTC) or with a prescription for lower cost
  - FDA approved up to 3 days, can be used up to 5 days postcoitally
- Ulipristal Acetate: Ella®
  - Requires a prescription
  - More effective than Plan B

Barrier Methods
- Male and female condom
  - Available OTC. Female condoms may be less readily accessible.
  - Can only be used once per sexual act.
  - Protects against sexually transmitting infections.
- Diaphragm
  - Some require fitting by a provider, a newer diaphragm, Caya, does not require fitting
  - Must be placed in vagina prior to each sexual act
  - Must be combined with spermicide for each sexual act

Behavioral Methods
Fertility Awareness or Natural Family Planning
- Patient tracks menstrual cycle, daily temperature, and/or vaginal mucous in order to predict fertile days and avoid sex on these days.
Withdrawal
- Sexual act is interrupted prior to ejaculation. If there is failure to properly interrupt sexual act emergency contraception can be used. Sperm are in the pre-ejaculate semen, failure rates are high.
Prevention/management of complications
- See "When to Hospitalize."
- Serious complications of most contraceptive methods are rare; all are safer than pregnancy.
- Side effects of hormonal contraception are a common reason for discontinuation. Hormones may cause a change in skin, hair, weight, and mood. These side effects are typically short term and well tolerated but cannot be predicted. Menstrual effects of hormonal contraception can be unpredictable. Irregular bleeding patterns are more commonly experienced with progestin-only methods.

Special populations
Pregnancy
- If a patient is using contraception and is found to be pregnant the contraception should be discontinued. The hormones in contraception are considered safe in pregnancy but do not provided added benefit to the pregnancy. An IUD should be removed as soon as pregnancy is confirmed if the IUD string is accessible.
- Pregnancy should be ruled out before initiating contraception. When it cannot be ruled out it is still recommended to start contraception. Patients should be adequately counseled that despite a negative urine pregnancy test they could already be pregnant and will need a repeat a pregnancy test in 2–3 weeks.
- For patients desiring an IUD for whom pregnancy cannot be reasonably ruled consider use of a bridge method (birth control pills, patch, or ring) or alternative method until IUD can be placed.

Children

- Adolescence is a high-risk time for pregnancy. Comprehensive education, access and use of highly effective LARC methods have been shown to decrease unintended pregnancy.
- State laws determine parental notification policies with minors. In New York State, minors can make their own decisions without parental consent or notification.

Elderly

- Postmenopausal women do not require contraception.

Others

- Postpartum: Contraception should be encouraged to promote birth spacing and improve maternal and child health outcomes. Avoid estrogen-containing contraceptives for a minimum of 6 weeks due to the added thrombosis risk that exogenous estrogen contributes to the already high thrombosis risk in the postpartum time. Estrogen may cause a decrease in milk supply and quality. Progestin-only pills can be used in the immediate postpartum period and do not affect milk supply. IUDs can be placed immediately postplacental at the time of a vaginal or cesarean delivery.
- Post-abortal: This period is an ideal time to initiate contraception. LARC devices can be placed at the time of surgical procedures. All hormonal methods can be started the same day as a surgical procedure in first or second trimester abortion.
- For patients who opt for a medication abortion, contraception is often delayed until confirmation of completion of the abortion.

Prognosis
Efficacy and continuation rates of methods

> **BOTTOM LINE/CLINICAL PEARLS**
> - LARC methods have low failure rates and highest continuation rates of all reversible methods, in every age group.
> - Contraceptive risks are significantly lower than risk of pregnancy.
> - Noncontraceptive benefits should be promoted in patient counseling.
> - Successful contraception is uncoupled from sexual activity and routine medical evaluation/testing.
> - Adolescents may be able to obtain sexual and reproductive health services without parental consent.

Reading list

ACOG committee opinion no. 774: Opportunistic salpingectomy as a strategy for epithelial ovarian cancer prevention. *Obstet Gynecol* 2019 Apr;133(4):e279-84.

American College of Obstetricians and Gynecologists. Salpingectomy for ovarian cancer prevention. Committee opinion no. 620. *Obstet Gynecol* 2015;125:279-81.

American College of Obstetricians and Gynecologists. Clinical challenges of long-acting reversible contraceptive methods. Committee opinion no. 672. *Obstet Gynecol* 2016;128:e69-77.

American College of Obstetricians and Gynecologists. Immediate postpartum long-acting reversible contraception. Committee opinion no. 670. *Obstet Gynecol* 2016;128:e32-37.

Centers for Disease Control and Prevention. United States medical eligibility criteria for contraceptive use. *MMWR Recomm Rep* 2016 Jul 29;65(3):1-103. Available from: https://www.cdc.gov/mmwr/volumes/65/rr/pdfs/rr6503.pdf.

Downey MM, Arteaga S, Villaseñor E et al. More than a destination: Contraceptive decision making as a Journey. *Womens Health Issues* 2017;Sep-Oct;27(5):539-45. doi: 10.1016/j.whi.2017.03.004.

Dreweke J. *Promiscuity propaganda: access to information and services does not lead to increases in sexual activity*. New York: Guttmacher Institute; 2019. Available from: https://www.guttmacher.org/gpr/2019/06/promiscuity-propaganda-access-information-and-services-does-not-lead-increases-sexual.

Finer LB, Zolna MR. Declines in unintended pregnancy in the United States, 2008–2011. *N Engl J Med* 2016;374:843-52.

Global Library of Women's Medicine, Category 6, Fertility Regulation: Breastfeeding, Fertility, and Family Planning. Available from: www.glowm.com.

Long-acting reversible contraception: implants and intrauterine devices. Practice bulletin no. 186. *Obstet Gynecol* 2017;130:e251-69.

Singh S1, Sedgh G, Hussain R. Unintended pregnancy: worldwide levels, trends, and outcomes. *Stud Fam Plann* 2010;41(4):241-50.

Sonfield A, Hasstedt K, Kavanaugh ML, et al. *The social and economic benefits of women's ability to determine whether and when to have children*. New York: Guttmacher Institute; 2013.

Whitaker AK, Chen BA. SFP clinical guideline: postplacental insertion of intrauterine devices. *Contraception* 2018; 97:2-13.

Suggested websites

Society of Family Planning. https://www.societyfp.org/resources/clinical-guidelines

United States Medical Eligibility Criteria for Contraceptive Use, 2016. https://www.cdc.gov/reproductivehealth/contraception/mmwr/mec/summary.html

The Guttmacher Institute. https://www.guttmacher.org/article/2019/06/over-counter-oral-contraceptives-getting-details-right

The Guttmacher Institute. https://www.guttmacher.org/state-policy/explore/overview-minors-consent-law (updated July 2019)

ACOG. https://www.acog.org/Womens-Health/Birth-Control-Contraception?IsMobileSet=false

Innovating Education in Reproductive Health. www.innovating-education.org

Contraceptive Tools for Educators. https://www.plannedparenthood.org/learn/for-educators

For patients. www.bedsider.org

Guidelines
National society guidelines

Title	Source	Date/full reference or URL
Society for Maternal-Fetal Medicine (SMFM) Consult Series #48: Immediate postpartum long-acting reversible contraception for women at high risk for medical complications	Society of Family Planning and Society of Maternal Fetal Medicine. On SFP guideline website and published in the *American Journal of Obstetrics and Gynecology*.	Feb 2019 https://www.societyfp.org/clinical-guidance https://www.ajog.org/article/S0002-9378(19)30352-7/pdf
Society of Family Planning clinical recommendations: contraception after surgical abortion	Society of Family Planning	SFP Guideline published August 2018 Roe AH, Bartz D. *Contraception* 2019 Jan;99(1):2-9. https://www.contraceptionjournal.org/article/S0010-7824(18)30425-6/pdf
Use of intrauterine devices in nulliparous women	Society of Family Planning	August 2017 Lohr PA, Lyus R, Prager S. *Contraception* 2017 Jun;95(6):529-37. https://www.contraceptionjournal.org/article/S0010-7824(16)30385-7/pdf
ACOG practice bulletin no. 208: Benefits and risks of sterilization	ACOG (American College of Obstetricians and Gynecologists)	American College of Obstetricians and Gynecologists. *Obstet Gynecol* 2019;133.
ACOG practice bulletin no. 206: Use of hormonal contraception in women with coexisting medical conditions	ACOG	American College of Obstetricians and Gynecologists. *Obstet Gynecol* 2019;133.

International society guidelines

Title	Source	Date/URL
Guidelines for contraceptive use	RCGP (Royal College of General Practitioners, UK) Comment: General guidelines for contraceptive use	May 2018 http://elearning.rcgp.org.uk/mod/page/view.php?id=6961
FSRH (Faculty of Sexual and Reproductive Healthcare of the Royal College of Obstetricians and Gynecologists) Guideline – Contraception after pregnancy	RCOG (Royal College of Obstetricians and Gynaecologists, UK) Comment: Postpartum contraception	January 2017 https://www.fsrh.org/news/new-fsrh-guideline--contraception-after-pregnancy/
Long-acting reversible contraception	NICE (National Institute for Health and Care Excellence, UK) Comment: Updated guidelines on Long-acting reversible contraception	July 2019 https://www.nice.org.uk/guidance/cg30

Evidence

Type of evidence	Title and comment	Date/URL
Medical eligibility criteria for contraceptive use	Centers for Disease Control and Prevention Comment: Dynamic document to guide the use of contraceptive methods with most medical conditions	Last updated in 2016, but the online document is updated annually. https://www.cdc.gov/mmwr/volumes/65/rr/pdfs/rr6503.pdf YouTube video: https://www.youtube.com/watch?v=Jl13ekl7rsM There is also a CDC Medical Eligibility Criteria app to download for free.

CHAPTER 45

Early Pregnancy Failure

Adam Jacobs, Britt Lunde, and Sharon Gerber
Division of Family Planning – Department of Obstetrics, Gynecology and Reproductive Science, Icahn School of Medicine at Mount Sinai, New York, NY

> **OVERALL BOTTOM LINE**
> - Early pregnancy failure affects 10% of all clinically recognized pregnancies.
> - 80% of all pregnancy loss occurs in the first trimester.
> - Clinicians can manage EPF with either conservative, medical, or surgical management.
> - Approximately 50% of EPF cases are due to chromosomal abnormalities.

Background

Definition of disease
- Early pregnancy failure (EPF) is defined as a nonviable intrauterine pregnancy within the first 12 6/7 weeks of gestation.

Disease classification
- Anembryonic gestation: (empty gestational sac)
- Missed abortion: (gestational sac with an embryo or fetus without fetal heart activity)

Prevalence
- −10% of all clinically recognized pregnancies

Etiology
- Chromosomal abnormalities approximately 50% of cases
- Thrombophilias
- Autoimmune disorders
- Luteal phase defect
- Idiopathic

Pathology/pathogenesis
- The full pathogenesis of EPF is not fully known.
- In regard to chromosomal abnormalities many are linked to an error in meiosis 1 separation, which is increased with maternal age.

Risk factors
- Advanced maternal age
- History of previous EPF
- History of thrombophilia
- History of autoimmune disease

Mount Sinai Expert Guides: Obstetrics and Gynecology, First Edition. Edited by Rhoda Sperling.
© 2020 John Wiley & Sons Ltd. Published 2020 by John Wiley & Sons Ltd.
Companion Website: www.wiley.com/go/sperling/mountsinai/obstetricsandgynecology

Prevention
- No interventions have been demonstrated to prevent the development of EPF.
- There are no data to support prophylactic bed rest, progesterone, aspirin, or anticoagulants.

Screening
- There are no known tests to help screen for EPF.

Primary prevention
- There are no known interventions to assist in preventing the first occurrence of EPF.

Secondary prevention
- Limited data shown to reduce EPF for women using aspirin or anticoagulants with a prior diagnosis of antiphospholipid syndrome.

Diagnosis
- The patient with EPF may present with vaginal bleeding or uterine cramping
- In most circumstances there are not any findings on clinical exam.
- Diagnosis of EPF can be made using ultrasonography or serum β-human chorionic gonadotropin (β-hCG) values.
- A single ultrasound or lab value may not be sufficient to make a diagnosis of EPF.

Differential diagnosis

Differential diagnosis	Features
Normal intrauterine pregnancy	Vaginal bleeding. Closed internal cervical os.
Ectopic pregnancy	Vaginal bleeding. Abdominal or pelvic pain.
Molar pregnancy	Vaginal bleeding. Enlarged uterus.

Typical presentation
- There is no typical presentation for a patient presenting with EPF.
- Some patients may experience vaginal spotting or bleeding.
- Some patients may experience uterine tenderness or cramping.

Clinical diagnosis
History
- Clinical history should include patient's first day of last menstrual period.
- Clinical history should include patient's prior pregnancy outcomes including prior diagnosis of EPF, molar pregnancy, or ectopic pregnancy.
- Clinicians should inquire about recent episodes of vaginal bleeding.

Physical examination
- In many circumstances a patient with EPF may present with no key clinical findings on physical exam
- Pelvic exam to assess vaginal bleeding, passage of pregnancy tissue, and cervical exam to assess if the internal cervical os is opened or closed.

Laboratory diagnosis
Serum β-hCG levels
- Single values may not be sufficient to diagnose EPF.
- A single value may be helpful in determining next steps and which diagnosis in the differential may be more likely.
- A normal intrauterine pregnancy should increase serum β-hCG values a minimum of 53% over 48 hours.

- A normal intrauterine pregnancy should increase serum β-hCG values based on the initial value at presentation.
- The following list are the minimum increases based on the initial value over 48 hours:
  - less than 1500: 49%
  - 1500–3000: 40%
  - greater than 3000: 33%

Serum progesterone levels
- A meta-analysis of 26 studies showed a single progesterone level between 3.2–6 ng/ml with a patient complaining of pain or bleeding and an inconclusive ultrasound had a 99.2% probability of a nonviable pregnancy.

List of imaging techniques
- Pelvic ultrasound

Diagnostic criteria of EPF
- Crown-rump length ≥ 7 mm without a heartbeat
- Mean gestational sac ≥ 25 mm without an embryo
- Absence of embryo with heartbeat ≥ 2 weeks after a scan that showed a gestational sac without a yolk sac
- Absence of embryo with heartbeat ≥ 11 days after a scan that showed a gestational sac with a yolk sac

Potential pitfalls
- Making the diagnosis on only one ultrasound or lab value
- Not following up with an ultrasound or lab value in a timely manner

Treatment
There are three treatment options for a patient with EPF. They are all appropriate first-line treatment options:
- Conservative management
- Medical management
- Surgical management

Table of treatment

Treatment	Comments
Conservative	Success rate: 66–90% Bleeding and cramping for 2–6 hours. Most likely will occur within 4 weeks No impact on future fertility No increase in risk of infection
Medical	Success rate 80–90% 800 ug of vaginal misoprostol only or 200 mg of mifepristone (PO) followed by 800 ug of vaginal misoprostol 24 hours later. Bleeding and cramping for 2–6 hours Follow-up recommended in 1–2 weeks to ensure success of the treatment No impact on future fertility
Surgical	Success rates 98–99% Suction aspiration procedure Light bleeding for 3–7 days post procedure. No impact on future fertility

Complications
- Hemorrhage. The patient should be seen in the office or emergency room to assess the need for medical or surgical management to complete the miscarriage.
- Infection. The patient should be evaluated in the office or emergency room to assess the need for antibiotics to treat posttreatment endometritis.
- Failed medical management. If the pregnancy is still present after medical management a discussion about next steps including either a second dose of medication or a surgical procedure.

Special populations
Minors
- The majority of pregnant minors, **regardless of pregnancy viability**, are medically emancipated. A total of 32 states and the District of Columbia have laws that enable pregnant minors to make medical decision in this situation without the need for parental consent.

Prognosis
- The use of medical management reduces the need for uterine aspiration by 80–90%.
- The success of complete uterine evacuation with aspiration approaches 99%.

Natural history of untreated pregnancy failure (conservative management)
- Patients will undergo moderate to heavy bleeding with cramping. Approximately 80% of women will complete expulsion of a nonviable pregnancy within 8 weeks of expectant management.
- No increased risk of infection seen in patients opting for conservative management.

Prognosis for treated patients (medical and surgical options)
- Patients who opt for medical management will undergo moderate to heavy bleeding with cramping. The need for surgical management is reduced by 80–90% and may need to be performed in case of medication failure.
- Medical management of EPF has a higher success rate in patients with complaints of vaginal bleeding prior to medical treatment.
- Medical management of EPF has a higher success rate when used with the diagnosis of missed abortions compared to anembryonic gestations.
- Surgical treatment spares patients prolonged bleeding and cramping with a success of uterine evacuation approaching 99%.

Follow-up tests and monitoring
- Follow-up 7–10 days after medical management is recommended. Ultrasound can be useful to document success of completion by the absence of a gestational sac. No interventions are needed in asymptomatic women with thickened endometrial linings.
- Serum β-hCG can be utilized if a follow-up visit is not possible. There is good evidence that a serum β-hCG value should drop by approximately 80% in 1 week after treatment. A drop of this level is associated with a 90% probability of complete passage of the gestational sac.
- There is limited but good evidence to identify complete passage of the gestational sac utilizing serial urine pregnancy tests, and follow-up phone calls.

Reading list
Baldwin MK, Edelman AB. Chapter 23. Pregnancy testing and assessment of early normal and abnormal pregnancy. In: RA Hatcher, AL Nelson, J Trussell, et al. *Contraceptive technology*. 21st ed. Atlanta, GA: Bridging the Gap Communications; 2018:747-78.

Goldstein SR, Reeves MF. Chapter 6. Clinical assessment and ultrasound in early pregnancy. In: Paul M, Lichtenberg S, Borgatta L, et al. eds. *Management of unintended and abnormal pregnancy*. Hoboken, NJ: Wiley-Blackwell; 2009: 63-77.

Porter TF, Branch DW, Scott JR. Chapter 4. Early pregnancy loss. In: Gibbs RS, Karlan BY, Haney AF, et al. *Danforth's obstetrics and gynecology*. 10th ed. Philadelphia: Lippincott, Williams & Wilkins; 2008:60-70.

Tulandi T, Al-Fozan HM. Spontaneous abortion: Risk factors, etiology, clinical manifestations, and diagnostic evaluation. *UpToDate*. Updated 19 January 2017.

Guidelines
National society guidelines

Title	Source	Date/URL
ACOG practice bulletin no. 200: Early pregnancy loss	ACOG	2018 https://www.acog.org/Clinical-Guidance-and-Publications/Practice-Bulletins/Committee-on-Practice-Bulletins-Gynecology/Early-Pregnancy-Loss?IsMobileSet=false
Medical treatments for incomplete miscarriage	Cochrane Review	2017 https://www.cochrane.org/CD007223/PREG_medical-treatments-incomplete-miscarriage

Evidence

Type of evidence	Title and comment	Date/full reference
Randomized controlled trial	Analysis of success rate using medical and surgical management for EPF	Zhang J, Gilles JM, Barnhart K, et al. A comparison of medical management with misoprostol and surgical management for early pregnancy failure. *N Engl J Med* 2005;353:761-9.
Retrospective review	Human chorionic gonadotropin rise in early pregnancy and value at presentation	Barnhart, K, Guo W, Cary MS, et al. Differences in serum human chorionic gonadotropin rise in early pregnancy by race and value at presentation. *Obstet Gynecol* 2016;128:504-11.
Retrospective review	Analysis of ultrasound diagnostic criteria for EPF	Doubilet P, Benson CB, Bourne T, et al. Diagnostic criteria for nonviable pregnancy in the first trimester. *N Engl J Med* 2013;Oct 10;369(15):1443-51.
Prospective review	Analysis of β-hCG levels in viable and non-viable early pregnancies	Barnhart K, Sammel MD, Rinaudo PF, et al. Symptomatic patients with early viable intrauterine pregnancy. hCG curves redefined. *Obstet Gynecol* 2004 Jul;104(1):50-5.
Prospective review	Analysis of β-hCG levels after medical treatment of EPF	Barnhart K, Bader T, Huang X, et al. Hormone pattern after misoprostol administration for a nonviable first trimester gestation. *Fertil Steril* 2004;Apr;81(4):1099-105.
Randomized controlled trial	Mifepristone and misoprostol for management of early pregnancy loss	Schreiber, C, Creinin MD, Atrio J, et al. Mifepristone pretreatment for the medical management of early pregnancy loss. *N Engl J Med* 2018;Jun 7;378(23):2161-70.

Additional material for this chapter can be found online at:
www.wiley.com/go/sperling/mountsinai/obstetricsandgynecology

This includes a case study, multiple choice questions, advice for patients, and ICD codes.

Index

Note: Page numbers in *italic* refer to figures.

Mount Sinai Expert Guides: Obstetrics and Gynecology, First Edition. Edited by Rhoda Sperling.
© 2020 John Wiley & Sons Ltd. Published 2020 by John Wiley & Sons Ltd.
Companion Website: www.wiley.com/go/sperling/mountsinai/obstetricsandgynecology